PET/CT and Patient Outcomes, Part II

Editor

RATHAN M. SUBRAMANIAM

PET CLINICS

www.pet.theclinics.com

Consulting Editor
ABASS ALAVI

July 2015 • Volume 10 • Number 3

ELSEVIER

1600 John F. Kennedy Boulevard • Suite 1800 • Philadelphia, Pennsylvania, 19103-2899

http://www.pet.theclinics.com

PET CLINICS Volume 10, Number 3
July 2015 ISSN 1556-8598, ISBN-13: 978-0-323-39111-5

Editor: John Vassallo (j.vassallo@elsevier.com)
Developmental Editor: Meredith Clinton

PET Clinics (ISSN 1556-8598) is published quarterly by Elsevier Inc., 360 Park Avenue South, New York, NY 10010-1710. Months of issue are January, April, July, and October. Periodicals postage paid at New York, NY, and additional mailing offices. Subscription prices per year are $225.00 (US individuals), $327.00 (US institutions), $115.00 (US students), $255.00 (Canadian individuals), $369.00 (Canadian institutions), $140.00 (Canadian students), $275.00 (foreign individuals), $369.00 (foreign institutions), and $140.00 (foreign students). To receive student and resident rate, orders must be accompanied by name of affiliated institution, date of term, and the signature of program/residency coordinator on institution letterhead. Orders will be billed at individual rate until proof of status is received. Foreign air speed delivery is included in all Clinics subscription prices. All prices are subject to change without notice. POSTMASTER: Send address changes to PET Clinics, Elsevier Health Sciences Division, Subscription Customer Service, 3251 Riverport Lane, Maryland Heights, MO 63043. **Customer Service: 1-800-654-2452 (U.S. and Canada); 314-447-8871 (outside U.S. and Canada). Fax: 314-447-8029. E-mail: journalscustomerservice-usa@elsevier.com (for print support); journalsonlinesupport-usa@elsevier.com (for online support).**

Reprints. For copies of 100 or more of articles in this publication, please contact the Commercial Reprints Department, Elsevier Inc., 360 Park Avenue South, New York, NY 10010-1710. Tel.: 212-633-3874; Fax: 212-633-3820; E-mail: reprints@elsevier.com.

PET Clinics is covered in MEDLINE/PubMed (Index Medicus).

Contributors

CONSULTING EDITOR

ABASS ALAVI, MD, PhD (Hon), Dsc (Hon)
Professor of Radiology, Division of Nuclear
Medicine, Department of Radiology, University
of Pennsylvania School of Medicine, Hospital
of the University of Pennsylvania, Philadelphia,
Pennsylvania

EDITOR

RATHAN M. SUBRAMANIAM, MD, PhD, MPH, FRANZCR, FACNM
Associate Professor, Russell H Morgan Department of Radiology and Radiological Sciences,
Department of Otolaryngology and Head and Neck Surgery, Department of Oncology, Sidney
Kimmel Comprehensive Cancer Center, Johns Hopkins School of Medicine; Department of Health
Policy and Management, Institute for Health Services and Outcome Research, Johns Hopkins
Bloomberg School of Public Health, Armstrong Institute for Patient Safety and Quality, Johns
Hopkins Medicine, Baltimore, Maryland

AUTHORS

SANDIP BASU, MBBS (Hons), DRM, DNB, MNAMS
Radiation Medicine Centre, Bhabha Atomic
Research Centre, Mumbai, Maharashtra,
India

KIRSTEN BOUCHELOUCHE, MD, DMSc
Chief Physician, Department of Nuclear
Medicine and PET Centre, Aarhus University
Hospital, Aarhus, Denmark

JACQUELINE C. BRUNETTI, MD
Director, Department of Radiology,
Holy Name Medical Center, Teaneck,
New Jersey; Associate Clinical Professor,
part-time, Department of Radiology,
Columbia University Medical Center,
New York, New York

PETER L. CHOYKE, MD, FACR
Chief, Molecular Imaging Program, Center for
Cancer Research, National Cancer Institute
(NCI), Bethesda, Maryland

NIMA HAFEZI-NEJAD, MD, MPH
Postdoctoral Research Fellow, Russell H
Morgan Department of Radiology and
Radiological Sciences, Johns Hopkins School
of Medicine, Baltimore, Maryland

MARC HICKESON, MD, FRCP
Nuclear Medicine, Royal Victoria Hospital,
Montreal, Quebec, Canada

ABHISHEK KUMAR, MD
Diagnostic Nuclear Medicine Division,
Department of Nuclear Medicine, All India
Institute of Medical Sciences, New Delhi, India

RAKESH KUMAR, MD, PhD
Professor and Head, Diagnostic Nuclear
Medicine Division, Department of Nuclear
Medicine, All India Institute of Medical
Sciences, New Delhi, India

SANDER THOMAS LAURENS, MD
Department of Radiology and Nuclear
Medicine, Radboud University Medical Center,
Nijmegen, The Netherlands

ROBERT LISBONA, MD
Nuclear Medicine, Royal Victoria Hospital, Montreal, Quebec, Canada

NOUF MALIBARI, MD
Nuclear Medicine, Royal Victoria Hospital, Montreal, Quebec, Canada

CHARLES MARCUS, MD
Postdoctoral Research Fellow, Russell H Morgan Department of Radiology and Radiological Sciences, Johns Hopkins School of Medicine, Baltimore, Maryland

ESTHER MENA, MD
Russell H Morgan Department of Radiology and Radiological Sciences, Johns Hopkins School of Medicine, Baltimore, Maryland

AVNER MEODED, MD
Russell H Morgan Department of Radiology and Radiological Sciences, Johns Hopkins School of Medicine, Baltimore, Maryland

WIM J.G. OYEN, MD, PhD
Department of Radiology and Nuclear Medicine, Radboud University Medical Center, Nijmegen, The Netherlands

UJAS PARIKH, MA
Medical Student, Russell H Morgan Department of Radiology and Radiological Sciences, Johns Hopkins School of Medicine, Baltimore, Maryland

ALOK S. PAWASKAR, MBBS, DRM, DNB
Radiation Medicine Centre, Bhabha Atomic Research Centre, Mumbai, Maharashtra, India; Department of Nuclear Medicine and PET-CT, Curie-Manavata Cancer Centre, Nashik, Maharashtra, India

ROHIT RANADE, MBBS, DRM
Radiation Medicine Centre, Bhabha Atomic Research Centre, Mumbai, Maharashtra, India

RUTUPARNA SARANGI, MA
Medical Student, Russell H Morgan Department of Radiology and Radiological Sciences, Johns Hopkins School of Medicine, Baltimore, Maryland

THOMAS HELLMUT SCHINDLER, MD
Director of Nuclear Cardiovascular Imaging; Associate Professor, Division of Nuclear Medicine, Department of Radiology SOM, Johns Hopkins University School of Medicine, Baltimore, Maryland

SHAMIM AHMED SHAMIM, MD
Assistant Professor, Therapeutic Nuclear Medicine Division, Department of Nuclear Medicine, All India Institute of Medical Sciences, New Delhi, India

SARA SHEIKHBAHAEI, MD, MPH
Postdoctoral Research Fellow, Russell H Morgan Department of Radiology and Radiological Sciences, Johns Hopkins School of Medicine, Baltimore, Maryland

LILJA SOLNES, MD
Russell H Morgan Department of Radiology and Radiological Sciences, Johns Hopkins School of Medicine, Baltimore, Maryland

RATHAN M. SUBRAMANIAM, MD, PhD, MPH, FRANZCR, FACNM
Associate Professor, Russell H Morgan Department of Radiology and Radiological Sciences, Department of Otolaryngology and Head and Neck Surgery, Department of Oncology, Sidney Kimmel Comprehensive Cancer Center, Johns Hopkins School of Medicine; Department of Health Policy and Management, Institute for Health Services and Outcome Research, Johns Hopkins Bloomberg School of Public Health, Armstrong Institute for Patient Safety and Quality, Johns Hopkins Medicine, Baltimore, Maryland

MEHDI TAGHIPOUR, MD
Postdoctoral Research Fellow, Russell H Morgan Department of Radiology and Radiological Sciences, Johns Hopkins School of Medicine, Baltimore, Maryland

RICK WRAY, MD
Russell H Morgan Department of Radiology and Radiological Sciences, Johns Hopkins School of Medicine, Baltimore, Maryland

Contents

FDG-PET/CT is a potentially useful imaging modality in the setting of Carcinoma of Unknown Primary (CUP) from various aspects. The central question is detection of site of primary, where most studies have documented the pooled sensitivity and specificity of FDG PET/CT in the range of 80%–85% and a tumor detection rate (after the failure of conventional imaging procedures) between 30%–37%. The heterogeneity in the (i) population studied and (ii) criteria used for labelling patient as of unknown primary, have been the prime reason for widely varying result amongst various studies. Initiating appropriate treatment strategies owing to simultaneous whole body disease staging can be regarded an added utility PET/CT, even in the case of failure of primary tumor detection. FDG-PET/CT changed the patient management in around 35% of patients (studies reporting heterogeneous results ranging from 18.2% to 60%). The futuristic approach will be to monitor molecular targeted and cystostatic therapies with FDG-PET/CT which obviously has advantages than anatomical imaging alone.

Although there has been a reduction of the incidence and mortality of gastric cancer, it remains among the most common causes of cancer-related death. Accurate staging and evaluation of treatment response are vital for management. PET is used to complement anatomic imaging in cancer management. PET/computed tomography (CT) has demonstrated its potential value for preoperative staging, evaluation of response to therapy, and detection of recurrence. Not all types of gastric cancers have a high affinity for fluorodeoxyglucose. PET/CT in the evaluation and staging of gastric cancer is not established, but studies indicate that there may be an evolving role for this imaging modality.

Fludeoxyglucose F 18 (^{18}F-FDG) PET/CT has not been shown to offer additional benefit in the initial diagnosis of pancreatic cancer, but studies show benefit of ^{18}F-FDG PET/CT in initial staging and patient prognosis. There is evidence for ^{18}F-FDG PET and ^{18}F-FDG PET/CT in staging and prognosis of cholangiocarcinoma and gallbladder cancer. ^{18}F-FDG PET/CT has shown promise in staging liver malignancies by detecting extrahepatic metastasis. There is evidence supporting the ability of PET/CT in predicting prognosis in patients with hepatocellular carcinoma.

endometrial, ovarian, and cervical malignancies, with emphasis on the impact of imaging on treatment stratification and prognosis.

PET/Computed Tomography in Neuroendocrine Tumor: Value to Patient Management and Survival Outcomes

411

Shamim Ahmed Shamim, Abhishek Kumar, and Rakesh Kumar

PET/computed tomography evaluation of neuroendocrine tumors is gaining prominence with the availability of novel pet radiotracers, such as ^{18}F-DOPA and gallium 68 somatostatin peptide derivatives. These tumors have unique properties and have become the basis of use of these new radiotracers. Prominent centers worldwide have reported the usefulness of these PET tracers in diagnosis and clinical decision making. Portability of 68Ge/68Ga generators has also helped in more widespread use of these somatostatin peptide derivatives as PET radiotracers. This article reviews established and potential roles of these novel PET radiotracers in diagnosis, management, and prognosis of neuroendocrine tumors.

[18]F-Flourodeoxy-Glucose PET/Computed Tomography in Brain Tumors: Value to Patient Management and Survival Outcomes

423

Rick Wray, Lilja Solnes, Esther Mena, Avner Meoded, and Rathan M. Subramaniam

[18]F-flourodeoxy-glucose (FDG) PET/computed tomography (CT) is most useful in the evaluation of primary central nervous system (CNS) lymphoma, important in diagnosis, pretherapy prognosis, and therapy response evaluation. Utility in working up gliomas is less effective, and FDG PET/CT is most helpful when MR imaging is unclear. FDG avidity correlates with the grade of gliomas. FDG PET/CT can be used to noninvasively identify malignant transformation. Establishing this change in the disease process has significant effects on patient management and survival outcome.

18-Fluoro-deoxyglucose–PET/Computed Tomography in Infection and Aseptic Inflammatory Disorders: Value to Patient Management

431

Sandip Basu and Rohit Ranade

This communication is aimed specifically at exploring the possible practical advantages and potentials of 18-fluoro-deoxyglucose (FDG)–PET/computed tomography (CT) that could translate into routine management of patients with infection and aseptic inflammatory disorders. From the viewpoint of patient management, the applications can be classified into two broad categories based upon primary intent of the investigation: [a] diagnostic (eg, pyrexia of unknown origin and other localized infectious processes) and [b] undertaking this as part of objective imaging assessment of early treatment response and thereby tailoring/altering therapy (eg, systemic infectious and non-infectious inflammatory diseases). Over the last decade, this promising FDG-PET/CT application has been debated and there is a need to make systematic approach for defining its value to patient management.

Cardiac PET/Computed Tomography Applications and Cardiovascular Outcome

441

Thomas Hellmut Schindler

Cardiac PET/computed tomography (CT) in conjunction with different blood flow tracers is increasingly applied for the assessment of myocardial perfusion and myocardial flow reserve (MFR) in the detection of coronary artery disease (CAD).

The ability of PET/CT to noninvasively determine regional myocardial blood flow at rest and during vasomotor stress allows the calculation of the MFR, which carries important prognostic information in patients with subclinical forms of cardiomyopathy. The measured MFR optimizes the identification and characterization of the extent and severity of CAD burden, and contributes to the flow-limiting effect of single lesions in multivessel CAD.

PET CLINICS

THE CLINICS ARE AVAILABLE ONLINE!
Access your subscription at:
www.theclinics.com

PET CLINICS

PROGRAM OBJECTIVE

The goal of the *PET Clinics* is to keep practicing radiologists and radiology residents up to date with current clinical practice in positron emission tomography by providing timely articles reviewing the state of the art in patient care.

TARGET AUDIENCE

Practicing radiologists, radiology residents, and other health care professionals who provide patient care utilizing radiologic findings.

LEARNING OBJECTIVES

Upon completion of this activity, participants will be able to:

1. Review the value of PET/CT imaging in the management and outcome of sarcomas, carcinomas, and other malignancies.
2. Discuss the use of FDG PET/CT in the management of infection and Aseptic Inflammatory disorders.
3. Recognize the applications of Cardiac PET/CT in cardiovascular outcome.

ACCREDITATION

The Elsevier Office of Continuing Medical Education (EOCME) is accredited by the Accreditation Council for Continuing Medical Education (ACCME) to provide continuing medical education for physicians.

The EOCME designates this enduring material for a maximum of 15 *AMA PRA Category 1 Credit*(s)™. Physicians should claim only the credit commensurate with the extent of their participation in the activity.

All other health care professionals requesting continuing education credit for this enduring material will be issued a certificate of participation.

DISCLOSURE OF CONFLICTS OF INTEREST

The EOCME assesses conflict of interest with its instructors, faculty, planners, and other individuals who are in a position to control the content of CME activities. All relevant conflicts of interest that are identified are thoroughly vetted by EOCME for fair balance, scientific objectivity, and patient care recommendations. EOCME is committed to providing its learners with CME activities that promote improvements or quality in healthcare and not a specific proprietary business or a commercial interest.

The planning committee, staff, authors and editors listed below have identified no financial relationships or relationships to products or devices they or their spouse/life partner have with commercial interest related to the content of this CME activity:

Abass Alavi, MD, PhD (Hon), Dsc (Hon); Sandip Basu, MBBS (Hons), DRM, DNB, MNAMS; Kirsten Bouchelouche, MD, DMSc; Jacqueline C. Brunetti, MD; Peter L. Choyke, MD, FACR; Anjali Fortna; Nima Hafezi-Nejad, MD, MPH; Kristen Helm; Marc Hickeson, MD, FRCP; Abhishek Kumar, MD; Rakesh Kumar, MD, PhD; Sander Thomas Laurens, MD; Robert Lisbona, MD; Nouf Malibari, MD; Charles Marcus, MD; Esther Mena, MD; Avner Meoded, MD; Mahalakshmi Narayanan; Wim J.G. Oyen, MD, PhD; Ujas Parikh, MA; Alok S. Pawaskar, MBBS, DRM, DNB; Rohit Ranade, MBBS, DRM; Rutuparna Sarangi, MA; Thomas Hellmut Schindler, MD; Shamim Ahmed Shamim, MD; Sara Sheikhbahaei, MD, MPH; Lilja Solnes, MD; Mehdi Taghipour, MD; John Vassallo; Rick Wray, MD.

The planning committee, staff, authors and editors listed below have identified financial relationships or relationships to products or devices they or their spouse/life partner have with commercial interest related to the content of this CME activity:

Rathan M. Subramaniam, MD, PhD, MPH, FRANZCR, FACNM participated in the board meeting for Phillips Healthcare Molecular Imaging, as well as a clinical trial for Bayer HealthCare AG.

UNAPPROVED/OFF-LABEL USE DISCLOSURE

The EOCME requires CME faculty to disclose to the participants:

1. When products or procedures being discussed are off-label, unlabelled, experimental, and/or investigational (not US Food and Drug Administration [FDA] approved); and
2. Any limitations on the information presented, such as data that are preliminary or that represent ongoing research, interim analyses, and/or unsupported opinions. Faculty may discuss information about pharmaceutical agents that is outside of FDA-approved labelling. This information is intended solely for CME and is not intended to promote off-label use of these medications. If you have any questions, contact the medical affairs department of the manufacturer for the most recent prescribing information.

TO ENROLL

To enroll in the *PET Clinics* Continuing Medical Education program, call customer service at 1-800-654-2452 or sign up online at http://www.theclinics.com/home/cme. The CME program is available to subscribers for an additional annual fee of USD $235.

METHOD OF PARTICIPATION

In order to claim credit, participants must complete the following:

1. Complete enrolment as indicated above.
2. Read the activity.
3. Complete the CME Test and Evaluation. Participants must achieve a score of 70% on the test. All CME Tests and Evaluations must be completed online.

CME INQUIRIES/SPECIAL NEEDS

For all CME inquiries or special needs, please contact elsevierCME@elsevier.com.

Preface
PET/CT: Defining Value to Patients and Health Systems

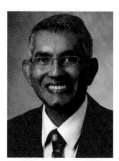

Rathan M. Subramaniam, MD, PhD, MPH,
FRANZCR, FACNM
Editor

As US health care reform is being implemented, it has become imperative that we demonstrate the value of PET/CT imaging to patients and health care systems. Value can be defined as the cost of delivering patient-related outcomes. However, value is not just about the cost alone; it also incorporates the patient and health care system perspectives to improve the quality of life of patients and their outcomes, delivering the most appropriate care, safely and efficiently, to the patient's satisfaction.

Imaging is a single node in a multiple node chain that influences patient outcomes. This care paradigm poses some challenges to directly link a single imaging test to traditional patient outcome endpoints: improvement in quality of life, progression-free survival, and overall survival. For these reasons, intermediate imaging-related value metrics must be developed, tested, validated, and proven to demonstrate value to patients and health care systems. For patients, these value metrics can be divided into five domains: appropriateness, safety, quality, efficiency, and patient satisfaction. Some of the value metrics include early diagnosis, right diagnosis, fewer mistakes and repeats, early and timely treatment, reduced cycle time from diagnosis to treatment, adding value to clinicians' judgment, and change in management and such.

In this issue of "PET/CT and Patient Outcomes II," a group of international authors demonstrates the value of PET/CT in human solid tumors, such as gastric cancers, neuroendocrine tumors, colorectal cancers, skeletal tumors, soft tissue tumors, brain tumors, infection and inflammation, myocardial perfusion. The evidence is evolving in rare tumors and infection/inflammation. This is a "work in progress" for the next decade. We must persist in these efforts to bring benefits to our patients and humanity.

Rathan M. Subramaniam, MD, PhD, MPH,
FRANZCR, FACNM
Russell H Morgan Department of
Radiology and Radiological Sciences
Johns Hopkins Medical Institutions
601 North Caroline Street/
JHOC 3235
Baltimore, MD 21287, USA

E-mail address:
rsubram4@jhmi.edu

PET Clin 10 (2015) xiii
http://dx.doi.org/10.1016/j.cpet.2015.04.001
1556-8598/15/$ – see front matter © 2015 Published by Elsevier Inc.

Preface

Role of 2-Fluoro-2-Deoxyglucose PET/Computed Tomography in Carcinoma of Unknown Primary

Alok S. Pawaskar, MBBS, DRM, DNB[a,b], Sandip Basu, DRM, DNB, MNAMS[a,*]

KEYWORDS

- Carcinoma of unknown primary • FDG PET/CT • Imaging

KEY POINTS

- Based on evidence in the literature, use of PET/computed tomography (CT) in patients with metastases to cervical nodes and unknown primary can be recommended.
- Although most of the studies and reviews support the use of 2-fluoro-2-deoxyglucose (FDG) PET/CT in extracervical malignancy with unknown primary, there is no clarity on investigative protocols.
- There is a need for prospective randomized trials to define the exact role of PET/CT in the management of patients with carcinoma of unknown primary (CUP).
- Advances in hybrid molecular imaging techniques along with advanced imaging are likely to lead the front for detection and management of patients with CUP in the future.

INTRODUCTION

Carcinoma of unknown primary (CUP) has been an area of challenge to the attending physicians and remains an enigma despite advances in diagnostics and imaging. By definition, CUP is a biopsy-proven malignancy whose organ of origin remains unidentified even after thorough investigations. There continues to be substantial variation in the extent to which investigations to detect the primary malignancy are carried out. In an early report published in the 1970s, some researchers even argued that a diagnosis of CUP origin could only be made if the primary tumor was not found at autopsy.[1] This argument has relatively less relevance as far as clinical management of these patients is concerned. It is imperative that the incidence of CUP depends on the number and type of investigations being undertaken; in most of the literature, it is estimated to be 3% to 5% of the total cancer diagnosis.[2,3] In the developed countries, such as the United States, there seems to be a decrease in the incidence of CUP as evidenced by 45,230 cases per year in 1995[4] to 31,000 per year in 2012.[5] This decrease may be attributable to the developments in immunohistochemistry and advances in medical imaging like better-quality computed tomography (CT) scanners, MR imaging, PET/CT, and so forth.

CUP is still not a very uncommon oncological diagnosis, being the seventh to eighth most frequently occurring cancer in the world.[6,7] The overall prognosis for patients with CUP is generally very poor with a median survival of 4 to 12 months, with about 50% of patients alive at 1 year and about

The authors have nothing to disclose.
[a] Radiation Medicine Centre, Bhabha Atomic Research Centre, Tata Memorial Centre Annexe, Jerbai Wadia Road, Parel, Mumbai, Maharashtra 400012, India; [b] Department of Nuclear Medicine and PET-CT, Curie-Manavata Cancer Centre, Mumbai Naka, Nashik, Maharashtra 422004, India
* Corresponding author. Radiation Medicine Centre, Bhabha Atomic Research Centre, Tata Memorial Hospital Annexe, Jerbai Wadia Road, Parel, Mumbai, Maharashtra 400012, India.
E-mail address: drsanb@yahoo.com

PET Clin 10 (2015) 297–310
http://dx.doi.org/10.1016/j.cpet.2015.03.004
1556-8598/15/$ – see front matter © 2015 Elsevier Inc. All rights reserved.

10% at 5 years from diagnosis.[8] There is a small subset of patients who show a more favorable prognosis owing to a well-differentiated and chemosensitive tumor and have better survival rates. However, most patients with CUP continue to have a worse prognosis and show resistance to standard therapy. In general it is postulated that if the primary becomes known in these patients, the patients would have a favorable prognosis, as therapy can then be optimized to the specific tumor type. Some studies have supported this postulation.[9,10]

Thus, as previously mentioned, finding out the primary offers the best hope for most patients with CUP; the initial diagnostic strategies are primarily toward this direction. The patients should undergo a thorough clinical history and clinical examination. Based on the suspicion and the laboratory and clinical investigations, various types of scopy examinations and imaging tests can be ordered. Besides these, female patients may have to undergo mammography and a vaginal ultrasonography (USG) scan, whereas prostate USG scan may be required in males. From a patient's perspective, undergoing these tests may be expensive, time consuming, and invasive to the extent that the search for the primary may become unpleasant and unnecessary for someone with a diagnosis of cancer and awaiting for appropriate treatment to be initiated at the earliest opportunity. Hence, a single test that is noninvasive, screens the whole body, and has a high yield will be highly desirable and can play a pivotal role in the given clinical setting. Whole-body PET/CT with 2-fluoro-2-deoxyglucose (FDG) has the potential to be one such investigation, and the present review discusses its role in patients with CUP.

WHY PET/COMPUTED TOMOGRAPHY?

As far as imaging tests for the diagnosis of unknown primary are concerned, radiographs and USG of the abdomen are initial tests generally ordered for screening and have obvious limitations for detection of the primary. The mainstay of imaging in oncology over the last few decades has been CT scan and MR imaging. Both of these modalities have 3-dimensional imaging capabilities with the ability to locate tumor in depths of the body tissue. CT scan is better for imaging lungs and bones and performs fairly well for the detection of soft tissue abnormalities. MR imaging is excellent for imaging brain and immobile soft tissue areas like head and neck and pelvis. Both are anatomic imaging modalities and depend on size, asymmetry and contrast enhancement for detection of tumor. However, a small-sized tumor may be missed, which is an important consideration for CUP whereby the primary tumor may be of small size.[7] The asymmetry and abnormal contrast enhancement may be seen in various benign conditions like infection and may be cause for false-positive findings. Further, if whole-body imaging with CT or MR imaging is done, then there are huge data to be analyzed for reporting an unknown primary tumor in these low-contrast images. This circumstance may reduce overall sensitivity of the study.

On the other hand, PET scan is a whole-body functional imaging whereby FDG is used as surrogate marker for glucose metabolism in the body. Most of the malignant tumors exhibit a shift toward glucose metabolism owing to the Warburg effect.[11] Hence, detection of metabolic changes is possible with PET, even when there is no or little change in the size of the organs. Further, high lesion-to-background contrast available in PET images increases sensitivity considerably. With widespread availability of state-of-the-art PET/CT scanners, accurate fusion of functional and anatomic images is now possible. This fusion has reduced the time for examination, eliminated problems associated with a lack of anatomic information on stand-alone PET scan, and improved attenuation-correction to a great degree. If contrast CT is performed along with PET, then it eliminates the need for a separate CT scan in most of the cases. However, it may add some artifacts in the images because of the higher density of contrast.

Initial Comparative Data of PET/PET-Computed Tomography and Computed Tomography Alone

There are several studies directly comparing PET scan against CT for the detection of an unknown primary. For example, Roh and colleagues[12] have shown that sensitivity of FDG PET/CT (87.5%) was significantly higher ($P = .016$) than that of CT alone (43.7%) in detecting primary tumors in 44 patients presenting with cervical metastases from an unknown origin. Nassenstein and colleagues[13] investigated 39 patients with cervical metastases of unknown origin; CT alone revealed the primary tumor in only 5 patients (13%), whereas FDG PET alone and combined FDG PET/CT detected a primary tumor in 10 patients (26%) and 11 patients (28%), respectively. In addition, Freudenberg and colleagues[14] evaluated 21 patients with cervical metastases and unknown primary. They showed that CT alone detected only 5 primary tumors (23%), whereas FDG PET alone and combined FDG PET/CT detected 11 primary tumors (52%) and 12 (57%) primary tumors, respectively, with a significant difference (P = .03) between CT alone and FDG PET/CT. These studies and many more show better sensitivity and specificity of PET/CT compared with CT or PET alone for the detection of an unknown primary. Several examples from routine clinical oncological settings (involving an unknown primary at different locations) have been illustrated in the figures found in this article (**Figs. 1** and **2**).

PROTOCOL FOR 2-FLUORO-2-DEOXYGLUCOSE PET/COMPUTED TOMOGRAPHY

The standard protocol for PET/CT imaging should be used.[15] It has been reported that focal intrapulmonary FDG uptake may occur as a result of iatrogenic pulmonary microembolism caused by aspiration of blood during intravenous FDG administration,[16] which should be avoided. Patients should be instructed to avoid chewing, swallowing, and talking immediately before and after FDG administration to avoid false-positive uptake in the oropharyngeal region. The time of imaging after tracer injection may be important for unknown primary detection. Some of the tumors may not show peak FDG uptake at 60- to 90-minute intervals and continue to show increase in FDG uptake over time.[17–19] Hence, delayed imaging at 3 to 4 hours may be recommended in selected patients, as this would improve the lesion-to-background ratio considerably. However, there is no consensus on a standard time for imaging in CUP as of today. Similarly, the issue of contrast administration for the CT component of PET/CT is unresolved. It may well seem that the use of intravenous and oral contrast agents should increase sensitivity/specificity of the PET/CT study. However, neither the study by of Fencl and colleagues[20] nor the meta-analysis by Kwee and Kwee[21] showed any beneficial effect of using contrast on diagnostic yield in patients with CUP compared with using no contrast agents at all. As mentioned earlier, high concentrations of contrast medium may artificially lead to overestimation of FDG uptake when using CT-based attenuation correction.[22] In addition, iodinated contrast agents may cause adverse reactions.[23] Hence, it may be of little use to perform a CT scan with contrast agents in this patient group with an unknown primary.

INTERPRETATION OF IMAGES
False-Positive/False-Negative Lesions

While reading PET/CT images, common false-positive and false-negative findings must be borne in mind. False-positive findings may lead to unnecessary biopsies or further investigations. The oropharynx and lungs are the most frequently reported locations with false-positive FDG PET/CT uptake.[21] Physiologic FDG uptake seen in the oropharynx in the lymphoid tissue of the adenoids and Waldeyer ring as well as a few muscles may cause false suspicion of malignancy. Reading CT images simultaneously may eliminate some of the false-positive results. Focal increased FDG uptake in the lungs may be characterized better on a CT scan, which may show the presence of a benign inflammatory or infectious lesion or a pulmonary embolism or infarction.[24–26] Infections and granulomatous lesions like tuberculosis and sarcoidosis are particularly notorious for mimicking malignancy; hence, any abnormal uptake on an FDG PET study should be confirmed with biopsy. Breast cancer is the most common cause of false-negative FDG PET/CT results.[21] This point may be explained by the fact that small (<1 cm) and slow-growing, low-grade (breast) cancers with low or no FDG uptake (eg, tubular carcinoma and noninvasive cancers, such as ductal or lobular carcinoma in situ) may be overlooked on FDG PET/CT.[27]

Important Clues for Interpreting 2-Fluoro-2-Deoxyglucose PET/Computed Tomography Studies

It should be kept in mind that the most frequently reported unknown primary tumor locations are the lung, pancreas, and oropharynx.[21,28–31] Hence, these areas should be carefully evaluated on PET/CT. In patients with involvement of the upper or midcervical lymph nodes, a primary site in the head and neck should be investigated.[8] In patients with poorly differentiated carcinoma and left supraclavicular lymphadenopathy (Virchow node), a primary gastrointestinal tumor may be detected.[8] In women with axillary lymph node metastases, primary breast cancer may be suspected. On the other hand, women with peritoneal carcinomatosis may have primary ovarian cancer.[8] Furthermore, in men with osteoblastic bone metastases, prostate cancer may be the primary tumor (**Figs. 3–5**).[8]

PERFORMANCE OF 2-FLUORO-2-DEOXYGLUCOSE PET/COMPUTED TOMOGRAPHY IN CARCINOMA OF UNKNOWN PRIMARY: A CRITICAL APPRAISAL

In up to 30% of patients with CUP, a primary site is identified ante mortem. Postmortem examinations reveal a putative primary site in 60% to 80% of patients with CUP, most often in the lung (27%) (see **Figs. 2** and **4**; **Fig. 6**), pancreas (24%), and hepatobiliary tree (8%).[32] It should be remembered that the antemortem diagnosis in 30%

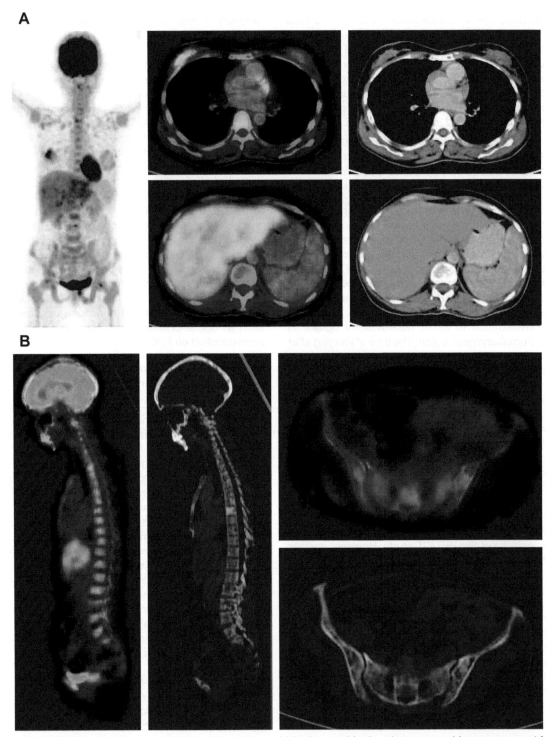

Fig. 1. A 35-year-old woman presented with per vaginal bleeding and had undergone total hysterectomy with right oophorectomy in a different center. The histopathology was suggestive of adenocarcinoma. She was referred to the authors' hospital with complaints of generalized weakness and pain. Clinically, the patient had bilateral breast fibroadenosis and her serum cancer antigen 125 level was 8.0 U/mL. She was advised to undergo a whole-body PET/CT scan with oral and intravenous contrast to find out the primary malignancy. PET/CT scan was suggestive of primary breast malignancy (A) with multiple hepatic and skeletal metastases (B). Biopsy from right breast lesion turned out to be infiltrative ductal carcinoma grade II. Hence, retrospectively it was concurred that adenocarcinoma detected in the oophorectomy specimen was actually a Krukenberg tumor.

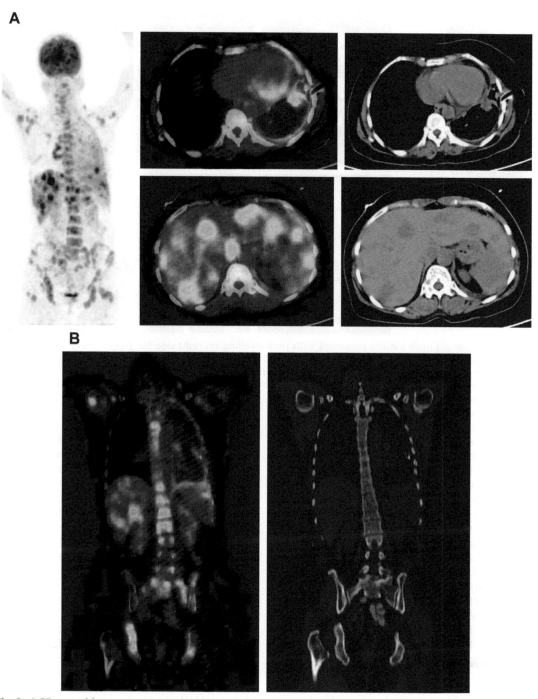

Fig. 2. A 55-year-old woman presented with cough for 8 days and reduced appetite. Her CT scan completed elsewhere showed patchy areas of consolidation with suspicious lymphangitis in left lung and left pleural effusion. It also demonstrated multiple lytic areas in skeleton and multiple hypodensities in liver. Intercostal drain was inserted, and pleural fluid cytology turned out to be positive for malignancy. She was referred for whole-body PET/CT scan for localization of primary malignancy. PET/CT scan showed primary lesion in lower lobe of left lung with lymphangitic changes in left lung. It also confirmed multiple mediastinal and hilar nodal metastases as well as multiple hepatic (*A*) and skeletal metastases (*B*). This finding was confirmed by CT-guided biopsy from left lower lobe lesion.

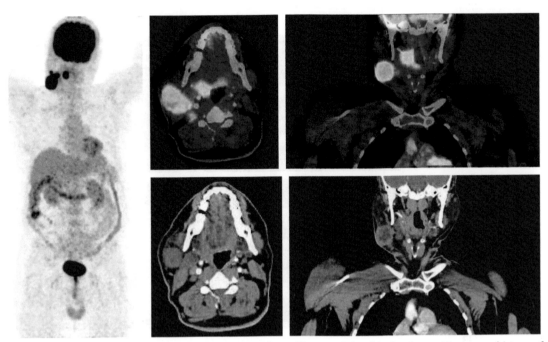

Fig. 3. A 53-year-old male patient presented with neck swelling on right side for 1 year. There was history of recent increase in the size of the swelling over last 15 days. Fine-needle aspiration cytology done from the swelling was positive for malignancy. Hence, he was referred for FDG PET/CT to locate the unknown primary malignancy. PET/CT scan showed primary malignancy in right tonsillar fossa with right level I, II, and III lymphadenopathy. There was no demonstrable distant metastasis.

of cases is after extensive diagnostic evaluation. These low numbers are still not well explained. Common hypotheses include spontaneous regression or immune-mediated destruction of the primary tumor or the inherent small size of the primary tumor (metastatic spread is favored above local tumor growth).[7,33,34]

Irrespective of the explanations provided for the primary remaining undiagnosed, it cannot be overemphasized that detection of the primary tumor improves survival of these patients.[9,10] Hence, it is important to know how PET/CT performs against conventional imaging modalities. In the review carried out by the National Collaborating Center for Cancer for the National Institute for Health and Care Excellence guideline development group, a total of 47 primary studies were analyzed (35 PET, 12 PET/CT); in 12 of these studies, data for extracervical metastatic presentations could be separately assessed. The pooled data showed a sensitivity of 0.80 (95% confidence interval [CI]: 0.72–0.86) and specificity of 0.81 (95% CI: 0.75–0.86) for either PET or PET/CT, with PET/CT having higher sensitivity and specificity than PET alone. The results of the individual studies, however, were significantly heterogeneous.[35]

Dong and colleagues,[36] in their review article, estimated the pooled sensitivity and specificity of

PET/CT as 81% (95% CI: 74%–87%) and 83% (95% CI: 78%–87%), respectively. The estimated tumor detection rate for PET/CT was 31% for Dong and colleagues.[36] Kwee and Kwee,[21] in their literature review, included 11 studies comprising a total sample size of 433 patients with CUP, with moderate methodological quality. The overall primary tumor detection rate, pooled sensitivity, and specificity of FDG PET/CT were 37%, 84% (95% CI 78%–88%), and 84% (95% CI 78%–89%), respectively. Other interesting conclusions of their review were that completeness of the diagnostic work-up before FDG PET/CT, location of metastases of unknown primary, administration of CT contrast agents, type of FDG PET/CT images evaluated, and way of FDG PET/CT review did not significantly influence the diagnostic performance. Hence, it seems that FDG PET/CT is a very useful test in the diagnosis of unknown primary. Although the emphasis of most of the studies is on finding out the primary site, the authors would like to bring out a new perspective that is the major advantage of PET/CT. PET/CT by nature is a whole-body imaging with high sensitivity. Apart from finding the primary, N and M staging is done in one go. There is usually no need for any additional investigations for staging once the primary diagnosis is established.

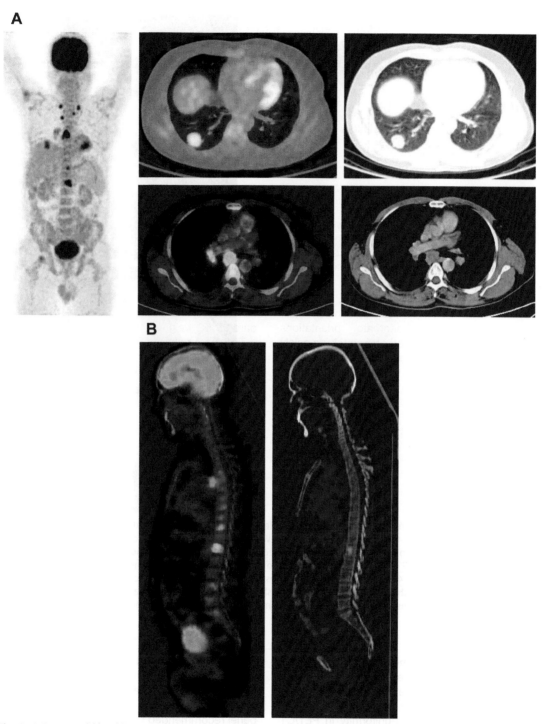

Fig. 4. A 51-year-old healthy man presented with backache of 2 months duration. His MR imaging spine done at a different center was suggestive of multiple areas of suspicious metastases. Biopsy was suggested. However, the patient refused any invasive procedure and was referred for FDG PET/CT scan. Whole-body PET/CT scan with oral and intravenous contrast was undertaken, which showed primary lesion in lower lobe of right lung (*A*) with hypermetabolic bilateral level IV, left supraclavicular, mediastinal and right hilar nodes, and multiple skeletal metastases (*B*). The biopsy from the lung lesion confirmed non–small-cell lung carcinoma.

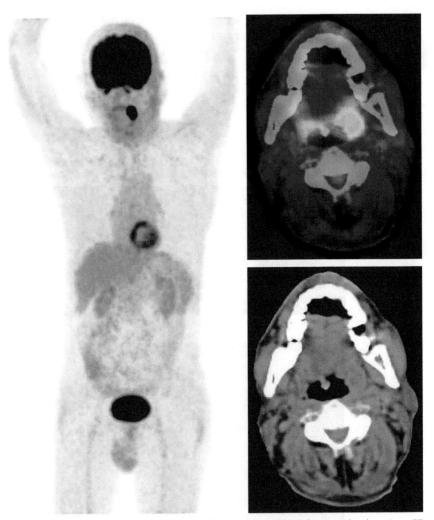

Fig. 5. A 72-year-old gentleman presented with left-sided neck swelling of 2 months duration. CT scan of neck was done elsewhere at that time, which showed left level II node and minimal thickening in upper esophagus. No other abnormality was noted in the head and neck region. Biopsy of left level II node was suggestive of poorly differentiated squamous cell carcinoma. However, patient did not receive any treatment because of financial constraints at that time. After 4 months of biopsy, he was referred to the authors' center for FDG PET/CT study. Whole-body PET/CT scan with contrast was done, which showed intensely hypermetabolic primary in left tonsillar fossa region with no demonstrable regional or distant metastases. PET/CT was able to detect primary as well as stage the disease in one go.

It should be noted that most of the studies in this domain were retrospective in nature. In addition, (1) there was significant heterogeneity in the population studied (criteria for labeling patients as of unknown primary), (2) non-uniformity in PET/CT protocols and interpretation of results, and (3) lack of prospective studies with a sufficient number of patients and with more uniform inclusion criteria. Despite the limited evidence regarding its utility, a multidisciplinary expert panel of oncologists, radiologists, and nuclear physicians with expertise in PET/CT concluded that using FDG PET/CT in the diagnostic work-up of patients with CUP is beneficial.[37] They also recommend that if FDG PET/CT findings are positive, confirmatory biopsy is necessary because of the risk of false-positive results.[37] Furthermore, the expert panel recommended that if the FDG PET/CT findings are negative in cases of a suspected unknown primary tumor in the head and neck region, further effort should be made to identify the primary tumor because of the chance of false-negative results.[37] Similar observations are made in international PET/CT-related guidelines[38] stating the studies of unknown primary malignancies are among the most appropriate indications for PET (see **Fig. 6**).

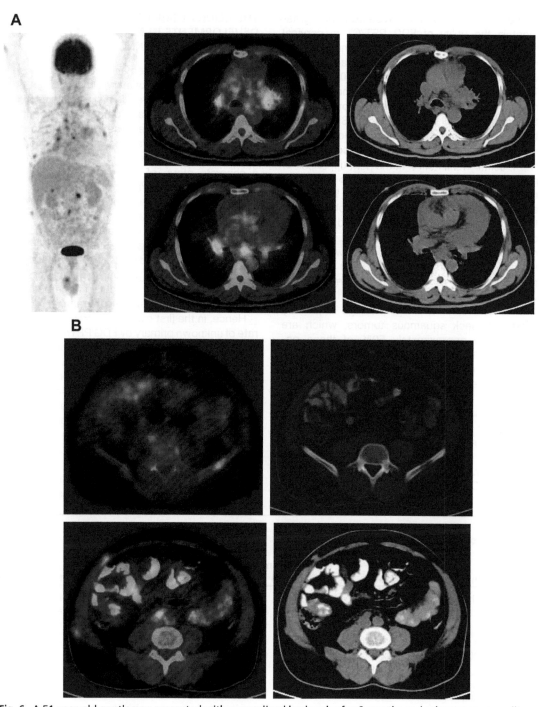

Fig. 6. A 51-year-old gentleman presented with generalized body ache for 6 months and subcutaneous swellings over skull, right arm, and neck. Excision of right arm and neck nodules was done. The histopathologic examination revealed metastatic adenocarcinoma. He was referred for evaluation of unknown primary. Whole-body PET/CT scan was done with oral and intravenous contrast. The scan showed primary malignancy in peribronchial region of left upper lobe (*A*) with metastatic mediastinal, hilar, and retroperitoneal adenopathy (*B*). Also noted were multiple osteolytic metastases, multiple subcutaneous nodules, and a deposit in right scrotal sac (*A*).

There seems to be more research and agreement in the utility of FDG PET/CT in cervical lymph node metastases from an unknown primary tumor. Rusthoven and colleagues[39] reviewed 16 studies with a total of 302 patients. The overall sensitivity, specificity, and accuracy rates of FDG PET in detecting unknown primary tumors were 88.3%, 74.9%, and 78.8%, respectively. Furthermore, FDG PET detected 24.5% tumors that were not apparent after conventional work-up. FDG PET also led to the detection of previously unrecognized metastases in 27.1% of patients (regional 15.9%; distant 11.2%).[39] In another article, by Fleming and colleagues,[40] the unknown primary site was found in 72.7% of patients with unknown primary head and neck cancer. Synchronous lesions were found in 8.1% of patients by PET/CT, with a positive predictive value of 66.6%. Distant metastases were detected in 15.4% of patients.[40] The other two reviews confirm similar findings in primary head and neck squamous tumors, which are identified in approximately 50% of these patients.[12,41] Also it should be noted that the synchronous primary is present in up to 20% of cases of head and neck cancer elsewhere in the body. Hence, it seems appropriate to perform whole-body PET/CT in this subgroup. In a recent review by Varadhachary,[42] PET/CT was recommended in patients with squamous cell cancer who present with malignant cervical adenopathy. The overall performance of FDG PET/CT in CUP is summarized in **Table 1**.

THE CLINICAL IMPACT: PROBABLE FUTURE DEVELOPMENTS IN MANAGEMENT OF CARCINOMA OF UNKNOWN PRIMARY

CUP may be considered as metastatic disease in patients in whom the primary tumor has not been detected and did not result in clinical signs of disease.[34,35] If this is the case, detection of the primary tumor is worthwhile because it may lead to more specific treatment planning and improve outcomes.[34,35] On the other hand, CUP may represent a separate group of cancers with genetic and phenotypic characteristics that underlie their unique clinical presentation.[34,35] In this case, detection of the primary tumor is of minor importance, and diagnostic evaluation should focus on the identification of treatable subsets.[34,35] In other words, research should focus on the metastatic genotype and phenotype and on the detection of specific biochemical or molecular targets for the development of CUP-specific therapy.[34,35]

Hence, in the first case, the increased detection rate of unknown primary by FDG PET/CT itself may improve survival with tumor-specific therapy being administered to patients. In patients with cervical nodal metastases with an unknown primary, FDG PET/CT is useful because it may help guide the biopsy of the suspected primary site; determine the extent of disease, including the radiation field and presence of metastatic disease elsewhere; and enable the appropriate treatment. In cases of extracervical CUP, PET/CT is useful when CUP manifests as localized disease or a single-site metastasis to find the primary site as well as to

Table 1
Summary of review articles on CUP origin

No.	Author	Data	Detection Rate (%)	Sensitivity (%)	Specificity (%)	Comments
1	Rusthoven et al,[39] 2004	16 Studies, 302 patients	24.5	88.3	74.9	Cervical nodal metastases of CUP
2	Séve et al,[43] 2007	10 Studies, 221 patients	41.0	91.9	81.9	—
3	Dong et al,[36] 2008	13 Studies, 295 patients	31.0	81.0	82.0	—
4	Kwee & Kwee,[21] 2009	11 Studies, 433 patients	37.0	84.0	84.0	—
5	Moller et al,[44] 2011	4 Studies, 152 patients	39.5	87.0	88.0	Extracervical primary
6	Zhu & Wang,[45] 2013	7 Studies, 246 patients	44.0	97.0	68.0	Cervical nodal metastases of CUP

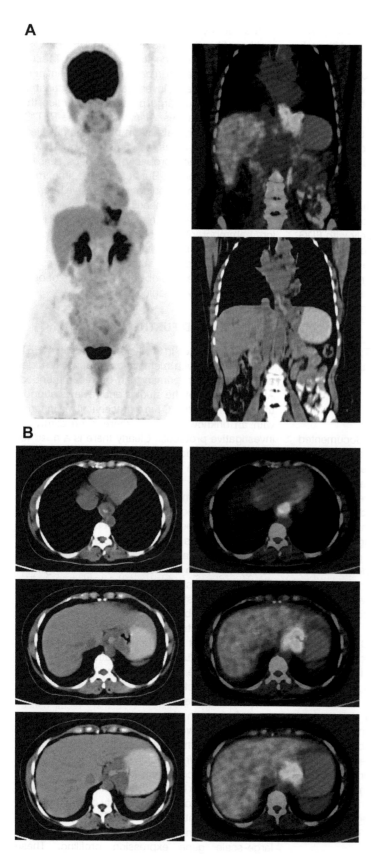

Fig. 7. A 44-year-old woman presented with 15- to 16-kg weight loss over last 6 months, weakness, and anorexia. She was evaluated earlier with blood tests, USG abdomen, and high-resolution CT scan of chest, both of which were reported normal, and refused any invasive tests like endoscopy. Hence, she was suggested for whole-body FDG PET/CT with oral and intravenous contrast by the attending oncologist. PET/CT scan showed primary hypermetabolic neoplastic thickening involving the lower thoracic esophagus (A), cardio-oesophageal junction, and proximal portion of gastric cardia with minimal ill-defined gastrohepatic adenopathy. Biopsy from the primary lesion confirmed adenocarcinoma of gastroesophageal junction. PET/CT scan not only detected the primary in this patient but staging was also done in the same scan (B).

determine the disease extent before locoregional treatment, such as surgery or radiation. Although in the second case it may not be important to find out the primary, finding other sites of metastatic disease would influence the management. Especially in the case of nodal disease, it would alter the radiation field owing to detection of additional sites of metastasis or it may avert unnecessary aggressive local therapy in the form of major surgery or radiotherapy. Thus, it could serve as a one-stop diagnostic and staging procedure. Furthermore, as there are advances in therapies targeted to particular molecule in tumor having mainly cytostatic effects, monitoring of these therapies may be possible more accurately with FDG PET/CT than anatomic imaging alone. A baseline FDG PET/CT may play a valuable role for planning treatment strategies and monitoring the following therapeutic intervention.[46] Indeed, PET/CT has been reported to change the patient management plan in 34.7% of patients with CUP.[2,43,47] Four individual studies in patients with CUP reported the therapeutic impact of FDG PET/CT; in these 4 studies, FDG PET/CT modified therapy in 18.2% to 60.0% of patients (**Fig. 7**).[48–51]

THE SHORTCOMINGS

Although multiple studies have documented impressive sensitivity and specificity of FDG PET/CT in CUP, these numbers are widely heterogeneous for several reasons. The extent to which these patients were investigated before undergoing PET/CT is highly varied among the study population groups. Further results of PET/CT scans had likely influenced the subsequent investigations that were performed. It would have also created bias regarding which patient would undergo biopsy (PET-positive patients are more likely to have a biopsy). On the other hand, in patients with extensive metastases, it may not be possible to distinguish the primary site from metastases.

The false-positive findings on PET/CT are not uncommon even in routine oncological cases. False-positive findings are also a concern in CUP. This fact becomes confounded as it leads to additional unnecessary investigations, which are usually invasive (scopies/biopsies). Considering the cost of PET/CT and additional investigations, it would significantly increase the economical burden. Also, a false-negative PET/CT study is likely to have a similar impact on finances. Even after the PET/CT scan, a considerable number of patients would still be labeled as having an unknown primary. However, with the advantages it offers with regard to treatment planning and monitoring, PET/CT could be of pivotal value in managing these cases.

In summary, to iterate that FDG PET/CT has a real benefit in the management of CUP, there is a need for clear evidence stating that PET/CT results in a favorable change in patient management or reduces the number of investigations. Unfortunately, there is a lack of large prospective studies that address these issues. Also, when to use PET/CT in the investigative algorithm of CUP is not clear. If it is used early on as recommended by a few investigators,[52] then probably other less sensitive tests can be avoided. But at the same time, many patients in whom the primary would have been detected by less costly means and by tests with less radiation exposure (eg, regional CT scan/MR imaging/mammography) would unnecessarily undergo PET/CT, which is a costly investigation. On the other hand, if it is used at the end of the investigative pathway, then the obvious advantage of being the most sensitive imaging test is lost.

SUMMARY AND FURTHER DIRECTIONS

Based on evidence in the literature, the use of PET/CT in patients with metastases to cervical nodes and an unknown primary can be recommended. Although most of the studies and reviews support the use of FDG PET/CT in extracervical malignancy with an unknown primary, there is no clarity on investigative protocols. Clearly there is a need for prospective randomized trials to define the exact role of PET/CT in the management of patients with CUP. Regarding increasing the detection rate of an unknown primary, the sensitivity of FDG PET/CT scanners needs to be improved. This improved sensitivity may be achieved with better-resolution PET/CT scanners, which includes advances in iterative algorithms and the use of time-of-flight technology. Although the use of contrast during PET/CT showed no significant impact on sensitivity, it would be interesting to know if it improves specificity and contributes to T staging, particularly in head and neck tumors. As mentioned earlier, delayed PET/CT at 3 to 4 hours may increase sensitivity in certain tumor types. Another issue worthy of mention is the use of dynamic FDG PET studies and PET parametric images, which can be particularly useful for the detection and characterization of small lesions in the oropharynx, lung, liver, or pancreas.[53] However, it is a technically demanding procedure and may not be applicable in busy clinical settings. Whole-body PET/MR imaging systems are now commercially available.[54] It would be interesting to know its usefulness with its superior soft tissue contrast and ability of functional imaging in patients with CUP. There are recent advances in molecular technology that allow large-scale gene expression profiling. These advances are useful in predicting the organ of origin in CUP. Thus, advances in molecular techniques along with advanced imaging are likely to lead the front for detection and management of patients with CUP in the future.

REFERENCES

1. Holmes FF, Fouts TL. Metastatic cancer of unknown primary site. Cancer 1970;26(4):816–20.

2. Greco FA, Hainsworth JD. Cancer of unknown primary site. In: DeVita TV, Hellman S, Rosenberg SA, editors. Cancer: principles and practice of oncology. 8th edition. Philadelphia: Lippincott, Williams & Wilkins; 2008. p. 2363–88.

3. Pavlidis N, Briasoulis E, Hainsworth J, et al. Diagnostic and therapeutic management of cancer of an unknown primary. Eur J Cancer 2003;39:1990–2005.

4. Wingo PA, Tong T, Bolden S. Cancer statistics, 1995. CA Cancer J Clin 1995;45:8–30.

5. Siegel R, Naishadham D, Jemal A. Cancer statistics, 2012. CA Cancer J Clin 2012;62:10–29.

6. Fizazi K, Greco FA, Pavlidis N, et al. Cancers of unknown primary site: ESMO clinical practice guidelines for diagnosis, treatment and follow-up. Ann Oncol 2011;22(Suppl 6):vi64–8.

7. Pavlidis N, Fizazi K. Carcinoma of unknown primary (CUP). Crit Rev Oncol Hematol 2009;69:271–8.

8. Hainsworth JD, Gereco FA. Treatment of patients with cancer of unknown primary site. N Engl J Med 1993;329(4):257–63.

9. Haas I, Hoffmann TK, Engers R, et al. Diagnostic strategies in cervical carcinoma of an unknown primary (CUP). Eur Arch Otorhinolaryngol 2002;259:325–33.

10. Raber MN, Faintuch J, Abbruzzese JL, et al. Continuous infusion 5-fluorouracil, etoposide and cisdiamminedichloroplatinum in patients with metastatic carcinoma of unknown primary origin. Ann Oncol 1991;2:519–20.

11. Rohren EM, Turkington TG, Coleman RE. Clinical applications of PET in oncology. Radiology 2004;231:305–32.

12. Roh JL, Kim JS, Lee JH, et al. Utility of combined (18)F-fluorodeoxyglucose-positron emission tomography and computed tomography in patients with cervical metastases from unknown primary tumors. Oral Oncol 2009;45:218–24.

13. Nassenstein K, Veit-Haibach P, Stergar H, et al. Cervical lymph node metastases of unknown origin: primary tumor detection with whole-body positron emission tomography/computed tomography. Acta Radiol 2007;48:1101–8.

14. Freudenberg LS, Fischer M, Antoch G, et al. Dual modality of 18F-fluorodeoxyglucosepositron emission tomography/computed tomography in patients with cervical carcinoma of unknown primary. Med Princ Pract 2005;14:155–60.

15. Kapoor V, McCook BM, Torok FS. An introduction to PET-CT imaging. Radiographics 2004;24:523–43.

16. Hany TF, Heuberger J, von Schulthess GK. Iatrogenic FDG foci in the lungs: a pitfall of PET image interpretation. Eur Radiol 2003;13:2122–7.

17. Kumar R, Dhanpathi H, Basu S, et al. Oncologic PET tracers beyond [(18)F]FDG and the novel quantitative approaches in PET imaging. Q J Nucl Med Mol Imaging 2008;52:50–65.

18. Basu S, Kung J, Houseni M, et al. Temporal profile of fluorodeoxyglucose uptake in malignant lesions and normal organs over extended time periods in patients with lung carcinoma: implications for its utilization in assessing malignant lesions. Q J Nucl Med Mol Imaging 2009;53:9–19.

19. Sanz-Viedma S, Torigian DA, Parsons M, et al. Potential clinical utility of dual time point FDG-PET for distinguishing benign from malignant lesions: implications for oncological imaging. Rev Esp Med Nucl 2009;28:159–66.

20. Fencl P, Belohlavek O, Skopalova M, et al. Prognostic and diagnostic accuracy of [18F]FDGPET/CT in 190 patients with carcinoma of unknown primary. Eur J Nucl Med Mol Imaging 2007;34:1783–92.

21. Kwee TC, Kwee RM. Combined FDG-PET/CT for the detection of unknown primary tumors: systematic review and meta-analysis. Eur Radiol 2009;19:731–44.

22. Ay MR, Zaidi H. Assessment of errors caused by X-ray scatter and use of contrast medium when using CT-based attenuation correction in PET. Eur J Nucl Med Mol Imaging 2006;33:1301–13.

23. Namasivayam S, Kalra MK, Torres WE, et al. Adverse reactions to intravenous iodinated contrast media: a primer for radiologists. Emerg Radiol 2006;12:210–5.

24. Metser U, Even-Sapir E. Increased (18)F-fluorodeoxyglucose uptake in benign, nonphysiologic lesions found on whole-body positron emission tomography/computed tomography (PET/CT): accumulated data from four years of experience with PET/CT. Semin Nucl Med 2007;37:206–22.

25. Shim SS, Lee KS, Kim BT, et al. Focal parenchymal lung lesions showing a potential of false-positive and false-negative interpretations on integrated PET/CT. AJR Am J Roentgenol 2006;186:639–48.

26. Wittram C, Scott JA. 18F-FDG PET of pulmonary embolism. AJR Am J Roentgenol 2007;189:171–6.

27. Lim HS, Yoon W, Chung TW, et al. FDG PET/CT for the detection and evaluation of breast diseases: usefulness and limitations. Radiographics 2007;27(Suppl 1):S197–213.

28. Al-Brahim N, Ross C, Carter B, et al. The value of postmortem examination in cases of metastasis of unknown origin-20-year retrospective data from a tertiary care center. Ann Diagn Pathol 2005;9:77–80.

29. Blaszyk H, Hartmann A, Bjornsson J. Cancer of unknown primary: clinicopathologic correlations. APMIS 2003;111:1089–94.

30. Mayordomo JI, Guerra JM, Guijarro C, et al. Neoplasms of unknown primary site: a clinicopathological study of autopsied patients. Tumori 1993;79: 321–4.

31. Le Chevalier T, Cvitkovic E, Caille P, et al. Early metastatic cancer of unknown primary origin at presentation. A clinical study of 302 consecutive autopsied patients. Arch Intern Med 1988;148:2035–9.

32. Pentheroudakis G, Greco FA, Pavlidis N. Molecular assignment of tissue of origin in cancer of unknown primary may not predict response to therapy or outcome: a systematic literature review. Cancer Treat Rev 2009;35:221–7.

33. Pentheroudakis G, Briasoulis E, Pavlidis N. Cancer of unknown primary site: missing primary or missing biology? Oncologist 2007;12:418–25.

34. van de Wouw AJ, Jansen RL, Speel EJ, et al. The unknown biology of the unknown primary tumour: a literature review. Ann Oncol 2003;14:191–6.

35. National Institute for Health and Clinical Excellence. Diagnosis and management of metastatic malignant disease of unknown primary origin (clinical guideline 104). London: National Institute for Health and Clinical Excellence; 2010. Available at: www.nice.org.uk/ CG104.

36. Dong MJ, Zhao K, Lin XT, et al. Role of fluorodeoxyglucose-PET versus fluorodeoxyglucose-PET/computed tomography in detection of unknown primary tumor: a meta-analysis of the literature. Nucl Med Commun 2008;29:791–802.

37. Fletcher JW, Djulbegovic B, Soares HP, et al. Recommendations on the use of 18F-FDG PET in oncology. J Nucl Med 2008;49:480–508.

38. Boellaard R, Doherty MJ, Weber WA, et al. FDG PET and PET/CT: EANM procedure guidelines for tumour PET imaging: version 1.0. Eur J Nucl Med Mol Imaging 2010;37(1):181–200.

39. Rusthoven KE, Koshy M, Paulino AC. The role of fluorodeoxyglucose positron emission tomography in cervical lymph node metastases from an unknown primary tumor. Cancer 2004;101:2641–9.

40. Fleming AJ Jr, Smith SP Jr, Paul CM, et al. Impact of [18F]-2-fluorodeoxyglucose-positron emission tomography–computed tomography on previously untreated head and neck cancer patients. Laryngoscope 2007;117:1173–9.

41. Ambrosini V, Nanni C, Rubello D, et al. 18F-FDG PET/CT in the assessment of carcinoma of unknown primary origin. Radiol Med 2006;111:1146–55.

42. Varadhachary GR. Carcinoma of unknown primary: focused evaluation. J Natl Compr Canc Netw 2011; 9:1406–12.

43. Sève P, Billotey C, Broussolle C, et al. The role of 2-deoxy-2-[F-18]fluoro-D-glucose positron emission tomography in disseminated carcinoma of unknown primary site. Cancer 2007;109:292–9.

44. Moller AK, Loft A, Berthelsen AK, et al. 18F-FDG PET/CT as a diagnostic tool in patients with extracervical carcinoma of unknown primary site: a literature review. Oncologist 2011;16(4):445–51.

45. Zhu L, Wang N. 18F-fluorodeoxyglucose positron emission tomography-computed tomography as a diagnostic tool in patients with cervical nodal metastases of unknown primary site: a meta-analysis. Surg Oncol 2013;22(3):190–4.

46. Basu S, Alavi A. FDG-PET in the clinical management of carcinoma of unknown primary with metastatic cervical lymphadenopathy: shifting gears from detecting the primary to planning therapeutic strategies. Eur J Nucl Med Mol Imaging 2007; 34:427–8.

47. Keller F, Psychogios G, Linke R, et al. Carcinoma of unknown primary in the head and neck: comparison between positron emission tomography (PET) and PET/CT. Head Neck 2011;33:1569–75.

48. Bruna C, Journo A, Netter F, et al. On the interest of PET with 18F-FDG in the management of cancer of unknown primary (CUP). Med Nucl 2007;31:242–9.

49. Wartski M, Le Stanc E, Gontier E, et al. In search of an unknown primary tumour presenting with cervical metastases: performance of hybrid FDG-PET-CT. Nucl Med Commun 2007;28:365–71.

50. Fakhry N, Barberet M, Lussato D, et al. Role of [18F]-FDG PET-CT in the management of the head and neck cancers. Bull Cancer 2006;93:1017–25.

51. Pelosi E, Pennone M, Deandreis D, et al. Role of whole body positron emission tomography/computed tomography scan with 18F-fluorodeoxyglucose in patients with biopsy proven tumor metastases from unknown primary site. Q J Nucl Med Mol Imaging 2006;50:15–22.

52. Kwee TC, Basu S, Cheng G, et al. FDG PET/CT in carcinoma of unknown primary. Eur J Nucl Med Mol Imaging 2010;37:635–44.

53. Anzai Y, Minoshima S, Wolf GT, et al. Head and neck cancer: detection of recurrence with three-dimensional principal components analysis at dynamic FDG PET. Radiology 1999;212:285–90.

54. von Schulthess GK, Schlemmer HP. A look ahead: PET/MR versus PET/CT. Eur J Nucl Med Mol Imaging 2009;36(Suppl 1):S3–9.

PET/Computed Tomography in the Diagnosis and Staging of Gastric Cancers

Nouf Malibari, MD, Marc Hickeson, MD, FRCP*,
Robert Lisbona, MD

KEYWORDS

- Gastric cancers • FDG • PET-CT

KEY POINTS

- The role of fluorodeoxyglucose (18F-FDG) PET in preoperative workup is limited owing to its low sensitivity for primary tumor and lymph node metastasis.
- PET and PET-computed tomography (CT) can decrease improper surgical resection, mainly because of the detection of distant metastases not diagnosed by conventional evaluation.
- In patients who have suspected recurrent disease, PET-CT can be helpful to detect sites of metastatic disease.

INTRODUCTION

Gastric cancer is among the most prevalent cancers worldwide and is among the commonest causes of cancer mortality, with approximately 750,000 deaths worldwide in 2010.[1] The overall 5-year survival rate of gastric cancer is less than 25%.[2] Gastric cancer is classified by its macroscopic appearance or histologic characteristics. The most common type of malignancy of the stomach is adenocarcinoma. Other tumors that will be discussed include gastric carcinoid, non-Hodgkin lymphoma, and gastrointestinal stromal tumors (GIST). Kaposi's sarcoma and metastatic disease from lung, breast, melanoma, esophageal, and colon primaries are less common.

GASTRIC ADENOCARCINOMA

Gastric adenocarcinomas comprise approximately 95% of all gastric cancers. There are 2 major subgroups—the intestinal type, which predominantly involves the distal stomach and is found most commonly in Asian patients, and the diffuse or signet ring type, which more commonly involves the proximal stomach and is found in Western patients. More than 80% of gastric cancer patients in the West are diagnosed at an advanced stage, resulting in a poor prognosis.[3] A variety of imaging modalities are used for the staging of gastric cancer. CT and endoscopic ultrasonography are used to determine the depth of involvement and presence of local and distant disease. In addition, staging laparoscopy is performed in patients who are thought to have resectable tumors or have imaging findings that are indeterminate for resectability to avoid surgery in patients with nonresectable tumor.[4,5] The only potential curative therapeutic modality of gastric adenocarcinoma is complete resection, which involves removal of part of or the entire stomach, in addition to lymph node dissection. Accurate staging and characterization of disease burden is of vital importance. The value of PET/CT has been of increasing interest among

The authors have nothing to disclose.
Nuclear Medicine, C02-8711, Royal Victoria Hospital, 1001 Decarie Boulevard, Montreal, Quebec H4A 3J1, Canada
* Corresponding author.
E-mail address: marc.hickeson@muhc.mcgill.ca

PET Clin 10 (2015) 311–326
http://dx.doi.org/10.1016/j.cpet.2015.03.008
1556-8598/15/$ – see front matter © 2015 Elsevier Inc. All rights reserved.

clinicians. Approximately one-third of the patients thought to have limited disease and to be candidates for surgery by conventional staging methods are found to have advanced disease at surgery. Multiple published studies evaluating gastric cancer with FDG-PET reported its potential value with regard to the staging of gastric cancer of intestinal type and nonmucinous tumors.[6]

IMAGING OF THE PRIMARY TUMOR

FDG-PET may normally show diffusely increased uptake, especially in the nondistended stomach. The use of oral contrast as well as the distention of the gastric walls will help to avoid this pitfall (Box 1).[7] Increased activity may be present in the gastroesophageal junction and this finding, in the absence of a CT abnormality, is also likely physiologic and secondary to normal muscular contraction of the lower esophageal sphincter.[8] This finding may also be seen in gastroesophageal reflux disease.[8]

INITIAL DIAGNOSIS

Studies have demonstrated a sensitivity of 93% to 94% of FDG-PET for the detection of gastric cancer,[9,10] which is similar to the sensitivity of CT (93%). FDG-PET has a higher specificity than CT (92% vs 62%).[10] In general, FDG-PET has a better sensitivity for more advanced disease (early gastric carcinoma, 63%; advanced gastric carcinoma, 98%).[10] Furthermore, a higher mean standardized uptake value (SUV; 7.7) is associated with the intestinal type of gastric adenocarcinoma.[10] A modest FDG activity is seen in mucinous and signet ring cell tumors (SUV mean, 4.2),[10] which is a function of the lower expression of GLUT-1 transporters on the cell membrane surface,[11] decreased cellularity, and an increased amount of intracellular mucin in mucinous and signet ring cell tumors.[12] Detection rates are higher when tumors are larger than 3.5 cm and have a deeper invasion (Fig. 1).[13]

DIFFERENTIAL DIAGNOSIS
Benign Ulcer

Benign ulcers appear on barium studies and CT scan as craters with sharply defined margin symmetric. They are confluent with healthy mucosa, and mucosal folds radiate from ulcer edge. Most

---

Box 1
Pitfalls and practical points in the use of fluorodeoxyglucose for the diagnosis of gastric cancers

Interactive pitfalls of fluorodeoxyglucose uptake in the stomach

1. Normal stomach uptake.

2. Inflammatory conditions (including gastritis, subclinical infection with *Helicobacter pylori*, or secondary to effects of chemotherapy).

Practical points

1. Normal stomach uptake

   - Although there may be elements of heterogeneity, in general, a physiologic pattern of activity has few or no discrete foci fusing to the gastric walls.
   - Water or food ingestion may decrease false positive from 31% to 8%.
   - Food has advantage of slower emptying from stomach resulting in a more prolonged duration of the gastric distension for imaging.
   - Misregistration artifacts can occur because of shifting gas/fluid volumes between CT and PET acquisition.
   - Additional single-field PET/CT acquisition can avoid misinterpretation.
   - In patients without a history of esophagogastric disease, a gastroesophageal SUV maximum of <4 is less likely to represent neoplasm. If the SUV is >4, further evaluation with endoscopy may be indicated.[8]

2. Inflammatory conditions

   - Usually demonstrate diffusely increased uptake that fuses to the wall on CT scan.
   - Clinical correlation is important in stratifying the differential diagnosis in that pattern of radiopharmaceutical distribution.
   - In addition to a thorough history and physical, blood counts and blood chemistries, abdominal CT, endoscopy, and pelvic ultrasonography or CT are important.

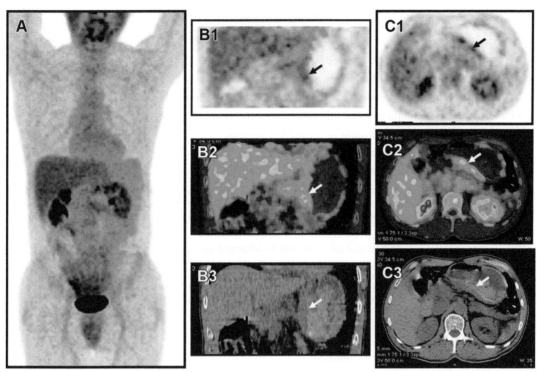

Fig. 1. This 61-year-old patient underwent an fluorodeoxyglucose (F-18 FDG) PET/CT scan. The maximal intensity projection image (*A*), the coronal PET images (*B1*), PET/CT fusion images (*B2*) and CT images (*B3*), and transaxial PET images (*C1*), PET/CT fusion images (*C2*) and CT images (*C3*) showed mild, ill-defined hypermetabolism in the stomach, mostly in the lesser curvature (*arrows*) associated with gastric wall thickening on imaging immediately after the patient drank water. The patient subsequently underwent total gastrectomy, which confirmed extensive tumor involvement of the lesser curvature. The histology was poorly differentiated diffuse type with Signet ring cells features.

are located in the lesser curve or posterior wall of antrum, or the body of the stomach.

GIST
Gastric lymphoma
Gastritis (see **Box 1**)
Physiologic FDG activity (see **Box 1**)

STAGING

The American Joint Committee on Cancer staging system is used widely to assess disease burden and prognosis in gastric cancer based on a TNM system. The 7th edition of American Joint Committee on Cancer guidelines designate tumor characteristic staging are delineated in **Box 2**. Pretreatment staging is essential to determine potential curability and to plan optimal therapy. The National Comprehensive Cancer Network staging guidelines now include PET/CT for staging of all patients with greater than T1 tumors and no clear-cut evidence of distant metastases.[14]

Primary Lesion (T) Staging

PET imaging is not particularly helpful for evaluation of the T stage.[15] In view of the limited spatial resolution, FDG-PET provides very limited information about the layer of the gastric wall involved and about invasion of adjacent organs.

Lymph Node (N) Staging

Lymph node metastases may initially involve the perigastric nodes, but regional lymph nodes along the celiac artery and its branch vessels may occur with some frequency as well (**Fig. 2**). According to the Japanese Gastric Cancer Association gastric lymph node classification, lymph nodes surrounding stomach are divided into 20 stations and are classified into 3 groups. In this grouping system, group 1 includes the most perigastric nodes (stations 1–6), group 2 includes stations 7 to 9, 11, and 12, and group 3 includes stations 10 and 13 through 20. D1 dissection is defined as a dissection of all the group 1 nodes and some of the station 7 nodes, depending on whether a total or partial gastrectomy is performed. D2 dissection is defined as dissection of all the group 1 and group 2 nodes, whereas D3 is defined as dissection of all the group 1, group 2, and group 3 nodes.[16]

Box 2
American Joint Committee on Cancer TNM staging system for gastric cancer

T—Primary tumor

- TX—Primary tumor cannot be assessed.
- T0—No evidence of primary tumor.
- Tis—Carcinoma in situ: intraepithelial tumor without invasion of the lamina propria.
- T1—Tumor invades lamina propria, muscularis mucosae, or submucosa.
- T1a—Tumor invades lamina propria or muscularis mucosa.
- T1b—Tumor invades submucosa.
- T2—Tumor invades muscularis propria.
- T3—Tumor penetrates subserosal connective tissue without invasion of visceral peritoneum or adjacent structures. T3 tumors also include those extending into the gastrocolic or gastrohepatic ligaments, or into the greater or lesser omentum, without perforation of the visceral peritoneum covering these structures.
- T4—Tumor invades serosa (visceral peritoneum) or adjacent structures.
- T4a—Tumor invades serosa (visceral peritoneum).
- T4b—Tumor invades adjacent structures such as spleen, transverse colon, liver, diaphragm, pancreas, abdominal wall, adrenal gland, kidney, small intestine, and retroperitoneum.

N—Regional lymph node

- NX—Regional lymph node(s) cannot be assessed.
- N0—No regional lymph node metastasis.
- N1—Metastasis in 1–2 regional lymph nodes.
- N2—Metastasis in 3–6 regional lymph nodes.
- N3—Metastasis in ≥7 regional lymph nodes.

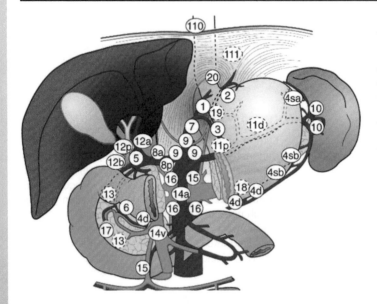

Fig. 2. Lymph node station numbers as defined by the Japanese Gastric Cancer Association. Stations 1/2, right/left pericardium; station 3, along the lesser curvature; station 4, along the greater curvature (4sa, along the short gastric vessels; 4sb, along the left gastroepiploic vessels; 4d, along the right gastroepiploic vessels); station 5, suprapylorum; station 6, infrapylorum; station 7, along the left gastric artery; station 8, along the common hepatic artery (8a, anterosuperior group; 8p, posterior group); station 9, along the celiac artery; station 10, at the splenic hilum; station 11, along the splenic artery (11p, along the proximal splenic artery; 11d, along the distal splenic artery); station 12, in the hepatoduodenal ligament (12a, along the hepatic artery; 12b, along the bile duct; 12p, posterior to the portal vein); station 13, on the posterior surface of the pancreatic head; station 14, along the superior mesenteric vessels (14a, along the superior mesenteric artery; 14v, along the superior mesenteric vein); station 15, along the middle colic vessels; station 16, around the abdominal aorta; station 17, on the anterior surface of the pancreatic head; station 18, along the inferior margin on the pancreas; station 19, infradiaphragmatic region; station 20, in the esophageal hiatus; station 110, paraesophageal region in the lower thorax and station 111, supradiaphragmatic region. (*From* Japanese Gastric Cancer Association. Japanese Classification of Gastric Carcinoma - 2nd English edition. Gastric Cancer 1998;1(1):16; with permission.)

The N1 disease status may not influence the surgical management of patients with gastric adenocarcinoma, because all will undergo at least D1 dissection.[16] What seems to be of greater clinical significance is the determination of N2 or N3 disease status, because the presence of N2 disease may increase the extent of lymph node dissection from D1 to D2 or greater. In view of the low sensitivity of PET/CT for the evaluation of N2 and N3 disease,[10] the absence of evidence of hypermetabolic lymph node metastases in N2 or N3 groups on PET/CT is insufficient for determining the extent of lymph node dissection. However, PET/CT is associated with high specificity for N2 and N3 disease.[10] As such, with the evidence of N2 disease on PET/CT, at least D2 lymph node dissection is required to achieve potentially curative resection.[10] The same holds true for evidence of N3 disease on PET/CT. Owing to its high specificity, PET/CT potentially has value for the determination of lymphadenectomy or reducing futile laparotomies in cases of unresectable lymph node metastases (**Fig. 3**).

Distant Metastases (M) Staging

The most common sites of distant metastases from gastric adenocarcinomas are within the abdominal cavity (including the peritoneal surfaces, liver, adrenals, kidneys, ovaries, and spleen) and in the left supraclavicular lymph nodes.[17] Metastatic disease beyond the abdomen and left supraclavicular nodes is uncommonly seen as a first site of recurrence. Distant metastatic disease associated with peritoneal dissemination is a common late manifestation of gastric adenocarcinoma (**Box 3**). FDG-PET has low sensitivity and CT has low specificity, but similar accuracy overall. Signet ring adenocarcinoma of the stomach may metastasize to the ovaries, which are sometimes referred to as Krukenberg's tumors. Overall, PET may be valuable for the detection of metastatic

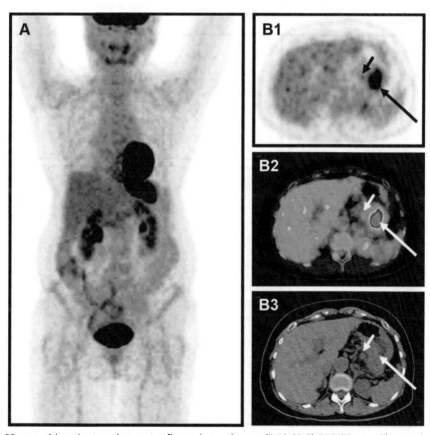

Fig. 3. This 66-year-old patient underwent a fluorodeoxyglucose (F-18 FDG) PET/CT scan. The maximal intensity projection image (*A*), the transaxial PET images (*B1*), PET/CT fusion images (*B2*), and CT images (*B3*) showed a hypermetabolic mass arising from the lesser curvature of the stomach (*long arrow*) with a maximal standardized uptake value (SUV) of 11.1. A small mildly hypermetabolic focus is demonstrated corresponds to a mildly enlarged gastrohepatic ligament lymph node with a maximal SUV of 3.0 (*small arrow*). Subsequent biopsy of the stomach revealed a diffuse type poorly differentiated gastric adenocarcinoma.

<table>
<tr><td colspan="2">Box 3
Anatomic stage/prognostic groups, gastric cancer</td></tr>
</table>

Stage 0	Tis N0 M0
Stage IA	T1 N0 M0
Stage IB	T2 N0 M0
	T1 N1 M0
Stage IIA	T3 N0 M0
	T2 N1 M0
	T1 N2 M0
Stage IIB	T4a N0 M0
	T3 N1 M0
	T2 N2 M0
	T1 N3 M0
Stage IIIA	T4a N1 M0
	T3 N2 M0
	T2 N3 M0
Stage IIIB	T4b N0 or N1 M0
	T4a N2 M0
	T3 N3 M0
Stage IIIC	T4b N2 or N3 M0
	T4a N3 M0
Stage IV	Any T Any N M1

to the liver, lungs, and distant lymph nodes, but has low sensitivity for the detection of osseous metastases and also peritoneal carcinomatosis owing to the limited spatial resolution (**Fig. 4**).[18]

PROGNOSIS

Lee and colleagues[19] reported that, on fluorodeoxyglucose (18F-FDG) PET, a maximum SUV (SUV_{max}) of equal or greater than 8.2 is an independent and poor prognostic factor associated with a 2-fold increase of the risk of cancer recurrence after curative surgical resection for patients with gastric cancer who did not receive any neoadjuvant therapy. Preoperative 18F-FDG-PET/CT could provide effective information on the prognosis after surgical resection in patients with gastric cancer.

THERAPY

Total gastrectomy is the preferred procedure for advanced gastric cancer of the proximal or middle

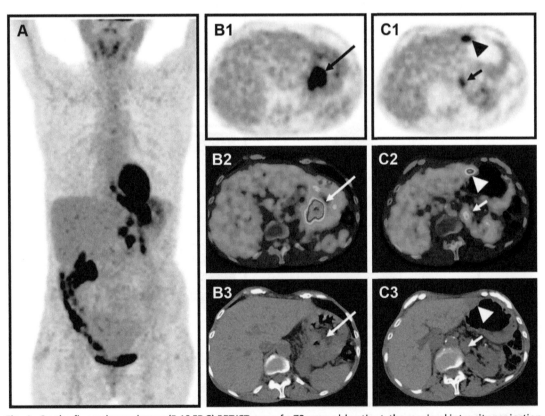

Fig. 4. On the fluorodeoxyglucose (F-18 FDG) PET/CT scan of a 72-year-old patient, the maximal intensity projection image (*A*), the transaxial PET images (*B1, C1*), PET/CT fusion images (*B2, C2*), and CT images (*B3, C3*) showed a hypermetabolic mass arising from the gastroesophageal junction (*long arrow*) with a maximal standardized uptake value (SUV) of 8.3 and hypermetabolic metastatic lesions in the left hepatic lobe (*arrow head*) with a maximal SUV of 4.9 and in the left adrenal gland (*short arrow*) with a maximal SUV of 3.5. Biopsy of the lesions in the gastroesophageal junction and in the liver confirmed the diagnosis of metastatic moderately differentiated adenocarcinoma.

third of the stomach, to eliminate the possibility of recurrence in the gastric stump or the surrounding lymph nodes.[20] Subtotal gastrectomy seems to be performed more commonly on patients with distal gastric tumors because there are no proven survival benefits compared with total or subtotal gastrectomy.[21] When tumor recurs in the remnant stomach, any treatments with curative intent are usually considered futile.[7,22]

RESPONSE TO THERAPY

PET has demonstrated usefulness for the evaluation of the response to neoadjuvant chemotherapy in gastric cancer.[23] Ott and colleagues[24] showed that a 35% decrease in uptake between prechemotherapy and PET scan taken 2 weeks after initiation of therapy predicted response with accuracy of 85%. The 2-year survival rate was 90% in responders (**Figs. 5** and **6**), and 25% in nonresponders (**Figs. 7** and **8**) using this criteria with $P = .002$.[24] Wahl and colleagues[25] have proposed a PET Response Criteria in Solid Tumors (PERCIST). PERCIST criteria propose a 30% or greater decline as indicative of "medically relevant beneficial changes." Per the criteria, normal reference tissue values are designated within a scan by using a consistent protocol based on regions of interest in the liver and the most active tissues. Wahl and

associates suggest that the PERCIST criteria be used as a starting point for clinical trials and clinical reporting. In some gastric cancers having low affinity to FDG, repeat imaging does not provide additional useful imaging for these patients. Wahl and colleagues recommend then the use of RECIST 1.1 in such cases. Ott and colleagues[24] reported that patient with non–FDG-avid gastric adenocarcinomas had a similar prognosis compared with nonresponders. Metabolic responders had a 69% histopathologic response rate, whereas the metabolic nonresponders had only a 17% histopathologic response rate, which was not different compared with that of the metabolic nonreponders, with a 24% histopathologic response rate. Survival was also similar between the nonavid group and the nonresponding group, but significantly different from the responding group.

DETECTION OF RECURRENCE

Despite complete resection with curative intent, tumor is known to recur in more than one-half of patients with gastric adenocarcinomas.[20,22] Systemic recurrence occurs more frequently than locoregional recurrence.[26] The most common sites of systemic recurrences are the liver and the peritoneal cavity, whereas for local recurrences, the most common sites are the luminal margin, the gastric

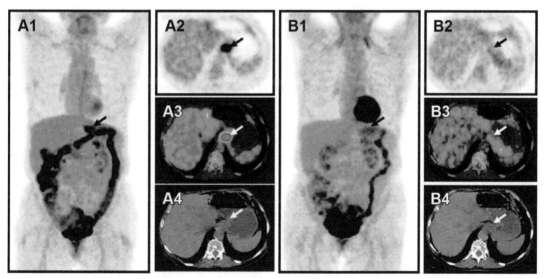

Fig. 5. This 64-year-old patient with adenocarcinoma of the gastroesophageal junction was treated with 3 months of neoadjuvant chemotherapy before resection of the distal esophagus and proximal stomach. On the baseline fluorodeoxyglucose (FDG)-PET study (*A*), the maximal intensity projection (*A1*), FDG-PET images (*A2*), PET/CT fusion images (*A3*), and CT images (*A4*) demonstrated a hypermetabolic mass measuring up to approximately 3.0 cm with a maximal standardized uptake value of 6.2 in the gastroesophageal junction (*arrow*). On the postchemotherapy FDG-PET study (*B*), the maximal intensity projection (*B1*), FDG-PET images (*B2*), PET/CT fusion images (*B3*), and CT images (*B4*) showed complete resolution of the hypermetabolic mass (*arrow*). These findings indicate complete metabolic response. After operative resection, the pathology report described a complete pathologic response to neoadjuvant chemotherapy.

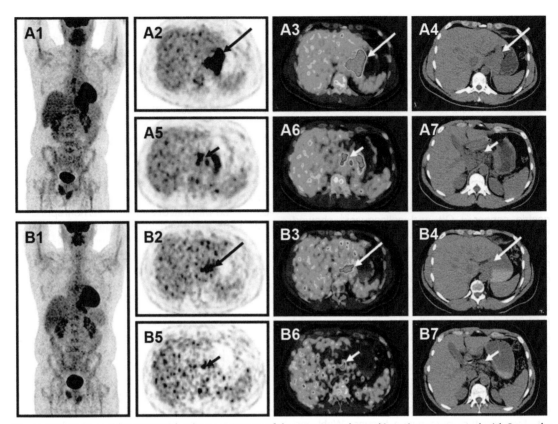

Fig. 6. This 41-year-old patient with adenocarcinoma of the gastroesophageal junction was treated with 3 months of neoadjuvant chemotherapy before resection of the distal esophagus and proximal stomach. On the baseline fluorodeoxyglucose (FDG)-PET study (*A*), the maximal intensity projection (*A1*), FDG-PET images (*A2, A5*), PET/CT fusion images (*A3, A6*), and CT images (*A4, A7*) demonstrated a hypermetabolic mass measuring up to approximately 8.8 cm with a maximal standardized uptake value (SUV) of 21.2 in the gastroesophageal junction (*long arrow*) and multiple lymph node metastases in the mediastinum and gastrohepatic ligament (*short arrow*). On the postchemotherapy FDG-PET study (*B*), the maximal intensity projection (*B1*), FDG-PET images (*B2, B5*), PET/CT fusion images (*B3, B6*), and CT images (*B4, B7*) showed a partial resolution of the hypermetabolic mass in the gastroesophageal junction (*long arrow*), with the maximal SUV decreasing to 7.8. There has been interval metabolic resolution of the mediastinal lesions, but residual focal hypermetabolism remaining in a gastrohepatic ligament lymph node (*short arrow*). These findings indicate a partial metabolic response. After operative resection, the pathology report described invasive moderately differentiated adenocarcinoma associated with minimal regression (fibrosis constitutes <25% of the tumor mass) and metastatic disease was present in 29 of the 39 lymph nodes sampled.

bed and locoregional lymph nodes.[27] Other than periodic surveillance using endoscopy, noninvasive anatomic imaging studies, such as a barium study or CT, have been used in detecting recurrent tumors of the remnant stomach. The main limitation with CT is its lack of specificity in differentiating recurrent tumor in the remnant stomach from improperly distended bowel loops, surgical plication, bowel adhesion, or stomal polypoid hypertrophic gastritis. Although 18F-FDG PET has been demonstrated to be useful for detecting recurrent diseases of various cancers, its usefulness for evaluating the remnant stomach is limited. A low level of 18F-FDG uptake is seen commonly in the normal stomach, although it can also have a high SUV.[27] Gastric distension makes it easier to delineate subtle mucosal

abnormalities of the stomach and decreases the possibility of misinterpretation.[28] Similar results were found in a study by Yun and colleagues.[7] Gastric distension by imaging the stomach immediately after a patient drinks a glass of water seems to be a simple, cost-effective method of increasing the diagnostic accuracy of 18F-FDG PET in suspected recurrence in the stomach remnant. Visual analysis with special attention to the configuration of 18F-FDG activity after water ingestion seems to be more accurate than a decrease of the SUV in evaluating the stomach remnant (**Fig. 9**).[7] De Potter and coworkers studied 33 patients with clinical suspicion for recurrent gastric carcinoma after operative intervention with curative intent. The study demonstrated a sensitivity of 70%, a specificity of

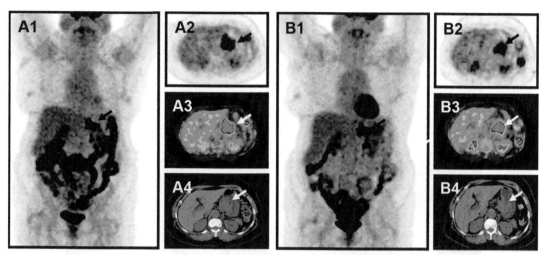

Fig. 7. This 73-year-old patient with gastric adenocarcinoma was treated with 3 months of neoadjuvant chemotherapy before undergoing partial gastrectomy. On the baseline fluorodeoxyglucose (FDG)-PET study (A), the maximal intensity projection (A1), FDG-PET images (A2), PET/CT fusion images (A3), and CT images (A4) demonstrated a hypermetabolic mass measuring up to approximately 7.5 cm with a maximal standardized uptake value (SUV) of 8.8 in the lesser curvature of the stomach (arrow). On the postchemotherapy FDG-PET study (B), the maximal intensity projection (B1), FDG-PET images (B2), PET/CT fusion images (B3), and CT images (B4) showed no change of the hypermetabolic mass (arrow) with a maximal SUV of 10.3. These findings indicate stable disease.

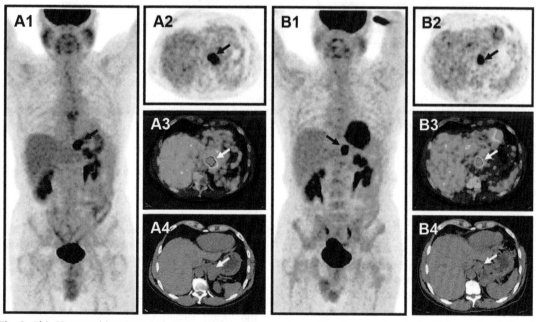

Fig. 8. This 63-year-old patient with cancer of the gastroesophageal junction was treated with 3 months of neoadjuvant chemotherapy before resection of the distal esophagus and proximal stomach. On the baseline fluorodeoxyglucose (FDG)-PET study (A), the maximal intensity projection (A1), FDG-PET images (A2), PET/CT fusion images (A3), and CT images (A4) demonstrated a hypermetabolic lesion with a maximal standardized uptake value (SUV) of 7.1 in the gastroesophageal junction (arrow). On the postchemotherapy FDG-PET study (B), the maximal intensity projection (B1), FDG-PET images (B2), PET/CT fusion images (B3), and CT images (B4) showed intensification of the hypermetabolic lesion (arrow) with the SUV increasing to 10.7. These findings indicate progressive disease. After surgical resection, the pathology report of that lesion described a viable poorly differentiated adenocarcinoma.

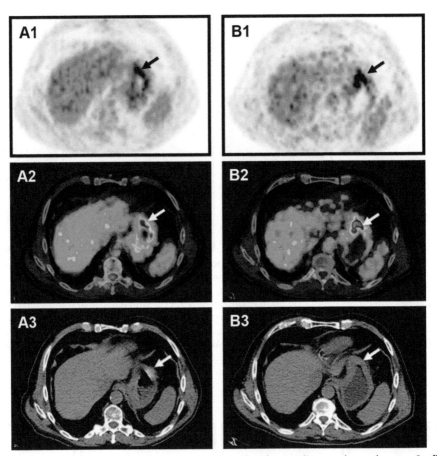

Fig. 9. This 67-year-old patient with gastric cancer was treated with neoadjuvant chemotherapy. On fluorodeoxyglucose PET/CT, the transaxial PET images (*A1*), PET/CT fusion images (*A2*), and CT images (*A3*) showed hypermetabolism in the stomach (*arrow*). On repeat PET imaging (*B1*), PET/CT fusion imaging (*B2*), and CT imaging (*B3*) obtained after the patient drank water, there was persistent hypermetabolism in the anterior gastric wall (*arrow*). This indicated residual tumor. The patient subsequently underwent total gastrectomy, which confirmed residual viable tumor in the stomach. The histology was mixed type consisting of poorly differentiated diffuse type and moderately differentiated intestinal type.

69%, a positive predictive value of 78%, and a negative predicted value of 60% in the detection of recurrent disease (**Fig. 10**).[29] In addition, they found a longer survival in patients with a negative PET scan (21.9 vs 19.0 months) compared with those with a positive PET scan (9.2 vs 8.2 months).[29] In recurrent disease with liver metastases, FDG-PET was shown in a metaanalysis to have a higher sensitivity (90%) than either CT (70%) or MRI (71%). PET/CT in comparison with CT alone has shown much greater sensitivity for mediastinal lymph node recurrences.[18]

OTHER RADIOTRACERS

18F-Fluorolevothymidine PET demonstrated a higher sensitivity than 18F-FDG PET and might serve as a useful diagnostic adjunct for the quantitative assessment of proliferation.[30]

GASTRIC LYMPHOMA

Primary gastric lymphoma (PGL) accounts for less than 5% of all gastric malignancies. It is, however, among the most common sites of extranodal lymphoma and occurs in 4 to 20% of patients.[31,32] PGL has a higher prevalence in men over the age of 50. The most common histologies of PGL are diffuse large B-cell lymphoma (**Fig. 11**), a high-grade or aggressive non-Hodgkin lymphoma (AGNHL), and low grade mucosal-associated lymphoid tissue (MALT; **Fig. 12**), also defined in the World Health Organization classification as extranodal marginal zone B-cell lymphoma.[32,33] Accurate staging of newly diagnosed PGL is important for the optimal treatment planning. Clinical presentation and radiologic features of PGL are in general nonspecific. In a retrospective study by Radan and colleagues,[34] 62 consecutive patients with newly diagnosed PGL by endoscopic biopsy were referred

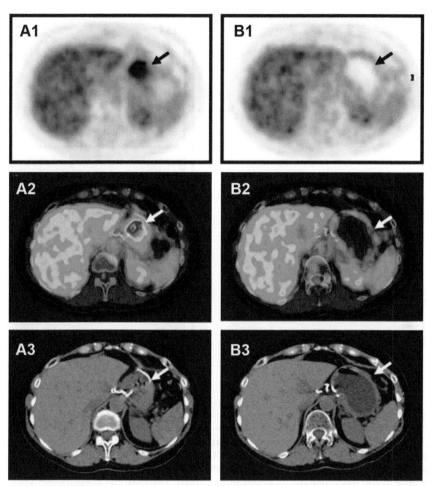

Fig. 10. This 55-year-old patient with gastric cancer had undergone partial gastrectomy. On fluorodeoxyglucose PET/CT, the transaxial PET images (*A1*), PET/CT fusion images (*A2*), and CT images (*A3*) showed moderate hypermetabolism in the remnant of the stomach (*arrow*) that is not apparent on delayed PET images (*B1*), PET/CT fusion images (*B2*), or CT images (*B3*) with the stomach distended after the patient drank water (*arrow*). These findings indicate physiologic activity of the stomach.

for FDG-PET/CT between February 2002 and August 2006.[28] Gastric FDG uptake was found in 55 of 62 of all cases (89%) of PGLs, including 100% of AGNHL versus 71% of MALT (*P*<.001) and 63% of controls. A diffuse pattern was found in 60% PGL (76% MALT vs 53% AGNHL; *P* = NS) and 47% controls. FDG uptake higher than liver was found in 82% PGL (58% MALT vs 97% AGNHL; *P*<.05) and 63% of controls. The SUV_{max} in FDG-avid PGLs was 15.3 ± 11.7 (5.4 ± 2.9 MALT vs 19.7 ± 11.5 AGNHL; *P*<.001) and 4.6 ± 1.4 in controls. CT abnormalities were found in 79% PGL (thickening, n = 49; ulcerations, n = 22). Extragastric FDG-avid sites were seen in none of MALT, but 61% of AGNHL (nodal, n = 18; nodal and extranodal, n = 5). The cause for the variable and lower FDG avidity in MALT lymphoma is unclear, but it has been hypothesized that it could be related to the heterogeneous cellular population in this lymphoma type

consisting of small or large B cells and plasma cells, as well as to their lower metabolic activity.[35] FDG uptake can be differentiated, in particular in AGNHL PGL from physiologic tracer activity by intensity, but not by pattern. Extragastric FDG-avid foci on PET and structural CT abnormalities are additional features that can improve PET/CT the evaluation of PGL. Defining FDG avidity and PET/CT patterns in AGNHL and a subgroup of MALT-PGL before treatment may be important for further monitoring of response to therapy. Although FDG imaging has a well-established role for the management of lymphoma in general, its value in assessing patients with PGL is still debated and challenging.

GASTROINTESTINAL STROMAL TUMOR

GIST (**Fig. 13**) is an uncommon tumor and accounts for only 0.1% to 3% of all gastrointestinal

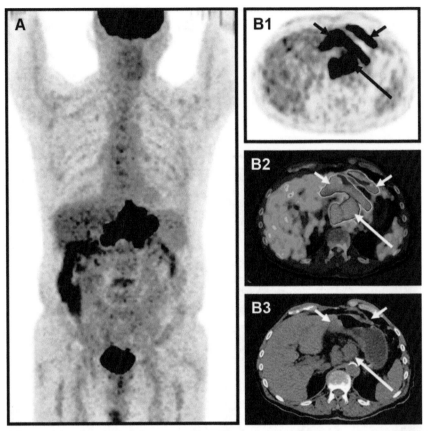

Fig. 11. This 81-year-old patient had undergone a fluorodeoxyglucose PET/CT scan. The maximal intensity projection image (*A*), the transaxial PET images (*B1*), PET/CT fusion images (*B2*), and CT images (*B3*) showed extensive hypermetabolism in the body and antrum of the stomach (*short arrow*) and bulky hypermetabolic lymphadenopathy in the gastrohepatic ligament (*long arrow*). The maximal standardized uptake value was approximately 27. The diagnosis of diffuse large B-cell lymphoma was subsequently established by a biopsy of the gastric antrum.

cancers and 6% of all sarcomas.[36] However, it is the most common mesenchymal neoplasm of the gastrointestinal tract[37] and up to 20% of small bowel malignancies are GIST.[38] Primary GISTs are usually solitary tumors that arise most frequently in the stomach (60%–70%) followed by small bowel (20%–25%), and rarely from the rectum (5%), esophagus, colon, and appendix.[39] The advents of immunochemistry and of electron microscopy made it possible to characterize GIST cells as originating from cells of Cajal and not from smooth muscle cells.[40–42] GISTs have been misclassified as leiomyomas, leiomyosarcomas, and leiomyoblastomas. Malignant GISTs tend to recur and metastasize, most often to the liver and peritoneum. Other metastatic sites include the lungs, pleura, retroperitoneum, bone, and subcutaneous tissues.[36] The unique feature of GIST is that approximately 95% of these tumors are immunoreactive with KIT (CD117), the c-kit receptor tyrosine kinase.

Staging

GISTs generally have greater FDG avidity than that of normal tissue. PET imaging of pulmonary and upper abdominal lesions often obscured by motion artifact and partial volume averaging on the CT portion of PET/CT requires careful scrutiny of these anatomic regions. More lesions are identified with contrast-enhanced CT alone than with FDG-PET alone, but FDG-avid lesions seem to be more clinically relevant.[43] PET/CT facilitates the identification of lesions in the majority of patients and provides a better evaluation of surgical resectability.[43] The sensitivity and positive predictive values were 93% and 100%, respectively, for CT and 86% and 98%, respectively, for 18F-FDG PET. No difference was found in CT and 18F-FDG PET sensitivity or positive predictive values ($P<.27$ and .25, respectively).[44] It has been recognized that not all GISTs are FDG avid; in 1 series of 34 patients, the sensitivity of FDG-PET on a per-patient basis was reported to be 79% (**Box 4**).[43]

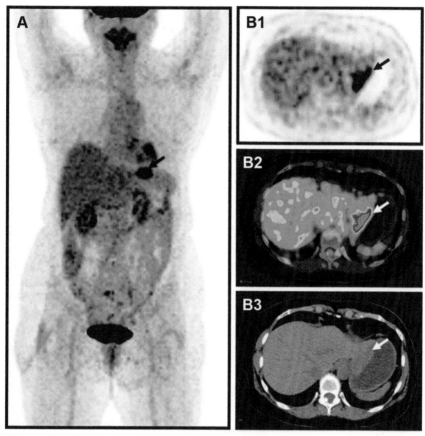

Fig. 12. This 66-year-old patient had undergone a fluorodeoxyglucose PET/CT scan. The maximal intensity projection image (*A*), the transaxial PET images (*B1*), PET/CT fusion images (*B2*), and CT images (*B3*) showed a hypermetabolic mass arising from the lesser curvature of the stomach (*arrow*) with a maximal standardized uptake value of 7. This mass is a biopsy-proven mucosa-associated lymphoid tissue lymphoma.

Prognosis

Important prognostic factors that have been suggested include tumor size of greater than 5 cm, ability to perform a complete initial resection of the tumor, and tumor grade and site.[38] It has been suggested of a correlation of the intensity of FDG uptake with the malignant potential and aggressiveness of a GIST.[43,45]

Therapy

Surgical resection and targeted therapy are the standard of care for the treatment of GIST. Imatinib mesylate (Gleevec, Novartis Pharmaceutical Corp., St Louis, MO), the first-line medication, acts as a tyrosine kinase inhibitor. This treatment was demonstrated to have an impressive response with the first single patient trial reported in 2001.[46,47] The second drug approved for the treatment of GIST is sunitinib (Sutent), which also interacts with vascular endothelial growth factor receptors 1 through 3, fluorolevothymidine-3, and RET receptors, resulting in a potential antiangiogenic effect. Sunitinib is reserved for patients with unresectable disease who have developed primary or secondary resistance to imatinib and who are progressing despite higher doses of imatinib mesylate.[48]

Response to Therapy

Some researchers believed that CT underestimated the therapeutic effect of imatinib mesylate during clinical trials of tyrosine kinase inhibitors,[49] because the tumor may even increase in size with a positive response to therapy. A positive response on FDG-PET may be evident as early as 24 hours after a single dose of imatinib. It might actually take weeks to months, even years, for tumors to start decrease in size as they undergo cystic and density changes on CT despite of a favorable pathologic response to the treatment.[50] FDG-PET was demonstrated to be useful to monitor for recurrence in surgically treated patient and may better predict response to imatinib at 1 week than CT at 2 months after initiating

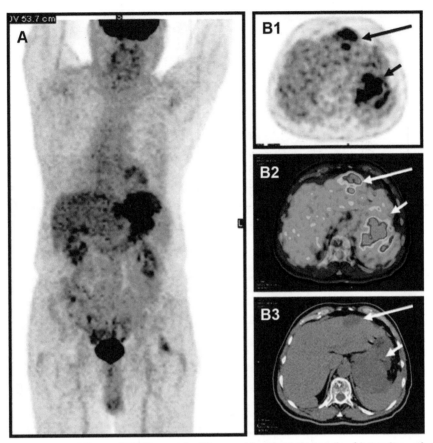

Fig. 13. On the fluorodeoxyglucose PET/CT scan of a 73-year-old patient, the maximal intensity projection image (*A*), the transaxial PET images (*B1*), PET/CT fusion images (*B2*), and CT images (*B3*) showed a heterogeneously hypermetabolic exophytic mass in the greater curvature of the stomach extending into the gastrosplenic ligament (*short arrow*) and a necrotic hypermetabolic metastasis in the left hepatic lobe (*long arrow*). The maximal standardized uptake value was approximately 13.6. The diagnosis of gastrointestinal stromal tumor was established by a biopsy of the stomach lesion.

treatment.[51–54] Choi and colleagues[52] suggested that the decrease of the SUV from baseline should be at least 65% and to an SUV of less than 2.5 to indicate response. On the other hand, Jager and associates found that a decrease of greater than 25% at 1 week correlated better with the response to treatment than tumor volume changes observed on CT at 2 months after initiation of therapy.[17] In addition, a good metabolic response predicts a significantly longer time to progression.[44,52,53] In contrast, it has been suggested that in a previously treated patient, low FDG avidity in newly recurrent GIST may be associated with a poor response to tyrosine kinase inhibitor therapy.[55]

Box 4
Diagnostic checklist

Bulky abdominal soft tissue mass without lymphadenopathy = common gastrointestinal stromal tumor presentation

Central necrosis/hemorrhage common

Usually highly fluorodeoxyglucose avid

REFERENCES

1. Lozano R, Naghavi M, Foreman K, et al. Global and regional mortality from 235 causes of death for 20 age groups in 1990 and 2010: a systematic analysis for the Global Burden of Disease Study 2010. Lancet 2012;380(9859):2095–128.
2. Chan AO, Wong BC, Lam SK. Gastric cancer: past, present and future. Can J Gastroenterol 2001;15(7): 469–74.
3. Roukos DH. Current status and future perspectives in gastric cancer management. Cancer Treat Rev 2000;26(4):243–55.
4. Abdalla EK, Pisters PW. Staging and preoperative evaluation of upper gastrointestinal malignancies. Semin Oncol 2004;31(4):513–29.

5. Weber WA, Ott K. Imaging of esophageal and gastric cancer. Semin Oncol 2004;31(4):530–41.

6. Stahl A, Ott K, Weber WA, et al. FDG PET imaging of locally advanced gastric carcinomas: correltion with endoscopic and histopathological findings. Eur J Nucl Med Mol Imaging 2003;30(2):288–95.

7. Yun M, Choi HS, Yoo E, et al. The role of gastric distention in differentiating recurrent tumor from physiologic uptake in the remnant stomach on 18F-FDG PET. J Nucl Med 2005;46(6):953–7.

8. Salaun PY, Grewal RK, Dodamane I, et al. An analysis of the 18F-FDG uptake pattern in the stomach. J Nucl Med 2005;46(1):48–51.

9. Yeung HW, Macapinlac H, Karpeh M, et al. Accuracy of FDG-PET in gastric cancer. preliminary experience. Clin Positron Imaging 1998;1(4):213–21.

10. Chen J, Cheong JH, Yun MJ, et al. Improvement in preoperative staging of gastric adenocarcinoma with positron emission tomography. Cancer 2005;103(11):2383–90.

11. Alakus H, Batur M, Schmidt M, et al. Variable 18F-fluorodeoxyglucose uptake in gastric cancer is associated with different levels of GLUT-1 expression. Nucl Med Commun 2010;31(6):532–8.

12. Berger KL, Nicholson SA, Dehdashti F, et al. FDG PET evaluation of mucinous neoplasms: correlation of FDG uptake with histopathologic features. AJR Am J Roentgenol 2000;174(4):1005–8.

13. Graziosi L, Evoli L, Cavazzoni E, et al. The role of 18FDG-PET in gastric cancer. Transl Gastrointest Cancer 2012;1(2):186–8.

14. Ajani JA, Bentrem DJ, Besh S, et al. Gastric cancer, version 2.2013: featured updates to the NCCN Guidelines. J Natl Compr Canc Netw 2013;11(5):531–46.

15. Yoon NR, Park JM, Jung HS, et al. Usefulness of (1)(8)F-fluoro-2-deoxyglucose positron emission tomography in evaluation of gastric cancer stage. Korean J Gastroenterol 2012;59(5):347–53 [in Korean].

16. Tamura S, Takeno A, Miki H. Lymph node dissection in curative gastrectomy for advanced gastric cancer. Int J Surg Oncol 2011;2011:748745.

17. Landry J, Tepper JE, Wood WC, et al. Patterns of failure following curative resection of gastric carcinoma. Int J Radiat Oncol Biol Phys 1990;19(6):1357–62.

18. Kinkel K, Lu Y, Both M, et al. Detection of hepatic metastases from cancers of the gastrointestinal tract by using noninvasive imaging methods (US, CT, MR imaging, PET): a meta-analysis. Radiology 2002;224(3):748–56.

19. Lee JW, Lee SM, Lee MS, et al. Role of (1)(8)F-FDG PET/CT in the prediction of gastric cancer recurrence after curative surgical resection. Eur J Nucl Med Mol Imaging 2012;39(9):1425–34.

20. Roukos DH. Extended (D2) lymph node dissection for gastric cancer: do patients benefit? Ann Surg Oncol 2000;7(4):253–5.

21. Gouzi JL, Huguier M, Fagniez PL, et al. Total versus subtotal gastrectomy for adenocarcinoma of the gastric antrum. A French prospective controlled study. Ann Surg 1989;209(2):162–6.

22. Lehnert T, Rudek B, Buhl K, et al. Surgical therapy for loco-regional recurrence and distant metastasis of gastric cancer. Eur J Surg Oncol 2002;28(4):455–61.

23. Ferri LE, Ades S, Alcindor T, et al. Perioperative docetaxel, cisplatin, and 5-fluorouracil (DCF) for locally advanced esophageal and gastric adenocarcinoma: a multicenter phase II trial. Ann Oncol 2012;23(6):1512–7.

24. Ott K, Herrmann K, Krause BJ, et al. The value of PET imaging in patients with localized gastroesophageal Cancer. Gastrointest Cancer Res 2008;2(6):287–94.

25. Wahl RL, Jacene H, Kasamon Y, et al. From RECIST to PERCIST: evolving considerations for PET response criteria in solid tumors. J Nucl Med 2009;50(Suppl 1):122S–50S.

26. Wanebo HJ, Kennedy BJ, Chmiel J, et al. Cancer of the stomach. A patient care study by the American College of Surgeons. Ann Surg 1993;218(5):583–92.

27. Shreve PD, Anzai Y, Wahl RL. Pitfalls in oncologic diagnosis with FDG PET imaging: physiologic and benign variants. Radiographics 1999;19(1):61–77 [quiz: 150–1].

28. Horton KM, Fishman EK. Helical CT of the stomach: evaluation with water as an oral contrast agent. AJR Am J Roentgenol 1998;171(5):1373–6.

29. De Potter T, Flamen P, Van Cutsem E, et al. Whole-body PET with FDG for the diagnosis of recurrent gastric cancer. Eur J Nucl Med Mol Imaging 2002;29(4):525–9.

30. Herrmann K, Ott K, Buck AK, et al. Imaging gastric cancer with PET and the radiotracers 18F-FLT and 18F-FDG: a comparative analysis. J Nucl Med 2007;48(12):1945–50.

31. d'Amore F, Brincker H, Gronbaek K, et al. Non-Hodgkin's lymphoma of the gastrointestinal tract: a population-based analysis of incidence, geographic distribution, clinicopathologic presentation features, and prognosis. Danish Lymphoma Study Group. J Clin Oncol 1994;12(8):1673–84.

32. Zucca E, Conconi A, Cavalli F. Treatment of extranodal lymphomas. Best Pract Res Clin Haematol 2002;15(3):533–47.

33. Al-Akwaa AM, Siddiqui N, Al-Mofleh IA. Primary gastric lymphoma. World J Gastroenterol 2004;10(1):5–11.

34. Radan L, Fischer D, Bar-Shalom R, et al. FDG avidity and PET/CT patterns in primary gastric lymphoma. Eur J Nucl Med Mol Imaging 2008;35(8):1424–30.

35. Maes B, De Wolf-Peeters C. Marginal zone cell lymphoma–an update on recent advances. Histopathology 2002;40(2):117–26.

36. Burkill GJ, Badran M, Al-Muderis O, et al. Malignant gastrointestinal stromal tumor: distribution, imaging features, and pattern of metastatic spread. Radiology 2003;226(2):527–32.

37. Miettinen M, Lasota J. Gastrointestinal stromal tumors–definition, clinical, histological, immunohistochemical, and molecular genetic features and differential diagnosis. Virchows Arch 2001;438(1):1–12.

38. Blanchard DK, Budde JM, Hatch GF 3rd, et al. Tumors of the small intestine. World J Surg 2000; 24(4):421–9.

39. Lau S, Tam KF, Kam CK, et al. Imaging of gastrointestinal stromal tumour (GIST). Clin Radiol 2004; 59(6):487–98.

40. Bucher P, Villiger P, Egger JF, et al. Management of gastrointestinal stromal tumors: from diagnosis to treatment. Swiss Med Wkly 2004;134(11–12): 145–53.

41. Hurlimann J, Gardiol D. Gastrointestinal stromal tumours: an immunohistochemical study of 165 cases. Histopathology 1991;19(4):311–20.

42. Walker P, Dvorak AM. Gastrointestinal autonomic nerve (GAN) tumor. Ultrastructural evidence for a newly recognized entity. Arch Pathol Lab Med 1986;110(4):309–16.

43. Kamiyama Y, Aihara R, Nakabayashi T, et al. 18F-fluorodeoxyglucose positron emission tomography: useful technique for predicting malignant potential of gastrointestinal stromal tumors. World J Surg 2005;29(11):1429–35.

44. Goerres GW, Stupp R, Barghouth G, et al. The value of PET, CT and in-line PET/CT in patients with gastrointestinal stromal tumours: long-term outcome of treatment with imatinib mesylate. Eur J Nucl Med Mol Imaging 2005;32(2):153–62.

45. Yamada M, Niwa Y, Matsuura T, et al. Gastric GIST malignancy evaluated by 18FDG-PET as compared with EUS-FNA and endoscopic biopsy. Scand J Gastroenterol 2007;42(5):633–41.

46. Joensuu H, Roberts PJ, Sarlomo-Rikala M, et al. Effect of the tyrosine kinase inhibitor STI571 in a patient with a metastatic gastrointestinal stromal tumor. N Engl J Med 2001;344(14):1052–6.

47. Tuveson DA, Willis NA, Jacks T, et al. STI571 inactivation of the gastrointestinal stromal tumor c-KIT oncoprotein: biological and clinical implications. Oncogene 2001;20(36):5054–8.

48. Demetri GD, van Oosterom AT, Garrett CR, et al. Efficacy and safety of sunitinib in patients with advanced gastrointestinal stromal tumour after failure of imatinib: a randomised controlled trial. Lancet 2006;368(9544):1329–38.

49. van Oosterom AT, Judson IR, Verweij J, et al. Update of phase I study of imatinib (STI571) in advanced soft tissue sarcomas and gastrointestinal stromal tumors: a report of the EORTC Soft Tissue and Bone Sarcoma Group. Eur J Cancer 2002;38(Suppl 5): S83–7.

50. Chen MY, Bechtold RE, Savage PD. Cystic changes in hepatic metastases from gastrointestinal stromal tumors (GISTs) treated with Gleevec (imatinib mesylate). AJR Am J Roentgenol 2002;179(4):1059–62.

51. Gayed I, Vu T, Iyer R, et al. The role of 18F-FDG PET in staging and early prediction of response to therapy of recurrent gastrointestinal stromal tumors. J Nucl Med 2004;45(1):17–21.

52. Choi H, Charnsangavej C, Faria SC, et al. Correlation of computed tomography and positron emission tomography in patients with metastatic gastrointestinal stromal tumor treated at a single institution with imatinib mesylate: proposal of new computed tomography response criteria. J Clin Oncol 2007; 25(13):1753–9.

53. Jager PL, Gietema JA, van der Graaf WT. Imatinib mesylate for the treatment of gastrointestinal stromal tumours: best monitored with FDG PET. Nucl Med Commun 2004;25(5):433–8.

54. Heinicke T, Wardelmann E, Sauerbruch T, et al. Very early detection of response to imatinib mesylate therapy of gastrointestinal stromal tumours using 18fluoro-deoxyglucose-positron emission tomography. Anticancer Res 2005;25(6C):4591–4.

55. Grimpen F, Yip D, McArthur G, et al. Resistance to imatinib, low-grade FDG-avidity on PET, and acquired KIT exon 17 mutation in gastrointestinal stromal tumour. Lancet Oncol 2005;6(9):724–7.

FDG PET/CT in Pancreatic and Hepatobiliary Carcinomas
Value to Patient Management and Patient Outcomes

Ujas Parikh, MA[a], Charles Marcus, MD[a],
Rutuparna Sarangi, MA[a], Mehdi Taghipour, MD[a],
Rathan M. Subramaniam, MD, PhD, MPH[a,b,c,*]

KEYWORDS

- ^{18}F-FDG PET/CT • Pancreatic cancer • Hepatocellular carcinoma

KEY POINTS

- Fludeoxyglucose F 18 (^{18}F-FDG) PET/CT has not been shown to offer additional benefit in the initial diagnosis of pancreatic cancer, but studies show benefit of ^{18}F-FDG PET/CT in staging, particularly in the detection of distant metastasis, and in patient prognosis.
- There is good evidence for ^{18}F-FDG PET and ^{18}F-FDG PET/CT in the staging and prognosis of both cholangiocarcinoma and gallbladder cancer.
- ^{18}F-FDG PET/CT has shown promise in the staging of liver malignancies by detecting extrahepatic metastasis.
- There is good evidence supporting the ability of PET/CT in predicting prognosis in patients with hepatocellular carcinoma (HCC).
- Evidence is evolving for the role of ^{18}F-FDG PET/CT in predicting prognosis and survival in patients with colorectal liver metastasis (CRLM).

INTRODUCTION

Pancreatic cancer is the tenth most common malignancy and fourth most common cause of cancer deaths in the United States, with a lifetime risk of 1.5%.[1] It was estimated that 46,420 people were expected to be diagnosed with pancreatic cancer in the United States in 2014. The average 5-year survival rate is drastically low at 6%, which is commonly attributed to the late presentation. At the time of diagnosis, only 20% of tumors are curative with resection.[2] Invasive ductal adenocarcinoma is the most common pancreatic malignancy, accounting for more than 80% of pancreatic cancers. Other less common malignancies include neuroendocrine tumors and exocrine acinar cell neoplasms.[3,4] Although smoking is the most highly studied risk factor, other factors include age, obesity, chronic pancreatitis, and

Disclosure: Dr Subramaniam – Phillips Health Care Molecular Imaging board meeting and Bayer Health Care – Clinical trials.
[a] Russell H Morgan Department of Radiology and Radiological Sciences, Johns Hopkins School of Medicine, JHOC 3230, 601 North Caroline Street, Baltimore, MD 21287, USA; [b] Department of Oncology, Johns Hopkins School of Medicine, 401 North Broadway, Baltimore, MD 21231, USA; [c] Department of Health Policy and Management, Johns Hopkins Bloomberg School of Public Health, 624 North Broadway, Baltimore, MD 21205, USA
* Corresponding author. Russell H Morgan Department of Radiology and Radiological Sciences, Johns Hopkins Medical Institutions, 601 North Caroline Street/JHOC 3235, Baltimore, MD 21287.
E-mail address: rsubram4@jhmi.edu

PET Clin 10 (2015) 327–343
http://dx.doi.org/10.1016/j.cpet.2015.03.001
1556-8598/15/$ – see front matter © 2015 Elsevier Inc. All rights reserved.

diabetes mellitus.[5] The National Comprehensive Cancer Center (NCCN) guidelines at this time recommend CT or MR imaging for evaluation, when there is clinical suspicion of pancreatic cancer and/or evidence of pancreatic ductal dilation.[6] The NCCN has stated that PET/CT is not a substitute for high-quality, contrast-enhanced CT (CECT).[6] Recently, the benefits of contrast-enhanced ^{18}F-FDG PET/CT, incorporating a 3-phase CECT and ^{18}F-FDG PET, have been shown in staging and treatment planning of pancreatic cancer.[3]

Two common cancers of the liver include HCC and liver metastasis, especially from colorectal cancers. HCC accounts for approximately three-fourths of all liver cancers. HCC is the sixth most common cancer and third most common cause of cancer deaths worldwide. It was estimated that 33,190 people were expected to be diagnosed with HCC in the United States in 2014.[1] The average 5-year survival rate (including intrahepatic bile duct cancer) is 16%, which is commonly attributed to the late presentation. In patients with either regional lymph node or distant metastasis, however, the survival rate decreases to approximately 10% and 3%, respectively.[1] Risk factors for HCC include alcohol-related cirrhosis, obesity, nonalcoholic steatohepatitis, and hepatitis B and C infections.[1] Current work-up for diagnosis and staging of HCC includes CT, MR imaging, ^{18}F-FDG PET, and bone scintigraphy, if clinically indicated.[7] Like pancreatic cancer, studies have suggested the benefit of ^{18}F-FDG PET/CT in the staging, treatment planning, and outcome of HCC.[8,9] CRLM, however, is common among patients with colorectal cancer. Metastasis to the liver is the most common location for stage IV colorectal cancer. The 5-year survival rate for patients who have resection of liver metastasis is approximately 25% to 40%.[10] ^{18}F-FDG PET/CT has been found to play a role in predicting prognosis and survival in patients with CRLM.

Biliary tract cancer commonly includes cholangiocarcinoma and gall bladder cancer. Cholangiocarcinoma is a malignancy arising from bile duct epithelial cells and can be divided into intrahepatic, extrahepatic, and the most common, perihilar cholangiocarcinoma, with an overall incidence of 1.67 per 100,000 in the United States.[11] Approximately 2000 to 3000 people in the United States are diagnosed with cholangiocarcinoma each year. Localized intrahepatic bile duct cancer has a 5-year survival rate of 15%, whereas the 5-year survival rate for extrahepatic bile duct cancer is 30%. With an average age of onset between 70 and 73, common risk factors for cholangiocarcinoma include primary sclerosing cholangitis, bile duct stones, and liver fluke infection, most commonly seen in Asia.[11] According to the NCCN guidelines, the conventional imaging work-up for diagnosis and staging of intrahepatic cholangiocarcinoma on suspicion and findings of an isolated intrahepatic mass includes CT or MR imaging, possible laparoscopy, esophagogastroduodenoscopy, and colonoscopy. Work-up for extrahepatic cholangiocarcinoma includes CT or MR imaging and noninvasive cholangiography. The only curative approach at this time is surgical resection.[6] Gallbladder carcinoma is also an uncommon malignancy that often presents late in the course of the disease. It was estimated that 6000 new cases of gallbladder cancer were expected to be diagnosed in the United States in 2014, with a 5-year survival rate ranging from 80% for stage 0 (TisN0M0) cancer to 2% in patients with stage IVB cancer. Common risk factors include gallstones, porcelain gallbladder, gall bladder polyps, and infection, among others. Likewise, both ^{18}F-FDG PET and ^{18}F-FDG PET/CT have been recently found to play a promising role in the staging, treatment planning, and outcome of gallbladder cancer.

^{18}F-FDG PET/CT is a valuable imaging test in the management of many human solid tumors.[3,12–19] In this review, the focus is on the value of ^{18}F-FDG PET/CT in the management and outcome of patients with pancreatic and hepatobiliary malignancies.

THE ROLE OF PET/COMPUTED TOMOGRAPHY IMAGING IN DIAGNOSIS, MANAGEMENT, AND OUTCOME

Fludeoxyglucose F 18 PET/Computed Tomography in the Diagnosis of Pancreatic Cancer

As discussed previously, the guidelines by the NCCN and the American College of Radiology suggest CT as the reference standard for the diagnosis and initial management of pancreatic cancer. There is no consensus that ^{18}F-FDG PET/CT is superior to CT in this regard, although debate exists. In 2014, a meta-analysis of 35 studies by Rijkers and colleagues[20] calculated pooled sensitivity (SN), specificity (SP), positive predictive value, and negative predictive value of 90%, 76%, 90%, and 76%, respectively, for ^{18}F-FDG PET, and 90%, 76%, 89%, and 78%, respectively, for ^{18}F-FDG PET/CT in the diagnosis. The investigators compared their values to pooled SN and SP of 91% and 85% for CT, and 84% and 82% for MR imaging, from a previous meta-analysis. The investigators, therefore, concluded that ^{18}F-FDG PET and ^{18}F-FDG PET/CT offered no additional benefit. Rijkers and colleagues discussed the promising role of ^{18}F-FDG PET/CT, however, in the diagnosis of pancreatic cancer in the future as advances in the modality occur. Conversely, in a 2009 study of 38 patients by Kauhanen and colleagues[21] comparing ^{18}F-FDG PET/CT to multidetector helical CT (MDCT) and MR imaging, the investigators found a higher diagnostic accuracy with PET/CT, with an SN of 85% and SP of 94%, whereas SN and SP for MDCT were 85% and 67%, respectively, and for MR imaging 85% and 72%, respectively. Casneuf and colleagues[22] discussed that although ^{18}F-FDG PET/CT may have higher SN and accuracy compared with CT, multidetector row CT is easily accessible with lower associated costs and radiation.

Although ^{18}F-FDG PET/CT may not be the first choice for diagnosis of pancreatic cancer at this time, it remains useful in early work-up. Numerous studies have shown benefit of ^{18}F-FDG PET/CT in differentiating carcinoma from inflammation.[3] One of the key differentiating features between pancreatic carcinoma and pancreatitis is the distribution of uptake detected by ^{18}F-FDG PET/CT: focal versus diffuse. Lee and colleagues[23] studied 17 patients with atypical image findings of autoimmune pancreatitis who then underwent ^{18}F-FDG PET/CT for further characterization. The investigators compared these readings to the ^{18}F-FDG PET/CT of 151 patients with known pancreatic carcinoma. Both diffuse pancreatic uptake and ^{18}F-FDG accumulation in the salivary gland on PET/CT were most commonly found in patients with autoimmune pancreatitis compared with those with pancreatic cancer ($P<.001$ and $P = .003$, respectively). ^{18}F-FDG accumulation was more localized in patients with pancreatic cancer. The investigators concluded that ^{18}F-FDG PET/CT is helpful in differentiating the 2.

Fludeoxyglucose F 18 PET/Computed Tomography in Staging and Therapy Planning of Pancreatic Cancer

TNM staging of pancreatic cancer by the American Joint Committee on Cancer (AJCC) remains the most widely accepted staging system. Staging is important in this aggressive disease to plan appropriate therapy and is done most commonly with CT, endoscopic ultrasound, MR imaging, and PET/CT. At this time, CT is the reference standard for staging.[6] Its value stems from the accurate delineation of anatomic structures, for example, the vessels (superior mesenteric artery) that pancreatic malignancies can invade.

Over the course of a decade, ^{18}F-FDG PET and ^{18}F-FDG PET/CT have shown promise in the staging of pancreatic malignancies. In earlier studies, ^{18}F-FDG PET was able not only to detect metastasis but also differentiate benign versus malignant tumors.[24,25] Recently, ^{18}F-FDG PET/CT has been on the forefront of research for clinical use. The addition of functional imaging to anatomic imaging has proved beneficial—altering staging, decreasing the need for exploratory surgery for staging, and changing clinical management. Specifically, ^{18}F-FDG PET/CT has been found to have high accuracy, SN, and SP in detecting distant metastasis, resulting in a change in therapy planning. In a 2005 study of 59 patients with suspected pancreatic cancer deemed surgically resectable after conventional imaging, the investigators[26] found that ^{18}F-FDG PET/CT detected distant metastasis in an additional 5 patients (8.5%) not detected by conventional staging measures, with an SN of 81% and SP of 100% (Fig. 1). ^{18}F-FDG PET/CT was also able to locate 2 patients (3.4%) with coexisting rectosigmoid cancer. Thus, ^{18}F-FDG PET/CT altered the management of 16% of patients with pancreatic cancer. In the study by Kauhanen and colleagues[21] discussed previously, the investigators found ^{18}F-FDG PET/CT more sensitive compared with MDCT and MR imaging in the detection of distant metastasis to the liver (88%, 38%, and 38% respectively). With evidence of distant metastases, management would have been altered in 29% of patients (11 of 38) with the use of ^{18}F-FDG PET/CT compared with MDCT. Surgical intervention would have thus been avoided in 6 patients. The investigators found no additional benefit using PET/CT to detect lymph node metastasis, with similar sensitivities of 30% for PET/CT and MR imaging (Fig. 2).

Other studies have shown, however, that PET/CT does play a role in distant as well as locoregional metastasis. In the study by Casneuf and colleagues[22] discussed previously, the investigators found ^{18}F-FDG PET/CT more accurate than CT or PET alone in locoregional staging (85.3% vs 83.8% vs 79.4%, respectively). In a 2013 study of 71 patients by Topkan and colleagues,[27] the investigators used ^{18}F-FDG PET/CT to restage patients (after conventional staging) with unresectable locally advanced pancreatic carcinoma prior to chemoradiotherapy; 19 patients (26.8%) were found to have distant metastases that were not found initially on conventional imaging. The treatment intent for these patients was changed from curative to palliative. ^{18}F-FDG PET/CT also detected 3 additional metastatic lymph nodes in 3 patients. Overall, management was changed in 36.6% of patients (26 of 71) (Fig. 3). In a study by Asagi and colleagues,[28] in 2013, the investigators evaluated the N and M staging of 31 patients with stage IVa pancreatic ductal cancer, comparing ^{18}F-FDG PET/CECT with abdominal CECT. The

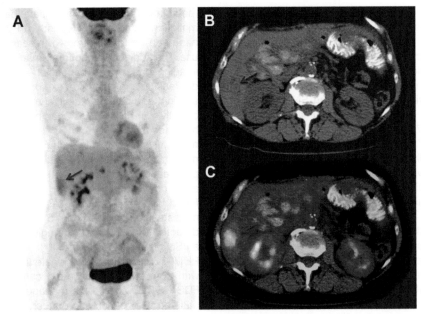

Fig. 1. Pancreas cancer–restaging of metastatic disease: anterior maximum intensity projection (*A*), axial CT (*B*), and axial fused PET/CT (*C*) of a 73-year-old woman with pancreatic adenocarcinoma post–Whipple surgery who underwent a restaging ^{18}F-FDG PET/CT study. The study demonstrates hypermetabolic (SUVmax 3.08) metastatic liver lesions (*red arrows*), which were confirmed to be metastatic pancreatic cancer by hisyopathology.

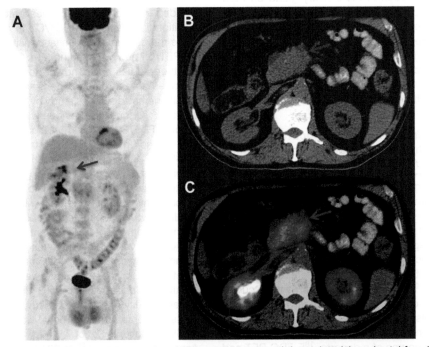

Fig. 2. Pancreas cancer staging: anterior maximum intensity projection (*A*), axial CT (*B*), and axial fused PET/CT (*C*) images of a 66-year-old man with newly diagnosed pancreatic adenocarcinoma who underwent a staging ^{18}F-FDG PET/CT study. The study demonstrates a moderately hypermetabolic (SUVmax 3.16), infilitrating mass (*red arrows*) in the head of the pancreas.

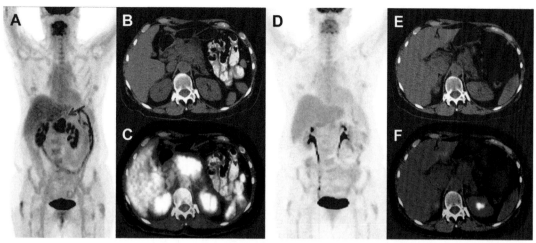

Fig. 3. Pancreas cancer—treatment response assessment: anterior maximum intensity projection (*A*), axial CT (*B*), and axial fused PET/CT (*C*) of a 59-year-old woman with pancreatic adenocarcinoma who underwent a staging ^{18}F-FDG PET/CT study. The study demonstrates a hypermetabolic (SUVmax 9.31) pancreatic body mass (*red arrows*). The patient underwent chemoradiation. The anterior maximum intensity projection (*D*), axial CT (*E*), and axial fused PET/CT (*F*) of the restaging PET/CT study shows significant interval response to treatment.

accuracies of N and M classifications were greater for PET/CECT compared with CECT. Although the accuracy of N staging was suboptimal for PET/CECT (42%), CECT performed worse (35%). PET/CECT proved beneficial in M staging with an accuracy of 94% (29 of 31 patients). A summary of the studies evaluating staging in pancreatic cancer is in **Table 1**.

Pancreatic Cancer: Patient Outcome and Prognosis

^{18}F-FDG PET/CT may play a role in the prognosis of patients with pancreatic cancer. Specifically, multiple studies have found that the use of ^{18}F-FDG PET/CT can help predict patient outcome, in terms of both overall survival (OS) and progression-free survival (PFS).[29–31] In a study of 122 patients with resectable pancreatic ductal adenocarcinoma by Xu and colleagues,[29] the investigators studied various volumetric parameters of ^{18}F-FDG PET/CT to determine factors that can predict OS and recurrence-free survival (RFS). Metabolic tumor volume (MTV) and total lesion glycolysis (TLG) were found independent risk factors. The hazard ratio for OS and RSF increased with larger values of MTV and TLG. A doubling of the MTV on ^{18}F-FDG PET/CT led to an increase in the hazard ratio of OS by 1.27 times and a decrease in RFS by 1.25 times. A more recent study in 2014 by Lee and colleagues[30] also showed the prognostic value of MTV and TLG on patient outcome. In a retrospective study, Schellenberg and colleagues[31] aimed to determine the impact of ^{18}F-FDG PET/CT on the outcome of

patients with unresectable pancreatic cancer undergoing stereotactic body radiotherapy (SBRT). The investigators concluded that both standardized uptake values (SUVs) and metabolic tumor burden (MTB) from PET scans are independent prognostic factors for both OS and PFS. The median OSs in months in patients with maximum SUV (SUVmax) below and above the median SUVmax value were 15.3 months and 9.8 months, respectively (*P*<.01). Likewise, a recent study by Moon and colleagues[32] showed the pretreatment SUVmax on ^{18}F-FDG PET/CT as a prognostic factor of PFS postpalliative chemotherapy (*P* = .046). Studies evaluating the role of PET and PET/CT in patient prognosis and outcome in pancreatic cancer are summarized in **Table 2 (Fig. 4)**.

FLUDEOXYGLUCOSE F 18 PET/COMPUTED TOMOGRAPHY IN STAGING AND THERAPY PLANNING OF BILIARY TRACT CANCERS

TNM staging for cholangiocarcinoma and gallbladder cancer by the AJCC is again the most widely used staging system. Staging can dramatically alter the therapy plan for a patient. ^{18}F-FDG PET and ^{18}F-FDG PET/CT have shown added benefit to the staging of cholangiocarcinoma. ^{18}F-FDG PET/CT is valuable in lymph node staging and in the detection of distant metastasis. In a prospective study by Kim and colleagues 2008,[33] 123 patients with suspected cholangiocarcinoma underwent work-up with conventional imaging, including CT, chest radiography, and MR imaging/MRCP with MR imaging angiography. These

Table 1
PET/CT in the staging of pancreas cancer

Study	N	Metastasis	Accuracy	SN (%)	SP (%)	% Change in Management	Description
Kauhanen et al,[21] 2009	38	Distant	—	85	94	29	SN and SP for ^{18}F-FDG PET/CT compared with MDCT and MR imaging. SN/SP for MDCT and MR imaging: 85%/67% and 85%/72%
Heinrich et al,[26] 2005	59	Distant	—	81	100	16	^{18}F-FDG PET/CT is more sensitive in diagnosing distant metastasis. ^{18}F-FDG PET/CT is important in staging.
Casneuf et al,[22] 2007	46	Locoregional	85.3	90	—	—	^{18}F-FDG PET/CT has higher accuracy and SN for locoregional staging compared with CT alone.
Topkan et al,[27] 2013	71	Distant and locoregional	—	—	—	36.6	^{18}F-FDG PET/CT has value in restaging of M0 patients with advanced pancreatic carcinoma.
Asagi et al,[28] 2013	31	Locoregional Distant	42 94	—	—	—	^{18}F-FDG PET/CT compared with CECT. CECT performed worse with accuracy of 35% for N staging.

Table 2
PET and PET/CT in patient prognosis and outcome in pancreatic cancer

Study	N	Study Type	Patients, Treatments	Description
Xu et al,[29] 2014	122	Retrospective	Resectable pancreatic ductal carcinoma	MTV and TLG are independent risk factors. Doubling of the MTV on ^{18}F-FDG PET/CT led to an increase in the hazard ratio of OS by 1.27 times, and a decrease in RFS by 1.25 times.
Lee et al,[30] 2014	87	Retrospective	Pancreatic carcinoma with surgical resection	TLG and MTV can help predict OS and RFS in patients with pancreatic cancer ($P<.05$).
Schellenberg et al,[31] 2010	55	Retrospective	Unresectable pancreatic cancer undergoing SBRT	SUVs and MTB from PET scans are independent prognostic factors for both OS and PFS.
Moon et al,[32] 2013	21	Retrospective	Metastatic pancreatic cancer prior to and after chemotherapy	Pretreatment SUVmax on ^{18}F-FDG PET/CT is a good prognostic factor of PFS postpalliative chemotherapy ($P = .046$)

patients also underwent ^{18}F-FDG PET/CT scanning, with the aim of comparing the 2 in both staging and management change. ^{18}F-FDG PET/CT was found to have a higher SP and accuracy in detecting lymph node metastasis compared with CT alone. The investigators calculated an SP and accuracy of 88.2% and 75.9%, respectively, compared with 64.7% and 60.9%, respectively, for CT. The SN for ^{18}F-FDG PET/CT was lower, however, at 31.6% compared with 47.4%. In

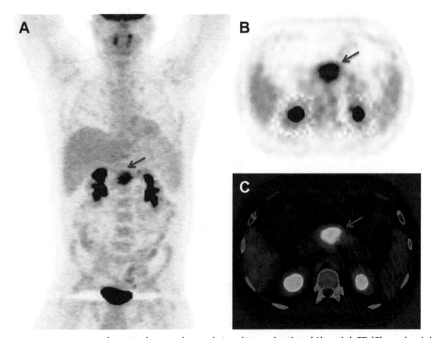

Fig. 4. Pancreas cancer—prognosis: anterior maximum intensity projection (A), axial CT (B), and axial fused PET/CT (C) of a 35-year-old man with newly diagnosed pancreatic adenocarcinoma. The study demonstrates an intensely ^{18}F-FDG avid (SUVmax 8.6, MTV 27.11 mL, TLG 134.41) pancreatic mass (*red arrows*). Despite aggressive treatment with chemoradiation, the disease progressed ending in death 18 months after the study.

regard to detection of distant metastasis, ^{18}F-FDG PET/CT was found superior. The calculated SN, SP, and accuracy for ^{18}F-FDG PET/CT were 58.3%, 92.7%, and 88.3%, respectively, compared with 0%, 90.2%, and 78.7%, respectively, for CT alone. PET/CT was, therefore, able to change management in 22.3% of patients (21 of 123). Seven patients (5.7%) were up-staged with treatment changing from curative to palliative and 8 patients (6.5%) were down-staged with treatment changing to surgical resection. In a study of 18 patients with pretreatment intrahepatic cholangiocarcinoma by Park and colleagues 2014,[34] ^{18}F-FDG PET/CT was found to have an SN and SP of 80% and 92.3%, respectively, in the detection of lymph node metastasis. In contrast, CT alone had an SN and SP of only 20% and 86.4%, respectively (**Fig. 5**).

Over the course of more than a decade, ^{18}F-FDG PET alone has shown to provide additional benefit in the staging of cholangiocarcinoma. In a study of 18 patients by Kluge and colleagues 2001,[35] ^{18}F-FDG PET was found to detect distant metastasis in 7 of the 10 cases (70%) of biopsy-proved cholangiocarcinoma, although ^{18}F-FDG PET was not suitable in detecting lymph node metastasis. In another study of 35 patients with intrahepatic cholangiocarcinoma, however, Seo and colleagues[36] found that ^{18}F-FDG PET was superior to CT and MR imaging in detecting lymph node metastasis. The accuracy, SN, and SP for detection of lymph node metastasis with ^{18}F-FDG PET were calculated as 86%, 43%, and 100%, respectively. The accuracy, SN, and SP for CT and MR imaging were 68%, 43%, and 76%, respectively and 57%, 43% and 64% respectively.

Likewise, ^{18}F-FDG PET and ^{18}F-FDG PET/CT may play a valuable role in the staging of gallbladder cancer, thus affecting treatment management. Studies, however, are scarce at this time. Conventional work-up for staging of gallbladder cancer includes CT, MR imaging, ultrasound, exploratory laparoscopy, and ^{18}F-FDG PET. ^{18}F-FDG PET alone remains, however, somewhat controversial, due to a lack of studies. A study by Leung and colleagues[37] in 2014 sought to identify the value of ^{18}F-FDG PET in staging patients with gallbladder cancer. In 63 with incidental gallbladder cancer postcholecystectomy, additional PET imaging to CT benefited 5 patients (8%). Of those 5 patients, PET imaging changed management to surgical resection in 3 patients and curative to palliative treatment in 2

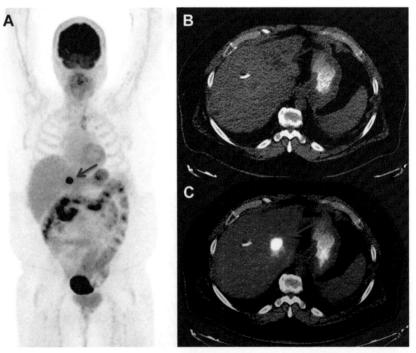

Fig. 5. Cholangiocarcinoma—staging and prognosis: anterior maximum intensity projection (*A*), axial CT (*B*), and axial fused PET/CT (*C*) of a 55-year-old man with cholangiocarcinoma, who underwent a staging ^{18}F-FDG PET/CT study. The study demonstrated an ^{18}F-FDG–avid (SUVmax 8.55) in the liver hilum (*red arrows*). Despite aggressive treatment the disease progressed, ending in death 1 year after the study.

Table 3
PET and PET/CT in biliary tract cancer staging

Study	Patients	Metastasis	Accuracy (%)	SN (%)	SP (%)	% Change in Management	Description
Kim et al,[33] 2008	123 patients with suspected cholangiocarcinoma	Locoregional lymph node, Distant	75.9 88.3	31.6 58.3	88.2 92.7	22.3	SN and SP for ^{18}F-FDG PET/CT compared with CT alone. 5.7% up-staged and 6.5% down-staged with treatment changes.
Park et al,[34] 2014	18 patients with pretreatment intrahepatic cholangiocarcinoma	Locoregional	—	80	92.3	—	^{18}F-FDG PET/CT detecting lymph nodes compared with CT alone with an SN and SP of 20% and 86.4%, respectively.
Kluge et al,[35] 2001	18 patients with biopsy-proved cholangiocarcinoma	Distant	70	—	—	—	^{18}F-FDG PET in detection of distant metastasis.
Seo et al,[36] 2008	35 patients with intrahepatic cholangiocarcinoma	Locoregional	86	43	100	—	^{18}F-FDG PET found superior to CT and MR imaging in detecting lymph nodes.

Table 4
PET and PET/CT in gallbladder cancer staging

Study	Patients	Metastasis	Accuracy (%)	SN (%)	SP (%)	% Change in Management	Description
Leung et al,[37] 2014	63 patients with incidental gallbladder carcinoma post cholecystectomy	Locoregional	—	56	94	8	^{18}F-FDG PET with correlation to CT/MR imaging scans. ^{18}F-FDG PET has added value as an addition to CT, and helps confirm suspicious nodal disease.
Butte et al,[38] 2009	32 patients with incidental gallbladder carcinoma	Locoregional, distant (disseminated)	—	—	—	38	^{18}F-FDG PET/CT superior in detecting lymph nodes compared with CT alone. ^{18}F-FDG PET/CT has value in staging in patients with T1b or greater.
Ramos-Font et al,[39] 2014	49 patients suspicious for gallbladder cancer	Locoregional Distant	85.7 95.9	—	—	22.4	^{18}F-FDG PET/CT has high diagnostic accuracy for staging using pathology report as reference standard.
Petrowsky et al,[40] 2006	14 patients with gallbladder carcinoma + 14 patients with cholangiocarcinoma	Locoregional Distant	—	12 100	96 100	—	^{18}F-FDG PET/CT found superior to CT alone in identifying distant metastasis. ^{18}F-FDG PET/CT showed no benefit in regional lymph node metastasis.

patients. An additional 12 patients had confirmation of equivocal CT findings with PET. ^{18}F-FDG PET alone, however, contributed to false-positive readings in 3% of patients. The investigators concluded that ^{18}F-FDG PET may be used as an adjunct to conventional CT, and its use is particularly valuable in patients with suspected nodal disease or other suspicious findings. Butte and colleagues,[38] in 2009, studied 32 patients with incidental gallbladder carcinoma and noted that ^{18}F-FDG PET/CT has value in staging and thus changing the management in patients with gallbladder cancer postcholecystectomy, specifically in patients with stage T1b cancer or greater. ^{18}F-FDG PET/CT was able to uncover both local and disseminated disease (either systemic disease or regional lymph node involvement) in the interaortacaval and para-aortic bed. Ten of 32 (31%) patients were found to have disseminated disease, altering surgical management in 25% of patients (8 of 32). Overall, ^{18}F-FDG PET/CT altered the pretest staging in 12 out of 32 patients (38%). In a recent study of 49 patients suspicious for gallbladder cancer by Ramos-Font and colleagues in 2014,[39] the investigators found that ^{18}F-FDG PET/CT had a diagnostic accuracy of 85.7% for lymph node detection and 95.9% for metastatic disease using pathology reports as the reference standard. ^{18}F-FDG PET/CT changed the management in 22.4% of patients. Moreover, in a study of 14 patients with gallbladder carcinoma, 14 patients with intrahepatic cholangiocarcinoma, and 33 patients with extrahepatic cholangiocarcinoma by Petrowsky and colleagues[40] 2006, the investigators concluded that ^{18}F-FDG PET/CT plays an important role in identifying distant metastasis from cholangiocarcinoma and gallbladder cancer. PET/CT was found to have an SN and SP of 100% and 100%, respectively compared with 25% and 100%, respectively, for CECT alone ($P = .001$). Therefore, PET/CT was able to detect every patient with distant metastasis. CECT failed to detect 9 patients with distant metastasis. This study, however, did not show a benefit in detection of regional lymph node metastasis. PET/CT was found to have an SN and SP of 12% and 96%, respectively, compared with 24% and 86% for CT alone. Larger multicenter prospective studies are indicated at this time to determine the benefit of ^{18}F-FDG PET/CT in detecting nodal and distant metastasis in gallbladder cancer. A summary of studies evaluating the role of ^{18}F-FDG PET and PET/CT in biliary tract cancer and gall bladder cancer staging has been described in **Tables 3** and **4**.

Cholangiocarcinoma: Patient Outcome and Prognosis

^{18}F-FDG PET/CT may play a role in the prognosis of patients with cholangiocarcinoma but has not been established. There are a few studies identifying the value of ^{18}F-FDG PET/CT in patient outcome, length of both OS, and PFS. Park and colleagues[34] evaluated 18 patients with intrahepatic cholangiocarcinoma and sought to determine the value of PET/CT to predict recurrence after surgical resection. The investigators found a positive correlation between PET/CT detection of lymph node metastasis and a 1-year recurrence of carcinoma ($P = .02$). In a study by Seo and colleagues,[36] the investigators compared SUVmax data to disease-free survival. Patients with high SUVmax had significantly lower disease-free survival compared with patients with low SUVmax ($P = .04$). OS was also statistically different when patients were stratified by detection of lymph node metastasis with ^{18}F-FDG PET. The investigators concluded that SUV data and lymph node metastasis detection from ^{18}F-FDG PET might be prognostic factors in cholangiocarcinoma for postoperative recurrence and disease-free survival (**Fig. 6**).

Gall Bladder Cancer: Patient Outcome and Prognosis

^{18}F-FDG PET/CT may also play a role in the prognosis of patients with gallbladder cancer. Currently, pathologic staging is the best predictive factor for survival in patients with gallbladder cancer.[41,42] In contrast to cholangiocarcinoma, several studies have now established the role of ^{18}F-FDG PET/CT in patient outcome. In a 2014 study of 50 patients with gallbladder cancer who underwent ^{18}F-FDG PET/CT imaging post-treatment by Hwang and colleagues,[43] the investigators concluded that SUVmax data from PET/CT imaging was prognostic and an independent predictor for OS. In the univariate analysis, a SUVmax cutoff of 6.0 was chosen. Patients with SUVmax greater than 6.0 had a median survival of 203 days versus 405 days in patients with SUVmax less than 6.0 ($P = .04$). In the multivariate analysis, SUVmax was found to have a hazard ratio of 3.05 with a P-value of .04. In a study of 44 patients with gallbladder cancer by Yoo and colleagues,[41] the investigators concluded that TLG, a volume-based metabolic parameter in ^{18}F-FDG PET/CT, was predictive of OS, superior to both MTV and SUV. In the univariate analysis, the mean OS was statistically significantly different with a TLG cutoff of 7090 g. The mean OS with a TLG greater than 7090 g was 36 months, whereas patients with a TLG less than or equal to 7090 g had

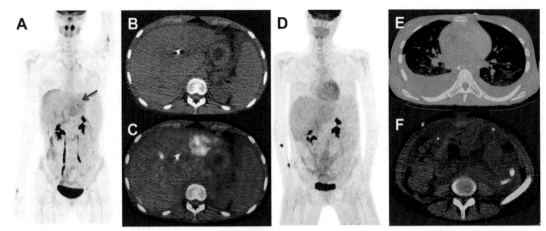

Fig. 6. Cholangiocarcinoma—restaging and prognosis: anterior maximum intensity projection (*A*), axial CT (*B*), and axial fused PET/CT (*C*) of 17-year-old woman with a recent diagnosis of cholangiocarcinoma who underwent a staging ^{18}F-FDG PET/CT study. The study demonstrates a moderately ^{18}F-FDG–avid (SUVmax 3.01) mass in the left lobe of liver (*red arrow*). The patient underwent chemotherapy. Anterior maximum intensity projection (*D*), axial CT (*E*), and axial fused PET/CT (*F*) of the restaging ^{18}F-FDG PET/CT study performed 2 months after the previous study demonstrates progressive disease involving the lungs and extensive omental/peritoneal involvement (*red arrow*). Despite aggressive treatment, the patient died 4 months after the study.

a mean OS of 8 months (*P* = .014). In the multivariate analysis, the hazard ratio for TLG was calculated to be 2.93 with a *P*-value of less than .05. In a study by Butte and colleagues,[38] the investigators concluded that ^{18}F-FDG PET/CT helps offer prognostic information. In 32 patients with incidental gallbladder carcinoma status postcholecystectomy, the findings on ^{18}F-FDG PET/CT correlated with median survival. In patients with a positive ^{18}F-FDG PET/CT showing disseminated disease, the median survival was approximately 4.9 months, whereas patients with a negative ^{18}F-FDG PET/CT had a median survival of 13.5 months. In a study by Redondo and colleagues,[44] the investigators also concluded that ^{18}F-FDG PET/CT holds valuable prognostic information. In 69 patients with incidental gallbladder carcinoma, the median survival in patients with a negative ^{18}F-FDG PET/CT was on average 115.3 months, whereas the medial survival for patients with a positive ^{18}F-FDG PET/CT was 35.3 months. Studies like these help establish ^{18}F-FDG PET/CT as a valuable tool in determining prognosis and survival in patients with gallbladder cancer.[38,41,43,44]

FLUDEOXYGLUCOSE F 18 PET/COMPUTED TOMOGRAPHY IN STAGING AND THERAPY PLANNING OF HEPATOCELLULAR CARCINOMA

Current work-up for diagnosis and staging of HCC includes CT, MR imaging, chest CT, and bone scintigraphy, if clinically indicated.[7] Although several staging systems exist, such as the Okuda system

and Barcelona Clinic Liver Cancer classification,[45,46] the AJCC TNM staging remains the most widely accepted system. Over the course of a decade, ^{18}F-FDG PET/CT has shown promise in the staging of liver malignancies by detecting extrahepatic metastasis. ^{18}F-FDG PET alone has been found to offer additional value to CT in identifying regional and distant metastasis, thereby changing therapy planning. In a study of 91 patients diagnosed with HCC by Wudel and colleagues,[47] ^{18}F-FDG PET detected distant metastasis in 5 patients. Ultimately, ^{18}F-FDG PET had an impact in the management plan in 26 of 91 patients with HCC. In a 2007 study of 18 patients with HCC by Yoon and colleagues,[48] ^{18}F-FDG PET detected all extrahepatic metastasis from HCC, including 19 lymph nodes, 12 lung, and 11 bone. ^{18}F-FDG PET was found superior to conventional imaging. Four lymph node metastases and 6 bone metastases were detected by ^{18}F-FDG PET that were not found on CT or MR imaging. Furthermore, ^{18}F-FDG PET changed management in 4 patients. With the addition of CT to provide anatomic localization, ^{18}F-FDG PET/CT has shown useful in detecting extrahepatic disease in patients with HCC. Lee and colleagues[49] found that ^{18}F-FDG PET/CT was more sensitive and specific for bone metastases compared with bone scans. Of the 11 patients with bone metastasis, ^{18}F-FDG PET/CT was found to have an accuracy, SN, and SP of 100%, 100% and 100%, respectively. Conversely, bone scan was found to have an accuracy, SN, and SP of 94.1%, 63.6%, and 96.8%, respectively. ^{18}F-FDG PET/CT was also found valuable in detecting lung metastasis greater than 1 cm in size. Kawaoka and colleagues[50] also found higher SN with ^{18}F-FDG PET/CT in the detection of bone metastasis compared with both bone scan and MDCT. The sensitivities for ^{18}F-FDG PET/CT, MDCT, and bone scan were 83.3%, 41.6%, and 52.7%, respectively. ^{18}F-FDG PET/CT also had higher SN and SP in the detection of lymph node metastasis: 66.7% and 91.7% for ^{18}F-FDG PET/CT compared with 62.5% and 79.2% for MDCT. Lin and colleagues[51] performed a meta-analysis of 8 studies and concluded that ^{18}F-FDG PET/CT helps rule in extrahepatic metastasis in patients with primary HCC. The investigators calculated pooled SN and SP of 76.6% and 98%, respectively. The positive likelihood ratio was calculated at 14.08 (**Fig. 7**).

Hepatocellular Carcinoma and Colorectal Liver Metastasis: Patient Outcome and Prognosis

^{18}F-FDG PET/CT plays an important role in the prognosis of patients with HCC. Studies have found that the use of ^{18}F-FDG PET/CT can help predict patient OS.[52–55] Xia and colleagues[53] determined that lymph node metastasis detected with ^{18}F-FDG PET/CT was the most important factor for OS. The median survival time for patients with lymph node metastasis was 5 months compared with 12 months for patients without lymph node metastasis ($P = .036$). In a recent study of 75 patients with cirrhosis and HCC by Sims and colleagues[52] the investigators also found that ^{18}F-FDG PET/CT is a predictor for OS in patients with HCC. In patients with positive ^{18}F-FDG uptake prior to treatment, the median survival was calculated to be 1038 days compared with 387 days in patients with negative ^{18}F-FDG uptake ($P = .0079$). Park and colleagues[54] studied 68 patients with resectable HCC and found that preoperative PET/CT markers, SUVmax, and tumor to background normal tissue ratios of SUVmax (TNR), were prognostic factors in OS. Increased SUVmax and TNR correlated with decreased OS with P values of .012 and .0005, respectively. Other studies have shown the prognostic value in terms of either OS or RFS of ^{18}F-FDG PET/CT after either radiation therapy or embolization.[56–58]

^{18}F-FDG PET/CT also may play an important role in predicting prognosis and survival in patients with CRLM.[1] Abbadi and colleagues,[59] in a retrospective study, found that staging CRLM by ^{18}F-FDG PET/CT improved OS compared with staging with CT. Survival rates for patients staged with ^{18}F-FDG PET/CT were 79.8% at 3 years and 54.1% at 5 years. Conversely, survival rates for patients staged with CT alone were 54.1% at

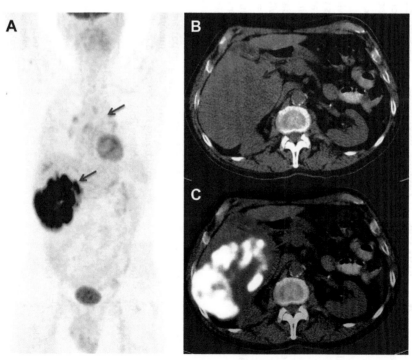

Fig. 7. HCC—staging: anterior maximum intensity projection (*A*), axial CT (*B*), and axial fused PET/CT (*C*) of a 76-year-old man with HCC who underwent a staging ^{18}F-FDG PET/CT study. The study demonstrates a large ^{18}F-FDG–avid (SUVmax 30.1) mass in the right lobe of liver (*red arrows*) with satellite lesions with multiple, moderately ^{18}F-FDG–avid, metastatic mediastinal lymphadenopathy.

Table 5
PET and PET/CT in prognosis and patient outcome in cholangiocarcinoma, gallbladder cancer, hepatocellular carcinoma, and colorectal liver metastasis

Study	N	Study Type	Patients, Treatments	Description
Park et al,[34] 2014	18	Retrospective	Intrahepatic cholangiocarcinoma status post-surgical resection	Positive correlation between PET/CT detection of lymph node metastasis and a 1-y recurrence of carcinoma ($P = .02$).
Seo et al,[36] 2008	35	Retrospective	Cholangiocarcinoma	Patients with high SUVmax had significantly lower disease-free survival compared with patients with low SUVmax ($P = .04$). SUV data and lymph node metastasis detection from ^{18}F-FDG PET might be prognostic factors in cholangiocarcinoma for postoperative RFS and disease-free survival.
Hwang et al,[43] 2014	50	Retrospective	Gallbladder cancer postcurative or palliative treatment	SUVmax data from PET/CT imaging was prognostic and an independent predictor for OS. Patients with SUVmax >6.0 had a median survival of 203 vs 405 d in patients with SUVmax <6.0 ($P = .04$).
Yoo et al,[41] 2012	44	Retrospective	Gallbladder carcinoma	TLG, a volume-based metabolic parameter in ^{18}F-FDG PET/CT, was predictive of OS, superior to both MTV and SUV. Mean clinical follow-up was 22.2 mo. The mean OS with a TLG >7090 g was 36 mo, whereas patients with a TLG less than or equal to 7090 g had a mean OS of 8 mo ($P = .014$).
Butte et al,[38] 2009	32	Retrospective	Incidental gallbladder carcinoma status postcholecystectomy	In patients with a positive ^{18}F-FDG PET/CT showing disseminated disease, the median survival was approximately 4.9 mo, whereas patients with a negative ^{18}F-FDG PET/CT had a median survival of 13.5 mo.
Redondo et al,[44] 2012	69	Retrospective	Incidental gallbladder carcinoma	The median survival in patients with a negative ^{18}F-FDG PET/CT was on average 115.3 mo, whereas the medial survival for patients with a positive ^{18}F-FDG PET/CT was 35.3 mo
Xia et al,[53] 2014	132	Retrospective	HCC with extrahepatic metastasis	Lymph node metastasis detected with ^{18}F-FDG PET/CT was the most important factor for OS. The median survival time for patients with lymph node metastasis was 5 mo, compared with 12 mo for patients without lymph node metastasis ($P = .036$).
Sims et al,[52] 2014	75	Retrospective	HCC and cirrhosis	^{18}F-FDG PET/CT is a predictor for OS in patients with HCC. In patients with positive ^{18}F-FDG uptake prior to treatment, the median survival was calculated to be 1038 d compared with 387 d in patients with negative ^{18}F-FDG uptake ($P = .0079$).
Abbadi et al,[59] 2014	131	Retrospective	CRLM undergoing hepatectomy	Staging CRLM by ^{18}F-FDG PET/CT improved OS compared with staging with CT. Survival rates for patients staged with ^{18}F-FDG PET/CT were 79.8% at 3 y and 54.1% at 5 y. Conversely, survival rates for patients staged with CT alone were 54.1% at 3 y and 37.3% at 5 y.

3 years and 37.3% at 5 years. Median survival lengths in years were calculated as 6.4 years for PET/CT and 3.9 years for CT alone (P = .018). A few large studies evaluating the value of PET and PET/CT in the prognosis and patient outcome in cholangiocarcinoma, gallbladder cancer, HCC, and CRLM are summarized in **Table 5**.

SUMMARY

Although ^{18}F-FDG PET/CT has not been shown to offer additional benefit in the initial diagnosis of pancreatic cancer, studies show benefit of ^{18}F-FDG PET/CT in staging, particularly in the detection of distant metastasis, and patient prognosis. Likewise, there is good evidence for ^{18}F-FDG PET and ^{18}F-FDG PET/CT in the staging and prognosis of both cholangiocarcinoma and gallbladder cancer. ^{18}F-FDG PET/CT has shown promise in the staging of liver malignancies by detecting extrahepatic metastasis. There is good evidence supporting the ability of PET/CT in predicting prognosis in patients with HCC. There is evolving evidence for ^{18}F-FDG PET/CTs role in predicting prognosis and survival in patients with CRLM.

REFERENCES

1. American Cancer Society. Cancer facts & figures 2014. Atlanta (GA): American Cancer Society; 2014.

2. Michl P, Pauls S, Gress TM. Evidence-based diagnosis and staging of pancreatic cancer. Best Pract Res Clin Gastroenterol 2006;20(2):227–51.

3. Dibble EH, Karantanis D, Mercier G, et al. PET/CT of cancer patients: part 1, pancreatic neoplasms. AJR Am J Roentgenol 2012;199(5):952–67.

4. Marsh Rde W, Hagler KT, Carag HR, et al. Pancreatic panniculitis. Eur J Surg Oncol 2005;31:1213–5.

5. Krejs GJ. Pancreatic cancer: epidemiology and risk factors. Dig Dis 2010;28(2):355–8.

6. National comprehensive cancer network website. NCCN guidelines version 1.2014: pancreatic adenocarcinoma. Available at: www.nccn.org/professionals/physician_gls/pdf/pancreatic.pdf. Accessed July 14, 2014.

7. Hennedige T, Venkatesh SK. Imaging of hepatocellular carcinoma: diagnosis, staging and treatment monitoring. Cancer Imaging 2013;12:530–47.

8. Sacks A, Peller PJ, Surasi DS, et al. Value of PET/CT in the management of liver metastases, part 1. AJR Am J Roentgenol 2011;197:W256–9.

9. Sacks A, Peller PJ, Surasi DS, et al. Value of PET/CT in the management of primary hepatobiliary tumors, part 2. AJR Am J Roentgenol 2011;197:W260–5.

10. Ismaili N. Treatment of colorectal liver metastases. World J Surg Oncol 2011;9:154.

11. Bragazzi MC, Cardinale V, Carpino G, et al. Cholangiocarcinoma: epidemiology and risk factors. Transl Gastrointest Cancer 2012;1:21–32.

12. Davison J, Mercier G, Russo G, et al. PET-based primary tumor volumetric parameters and survival of patients with non-small cell lung carcinoma. AJR Am J Roentgenol 2013;200(3):635–40.

13. Agarwal A, Chirindel A, Shah BA, et al. Evolving role of FDG PET/CT in multiple myeloma imaging and management. AJR Am J Roentgenol 2013;200(4):884–90.

14. Jackson T, Chung MK, Mercier G, et al. FDG PET/CT interobserver agreement in head and neck cancer: FDG and CT measurements of the primary tumor site. Nucl Med Commun 2012;33(3):305–12.

15. Paidpally V, Chirindel A, Lam S, et al. FDG-PET/CT imaging biomarkers in head and neck squamous cell carcinoma. Imaging Med 2012;4(6):633–47.

16. Hadiprodjo D, Ryan T, Truong MT, et al. Parotid gland tumors: preliminary data for the value of FDG PET/CT diagnostic parameters. AJR Am J Roentgenol 2012;198:W185–90.

17. Antoniou AJ, Marcus C, Tahari AK, et al. Follow-up or surveillance 18F-FDG PET/CT and survival outcome in lung cancer patients. J Nucl Med 2014;55(7):1062–8.

18. Karantanis D, Kalkanis D, Czernin J, et al. Perceived misinterpretation rates in oncologic 18F-FDG PET/CT studies: a survey of referring physicians. J Nucl Med 2014;55(12):1925–9.

19. Sridhar P, Mercier G, Tan J, et al. FDG PET metabolic tumor volume segmentation and pathologic volume of primary human solid tumors. AJR Am J Roentgenol 2014;202(5):1114–9.

20. Rijkers AP, Valkema R, Duivenvoorden HJ, et al. Usefulness of F-18-fluorodeoxyglucose positron emission tomography to confirm suspected pancreatic cancer: a meta-analysis. Eur J Surg Oncol 2014;40(7):794–804.

21. Kauhanen SP, Komar G, Seppänen MP, et al. A prospective diagnostic accuracy study of 18F-fluorodeoxyglucose positron emission tomography/computed tomography, multidetector row computed tomography, and magnetic resonance imaging in primary diagnosis and staging of pancreatic cancer. Ann Surg 2009;250(6):957–63.

22. Casneuf V, Delrue L, Kelles A, et al. Is combined 18F-fluorodeoxyglucose-positron emission tomography/computed tomography superior to positron emission tomography or computed tomography alone for diagnosis, staging and restaging of pancreatic lesions? Acta Gastroenterol Belg 2007;70(4):331–8.

23. Lee TY, Kim MH, Park do H, et al. Utility of 18F-FDG PET/CT for differentiation of autoimmune pancreatitis with atypical pancreatic imaging findings from pancreatic cancer. AJR Am J Roentgenol 2009;193(2):343–8.

24. Nakamoto Y, Higashi T, Sakahara H, et al. Delayed (18)F-fluoro-2-deoxy-D-glucose positron emission tomography scan for differentiation between malignant and benign lesions in the pancreas. Cancer 2000;89(12):2547–54.

25. Saif MW, Cornfeld D, Modarresifar H, et al. 18F-FDG positron emission tomography CT (FDG PET-CT) in the management of pancreatic cancer: initial experience in 12 patients. J Gastrointestin Liver Dis 2008; 17(2):173–8.

26. Heinrich S, Goerres GW, Schäfer M, et al. Positron emission tomography/computed tomography influences on the management of resectable pancreatic cancer and its cost-effectiveness. Ann Surg 2005; 242(2):235–43.

27. Topkan E, Parlak C, Yapar AF. FDG-PET/CT-based restaging may alter initial management decisions and clinical outcomes in patients with locally advanced pancreatic carcinoma planned to undergo chemoradiotherapy. Cancer Imaging 2013;13(3):423–8.

28. Asagi A, Ohta K, Nasu J, et al. Utility of contrast-enhanced FDG-PET/CT in the clinical management of pancreatic cancer: impact on diagnosis, staging, evaluation of treatment response, and detection of recurrence. Pancreas 2013;42(1):11–9.

29. Xu HX, Chen T, Wang WQ, et al. Metabolic tumour burden assessed by (1)(8)F-FDG PET/CT associated with serum CA19-9 predicts pancreatic cancer outcome after resection. Eur J Nucl Med Mol Imaging 2014;41(6):1093–102.

30. Lee JW, Kang CM, Choi HJ, et al. Prognostic value of metabolic tumor volume and total lesion glycolysis on preoperative 18F-FDG PET/CT in patients with pancreatic cancer. J Nucl Med 2014;55(6):898–904.

31. Schellenberg D, Quon A, Minn AY, et al. 18Fluorodeoxyglucose PET is prognostic of progression-free and overall survival in locally advanced pancreas cancer treated with stereotactic radiotherapy. Int J Radiat Oncol Biol Phys 2010;77(5): 1420–5.

32. Moon SY, Joo KR, So YR, et al. Predictive value of maximum standardized uptake value (SUVmax) on 18F-FDG PET/CT in patients with locally advanced or metastatic pancreatic cancer. Clin Nucl Med 2013;38(10):778–83.

33. Kim JY, Kim MH, Lee TY, et al. Clinical role of 18F-FDG PET-CT in suspected and potentially operable cholangiocarcinoma: a prospective study compared with conventional imaging. Am J Gastroenterol 2008;103(5):1145–51.

34. Park TG, Schmidt F, Caca K, et al. Implication of lymph node metastasis detected on 18F-FDG PET/CT for surgical planning in patients with peripheral intrahepatic cholangiocarcinoma. Clin Nucl Med 2014;39(1):1–7.

35. Kluge R, Schmidt F, Caca K, et al. Positron emission tomography with [(18)F]fluoro-2-deoxy-D-glucose for diagnosis and staging of bile duct cancer. Hepatology 2001;33(5):1029–35.

36. Seo S, Hatano E, Higashi T, et al. Fluorine-18 fluorodeoxyglucose positron emission tomography predicts lymph node metastasis, P-glycoprotein expression, and recurrence after resection in mass-forming intrahepatic cholangiocarcinoma. Surgery 2008;143(6): 769–77.

37. Leung U, Pandit-Taskar N, Corvera CU, et al. Impact of pre-operative positron emission tomography in gallbladder cancer. HPB (Oxford) 2014;16:1023–30.

38. Butte JM, Redondo F, Waugh E, et al. The role of PET-CT in patients with incidental gallbladder cancer. HPB (Oxford) 2009;11(7):585–91.

39. Ramos-Font C, Gómez-Rio M, Rodríguez-Fernández A, et al. Ability of FDG-PET/CT in the detection of gallbladder cancer. J Surg Oncol 2014;109(3):218–24.

40. Petrowsky H, Wildbrett P, Husarik DB, et al. Impact of integrated positron emission tomography and computed tomography on staging and management of gallbladder cancer and cholangiocarcinoma. J Hepatol 2006;45(1):43–50.

41. Yoo J, Choi JY, Lee KT, et al. Prognostic significance of volume-based metabolic parameters by (18)F-FDG PET/CT in gallbladder carcinoma. Nucl Med Mol Imaging 2012;46(3):201–6.

42. Donohue JH. Present status of the diagnosis and treatment of gallbladder carcinoma. J Hepatobiliary Pancreat Surg 2001;8(6):530–4.

43. Hwang JP, Lim I, Na II, et al. Prognostic value of suvmax measured by fluorine-18 fluorodeoxyglucose positron emission tomography with computed tomography in patients with gallbladder cancer. Nucl Med Mol Imaging 2014;48(2):114–20.

44. Redondo F, Butte J, Lavados H, et al. 18F-FDG PET/CT performance and prognostic value in patients with incidental gallbladder carcinoma. J Nucl Med 2012;53(515):515.

45. Okuda K, Ohtsuki T, Obata H, et al. Natural history of hepatocellular carcinoma and prognosis in relation to treatment. Study of 850 patients. Cancer 1985; 56(4):918–28.

46. Llovet JM, Fuster J, Bruix J, et al. The Barcelona approach: diagnosis, staging, and treatment of hepatocellular carcinoma. Liver Transpl 2004;10(2 Suppl 1):S115–20.

47. Wudel LJ Jr, Delbeke D, Morris D, et al. The role of [18F]fluorodeoxyglucose positron emission tomography imaging in the evaluation of hepatocellular carcinoma. Am Surg 2003;69(2):117–24 [discussion: 124–6].

48. Yoon KT, Kim JK, Kim do Y, et al. Role of 18F-fluorodeoxyglucose positron emission tomography in detecting extrahepatic metastasis in pretreatment staging of hepatocellular carcinoma. Oncology 2007;72:104–10.

49. Lee JE, Jang JY, Jeong SW, et al. Diagnostic value for extrahepatic metastases of hepatocellular carcinoma in positron emission tomography/computed tomography scan. World J Gastroenterol 2012;18(23): 2979–87.

50. Kawaoka T, Aikata H, Takaki S, et al. FDG positron emission tomography/computed tomography for the detection of extrahepatic metastases from hepatocellular carcinoma. Hepatol Res 2009;39(2): 134–42.

51. Lin CY, Chen JH, Liang JA, et al. 18F-FDG PET or PET/CT for detecting extrahepatic metastases or recurrent hepatocellular carcinoma: a systematic review and meta-analysis. Eur J Radiol 2012;81(9): 2417–22.

52. Sims J, Tann M, Baskin M. FDG PET/CT predicts overall survival in patiens with hepatocellular carcinoma. J Nucl Med 2014;54(Supplement 2):1478.

53. Xia F, Wu L, Lau WY, et al. Positive lymph node metastasis has a marked impact on the long-term survival of patients with hepatocellular carcinoma with extrahepatic metastasis. PLoS One 2014;9: e95889.

54. Park J, Lim I, Cho E, et al. Preoperative 18F-FDG PET/CT predicts the overall survival of patients with resectable hepatocellular carcinoma. J Nucl Med 2013;54(Supplement 2):574.

55. Pant V, Sen IB, Soin AS. Role of (1)(8)F-FDG PET CT as an independent prognostic indicator in patients with hepatocellular carcinoma. Nucl Med Commun 2013;34(8):749–57.

56. Sabet A, Ahmadzadehfar H, Bruhman J, et al. Survival in patients with hepatocellular carcinoma treated with 90Y-microsphere radioembolization. Prediction by 18F-FDG PET. Nuklearmedizin 2014; 53(2):39–45.

57. Kucuk ON, Soydal C, Araz M, et al. Prognostic importance of 18F-FDG uptake pattern of hepatocellular cancer patients who received SIRT. Clin Nucl Med 2013;38:e283–9.

58. Huang WY, Kao CH, Huang WS, et al. 18F-FDG PET and combined 18F-FDG-contrast CT parameters as predictors of tumor control for hepatocellular carcinoma after stereotactic ablative radiotherapy. J Nucl Med 2013;54(10):1710–6.

59. Abbadi RA, Sadat U, Jah A, et al. Improved long-term survival after resection of colorectal liver metastases following staging with FDG positron emission tomography. J Surg Oncol 2014;110(3):313–9.

Impact of Fluorodeoxyglucose PET/Computed Tomography on the Management of Patients with Colorectal Cancer

Sander Thomas Laurens, MD, Wim J.G. Oyen, MD, PhD*

KEYWORDS

- Colorectal carcinoma • FDG-PET/CT • Patient management • Survival outcome

KEY POINTS

- Studies show that fluorodeoxyglucose (FDG) PET/computed tomography (CT) can have a significant clinical impact in patients with colorectal cancer in various stages of the disease.
- In patients with suspected recurrent disease, and in patients with liver metastases who might be eligible for surgery, FDG-PET/CT has clinically relevant advantages compared with conventional imaging.
- The value of FDG-PET/CT for primary staging in patients with colorectal carcinoma is limited, but studies show that there may be added value in patients with more advanced disease.

INTRODUCTION

Colorectal cancer (CRC) is a common malignancy in the Western world. In 2012, it was the second most frequent cancer in Europe with 447,000 new cases, which represents 13.2% of all cases in men and 12.7% of all cases in women. The age-adjusted incidence rate was 59.0 per 100,000 per year and 36.1 per 100,000 per year for men and women, respectively. CRC was also the second most frequent cause of cancer-related death in 2012 with 215,000 deaths, which represents 11.6% of all cancer deaths in men and 13.0% of all cancer deaths in women.[1]

Various biochemical and radiological test are used to identify the optimal treatment strategy for patients with (metastatic) CRC. Molecular imaging with [18F]-fluorodeoxyglucose (FDG) PET combined with computed tomography (CT) is one of the most recent modalities used in different, usually more advanced stages of the disease. The glucose analogue FDG exploits the increased glucose consumption of cancer cells. Most CRCs exhibit increased FDG uptake, although in mucinous adenocarcinoma uptake may be limited. This article focuses on the role of FDG-PET/CT in patient management and outcome in patients with colorectal carcinoma. More specifically, it focuses on the value of FDG-PET/CT in (preoperative) staging of primary and recurrent disease, the staging of primary and recurrent liver metastases, and the assessment of therapy response.

SEARCH

We used the Preferred Reporting Items for Systematic Reviews and Meta-analysis (PRISMA) guidelines for our article-selection process (**Box 1**).

Disclosure: The authors have nothing to disclose.
Department of Radiology and Nuclear Medicine, Radboud University Medical Center, PO Box 9101, Nijmegen 6500HB, The Netherlands
* Corresponding author.
E-mail address: wim.oyen@radboudumc.nl

PET Clin 10 (2015) 345–360
http://dx.doi.org/10.1016/j.cpet.2015.03.007
1556-8598/15/$ – see front matter © 2015 Elsevier Inc. All rights reserved.

Box 1
Search results from PRISMA

Main research question:

P: adult patients with colorectal carcinoma

I: FDG-PET/CT

C: survival outcome

Target condition: changes in patient management

Study design strategy: cohort studies, randomized controlled trials, and meta-analyses

Search query:

(((((((((((("Positron-Emission Tomography"[Mesh]) OR PET) OR PET/*) OR PETscan*) OR PET/CT*) OR PET-CT*) OR CT/PET*) OR CT-PET*) OR (((positron) AND emission) AND tomography)) OR "Fluoro-deoxyglucose F18"[Mesh]) OR FDG)) AND ((((("Colorectal Neoplasms"[Mesh]) OR colorect*) OR colon) OR rectal*) OR rectum*)) AND (((((((carcinom*) OR adenocarc*) OR cancer) OR neoplas*) OR tumor) OR tumour) OR tumors) OR tumours)

Data sources (13 December 2014):

PubMed by the National Institutes of Health: 2592 results

Library of the Cochrane collaborations: 642 results

OvidSP MEDLINE: 2113 results

OvidSP MEDLINE in process and other nonindexed citations and Ovid MEDLINE by Wolters Kluwer: 2352 results

Number of records after duplicates removed: 3317 records

Number of studies considered eligible for this review: 77

*, The asterix indicates a truncation.

Studies for this review were identified by a systematic search that was conducted using PubMed, MEDLINE, and the Cochrane Library. Our research question was defined using the target population, index test, comparator test, target condition, and study design strategy, which led to the following search string: (PET/CT OR PET) AND Colorectal AND Cancer. The search was performed on 13/12/2014 and was constructed using Medical Subject Headings, keywords, and truncated synonyms.

Animal studies, case reports, reviews without a meta-analysis, articles that included fewer than 15 patients, letters to the editor, PET tracers other than FDG, and all articles written in a language other than English were excluded. Studies on recurrence or treatment response without implicating a consequence for patient management or survival outcome were excluded.

Our search resulted in 77 articles that were considered eligible for this article.

PRIMARY STAGING

For patients with CRC it is important to determine the best treatment strategy, which may be surgical intervention, chemotherapy, or radiation therapy, or combinations thereof. When a patient is diagnosed with CRC, computed tomography (CT) and, in case of rectum carcinoma, MR imaging are the primary imaging modalities for staging. However, FDG-PET/CT may have added value in selected cases in patients with higher disease stage.

Colorectal Cancer

In colorectal carcinoma, FDG-PET/CT can influence patient management in 2%[2] to 30%[3] of cases. In a retrospective analysis, Petersen and colleagues[3] studied 67 patients with CRC who had undergone FDG-PET/CT in addition to conventional imaging for initial staging. Of these patients, 20 (30%) had a change in patient management. In one-third of these cases there was a change from intended curative to palliative therapy or vice versa, in the remaining two-thirds the change in patient management was more mixed. In contrast, a study on additional PET/CT from 2013 by Cipe and colleagues[4] revealed a change of surgical management in only 2 (3.2%) of 64 patients. In 1 patient a liver metastasis was identified that was not visible on conventional imaging and as a consequence a chemotherapy regimen was started. In the second patient an additional supraclavicular lymph node was detected by

FDG-PET/CT, which caused a change in management by performing both a total mesorectal excision and a supraclavicular lymph node excision. The large difference between the studies from Petersen and colleagues[3] and Cipe and colleagues[4] is probably caused by Cipe and colleagues[4] including patients regardless of stage, whereas Petersen and colleagues included patients with advanced disease stages. A large number of patients in the study of Cipe and colleagues[4] probably had only limited disease, which explains the low number of patients who benefited from the FDG-PET/CT scan. The studies from Lee and Lee,[5] Park and colleagues,[6] and Furukawa and colleagues[2] support this. Lee and Lee[5] conducted a retrospective study in which 266 patients with colon cancer were assessed with both FDG-PET/CT and conventional studies for staging of colon cancer. In this study FDG-PET/CT led to a change in management for 1 of 40 patients (2.5%) with clinical stage I, 0 of 25 patients (0%) with stage II, 9 of 138 patients (6.5%) with stage III, and 8 of 63 patients (12.7%) with stage 4 disease. In the study by Park and colleagues,[6] 100 patients with CRC were included, of whom 3 patients had stage I, 23 patients had stage II, 25 had stage III, and 49 had stage IV disease. In 27% of these patients FDG-PET/CT changed the surgical treatment plan; in 18 patients (18%) the extent of surgery was changed and in 9 patients (9%) treatment regarding preoperative chemoradiotherapy was changed. Furukawa and colleagues[2] showed a limited impact of FDG-PET/CT on clinical management. Forty-four patients with CRC were included and in only 1 patient (2%) patient management was changed because FDG-PET showed bone and distant lymph node metastases. The low-number of management changes was again attributed to the less advanced disease stage of the included patients. In a prospective study by Kantorova and colleagues,[7] FDG-PET led to a change of treatment in 6 (16%) out of 38 patients with colorectal carcinoma; treatment modality was changed in 3 patients (8%) and the extent of surgery was changed in 5 patients (13%). Veit-Haibach and colleagues[8] included 47 patients with suspicious lesions at colonoscopy and found that FDG-PET/CT led to a change of management in 9% of the patients compared with CT. Llamas-Elvira[9] included 104 patients with CRC referred for surgery. In this group FDG-PET/CT modified the scope of surgery in 12% of the cases. Eight patients (7.7%) did not receive surgery because of the extent of disease found on FDG-PET/CT, which was not detected by conventional imaging. Engelmann and colleagues[10] prospectively investigated the diagnostic accuracy of FDG-PET/CT

and CT in 66 patients for staging of primary CRC. The diagnostic accuracies for tumor, nodal disease, and metastasis staging by FDG-PET/CT were 82%, 66%, and 89% respectively. For CT the diagnostic accuracies were 77%, 60%, and 69%.

These studies indicate that routine FDG-PET/CT is generally not beneficial in the initial staging of CRC, but it may have added value in patients with stage 3 and stage 4 disease.

Rectal Cancer

In rectal cancer FDG-PET/CT can influence patient management in 12%[11] to 27%[12] of cases. Ozis and colleagues[13] included 97 patients with primary rectal adenocarcinoma who all underwent conventional imaging as well as FDG-PET/CT. More than half of the patients in this population had stage II disease or higher. In 14 patients (14.4%) FDG-PET/CT changed the stage of disease. Treatment strategy was changed in 10 patients (9.7%) and the type of operation was changed in 4 patients (4%). In a study by Eglinton and colleagues,[14] 20 patients with adenocarcinoma of the rectum underwent both PET/CT and CT conventional imaging. FDG-PET/CT resulted in minor management changes in 5 patients (25%), but no surgical management changes occurred. In a study by Davey and colleagues,[11] 10 out of a total of 83 patients (12%) with rectal cancer had a change of management because of findings on FDG-PET/CT. Another study by Bassi and colleagues[15] showed that in 24% of 25 patients with T3 to T4 rectal cancer FDG-PET/CT affected tumor staging or the assessment of treatment response. Gearhart and colleagues[12] prospectively evaluated the utility of PET/CT imaging in the initial evaluation of primary rectal cancer. Thirty-seven patients were included and received transrectal ultrasonography or MR imaging, spiral CT, and FDG-PET/CT. Discordant findings were identified in 14 patients (38%), which in 10 cases (27%) resulted in a deviation of the treatment plan. In a study by Heriot and colleagues,[16] 46 patients with stage II to IV rectal cancer were included. FDG-PET after conventional imaging changed the previously proposed patient management in 8 patients (17%), in 6 cases (13%) leading to cancellation of surgery because of metastatic disease and in the 2 other cases changing the radiotherapy field.

LIVER METASTASES

For patients with CRC, the liver is the most common site for distant metastases.[17] FDG-PET/CT is an accurate imaging modality for diagnosing patients with CRC with liver metastases. Resection of liver metastases is the only potentially curative therapy, but to achieve this it is important that all liver tumors are completely resected while maintaining sufficient hepatic function and that there is no extrahepatic spread. This article discuss the value of FDG-PET/CT in patients with potentially resectable colorectal liver metastases for staging, the added value of PET compared with conventional imaging, and the predictive value of preoperative FDG-PET/CT findings for survival. **Fig. 1** shows an example of a patient with colorectal liver metastases but no evidence of extrahepatic disease.

Can Fluorodeoxyglucose-PET/Computed Tomography Change Patient Management in the Primary Staging of Colorectal Metastases?

Two randomized controlled trials were identified.[18,19] Ruers and colleagues[18] included 150 patients with CRC liver metastases who received CT scanning and were selected for surgical treatment. Patients were randomized for either CT only (n = 75) or CT plus FDG-PET (n = 75). The primary outcome of the study was a significantly lower number of futile laparotomies in the FDG-PET group (28%) than in the control group (45%), with a relative risk reduction of 38% (P = .042). FDG-PET performed in the work-up for surgical resection could prevent futile laparotomy in 1 of 6 patients. The more recent randomized study by Moulton and colleagues[19] showed contradictory results. After baseline CT imaging, 263 patients were randomized to the FDG-PET/CT group and 121 patients to the no FDG-PET/CT group (control group). Of the 263 patients in the FDG-PET/CT group, 21 patients eventually had a change in patient management, of whom 7 patients had a cancellation of surgery, 4 patients had more extensive surgery, 9 patients had further nonhepatic surgery including biopsy, and 1 patient had more extensive and further nonhepatic surgery. In the FDG-PET/CT group, liver resection was performed

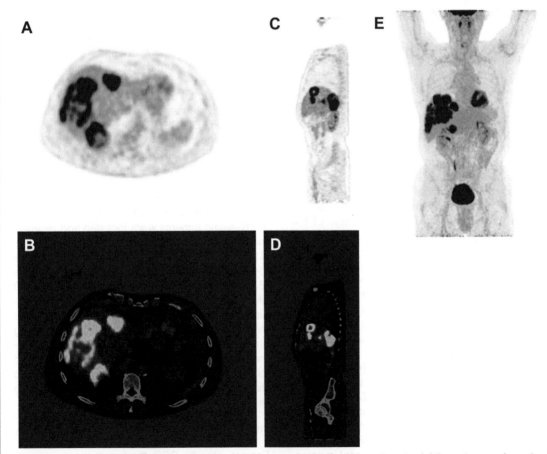

Fig. 1. Patient with colorectal liver metastases. FDG-PET transverse (A) and sagittal (C) sections and maximal intensity projection. (E) Fused FDG-PET/CT transverse (B) and sagittal (D) sections. Extensive involvement of the liver, but no evidence of extrahepatic disease.

in 91% of the cases and in the control group 92%. No significant difference was found in overall survival or disease-free survival. A significant limitation of this study is that about 70% of the patients received chemotherapy within 12 weeks of surgery, whereas none of the patients in the study by Ruers and colleagues[18] were treated with neoadjuvant chemotherapy before FDG-PET/CT. Chemotherapy significantly decreases FDG uptake in tumors, which results in less efficient detection of cancerous lesions.[20–22] Note that this may have caused false-negative FDG-PET/CT scans in a significant number of patients in the study by Moulton and colleagues.[19] Another important potential pitfall is that patients were included if they had resectable colorectal liver metastases on contrast-enhanced CT scans within the previous 30 days, whereas patients who were unresponsive to adjuvant therapy and continued to show extrahepatic disease were excluded. This difference could have led to selection bias, because this group of patients might have benefited from FDG-PET/CT scan before initiating therapy.

In a recent meta-analysis by Maffione and colleagues,[23] 4 studies were included for a patient-based analysis to examine the diagnostic performance of PET.[24–27] These studies provided a total number of 484 patients with a pooled sensitivity of 93% (range, 88%–96%), specificity of 93% (range, 84%–98%), and an area under the summary receiver operating characteristic (ROC) curve of 0.97. Another 4 studies[28–31] were included for a lesion-based analysis. These studies provided a total of 575 lesions with a pooled sensitivity of 50 (range, 55%–64%), specificity of 79% (range, 68%–87%), and an area under the ROC curve of 0.67.

Our search included 15 nonrandomized studies affecting patient management (**Table 1**). Ramos and colleagues[30] included 97 patients in a prospective study to determine whether FDG-PET/CT could improve accuracy of staging in patients with CRC liver metastases and to assess the impact on therapeutic staging. All patients received a preoperative contrast-enhanced CT scan (86 patients) or MR scan (11 patients) and an FDG-PET/CT scan. In 17 (17%) patients FDG-PET/CT would have changed the therapeutic strategy, and in only 8 (8%) patients the additional findings of FDG-PET/CT proved to be correct. FDG-PET/CT would have prevented 2 futile laparotomies (2%). A prospective study by Georgakopoulos and colleagues[32] showed that FDG-PET/CT detected extrahepatic disease in 7 (36.8%) out of 19 patients with CRC with liver metastases scheduled for hepatic surgery, which directly altered patient management.

They also showed that FDG-PET/CT detected extrahepatic disease in 4 (25%) out of 16 patients with CRC with liver metastases scheduled for radiofrequency ablation. In a retrospective study by Briggs and colleagues,[33] 102 patients with metastatic CRC were included, of whom 94 had liver metastases. All patients received FDG-PET/CT in addition to conventional imaging. FDG-PET/CT had a major impact on patient management in 31 patients (30%). Extrahepatic disease was found in 9 patients in addition to the known liver metastases, in 16 patients FDG-PET/CT correctly identified inoperable metastatic disease considered to be intermediate lesions on conventional imaging, in 3 patients a second primary tumor was identified, and 3 patients were correctly downstaged. Futile laparotomy was prevented in 16 patients (16%). McLeish and colleagues[34] suggested in a retrospective study that FDG-PET can greatly affect the management plan of patients with CRC liver metastases (n = 54) by showing that FDG-PET changed the patient management in 36 (66.7%) of the cases. In 24 cases (44.4%) hepatic surgery was canceled. Twelve patients were classified by conventional imaging as having the potential of future liver patients, and FDG-PET showed that all patients were suitable for resection. Another study by Wiering and colleagues[35] prospectively selected 203 patients with CRC and liver metastases. One-hundred patients (group A) were selected for hepatic surgery by CT and 103 patients (group B) were selected for hepatic surgery with CT plus FDG-PET/CT. There was no difference in futile laparotomy between the groups (28% vs 19.4%; $P = .186$). However, significantly less extrahepatic disease was seen during surgery in group B (1.9% vs 10%; $P = .017$). Chua and colleagues[25] included 131 patients (of whom 75 patients had CRC) with suspected metastatic liver disease in a retrospective study. They suggested that FDG-PET/CT changed patient management in 25% of the cases. Teague and colleagues[36] reported an influence of management by FDG-PET of 25% out of 16 patients undergoing investigation of known or suspected CRC. Selzner and colleagues[26] prospectively included 76 patients with CRC who were evaluated for resection of liver metastases by contrast-enhanced CT and FDG-PET/CT. FDG-PET/CT changed therapeutic strategy in 21% of the patients. Arulampalam and colleagues[37] prospectively studied 28 patients who were referred for hepatic resection of CRC liver metastases and all underwent spiral CT and an FDG-PET scan. FDG-PET altered management in 12 patients and avoided inappropriate surgery in 7 patients (25%). Ruers and colleagues[38] prospectively analyzed 51 patients for resection of colorectal liver

Table 1
Management changes by FDG-PET or FDG-PET/CT of patients with colorectal liver metastases

Study, Year	Number of Patients	Design	Management Changes (%)	Investigators' Conclusions
Ruers et al,[38] 2002	51	Prospective	20	FDG-PET as a complementary staging method improves the therapeutic management of patients with colorectal liver metastases, especially by detecting unsuspected extrahepatic disease
Teague et al,[36] 2004	16	Retrospective	25	The results support the use of FDG-PET for selecting patients with colorectal liver metastases
Selzner et al,[26] 2004	76	Prospective	21	PET/CT provides important additional information in patients with presumed resectable colorectal metastases to the liver, resulting in a change of therapy in a fifth of patients
Arulampalam et al,[86] 2004	28	Prospective	42	FDG-PET confers clinical benefit through altered patient management
Joyce et al,[41] 2006	64	Prospective	24	PET provides useful information in the selection of patients with hepatic metastases from CRC being considered for surgical therapy
Sorensen et al,[39] 2007	54	Prospective	19	Pretreatment FDG-PET, used supplementary to CT, improved the treatment plan in one-fifth of patients with colorectal liver metastases
Briggs et al,[33] 2011	102 (94 liver metastases)	Retrospective	30	FDG-PET/CT can improve staging accuracy, characterize intermediate lesions, and help triage patients with metastatic CRC to the appropriate treatment
Ramos et al,[30] 2011	97	Prospective	17	FDG-PET/CT has limited use in hepatic staging in patients with colorectal liver metastases. It provided additional information in 8% of the cases and potential harmful information in 9% of the cases

(continued on next page)

Table 1
(continued)

Study, Year	Number of Patients	Design	Management Changes (%)	Investigators' Conclusions
Engledow et al,[40] 2012	64	Prospective	34	The addition of PET/CT led to management changes in more than one-third of patients but there was no correlation between alterations in staging or management and the Fong clinical risk score, suggesting that PET/CT should be used, where available, in the preoperative staging of patients with colorectal liver metastases
McLeish et al,[34] 2012	54	Retrospective	67	FDG-PET can profoundly affect the management plan of patients with colorectal liver metastases suitable for surgery
Georgakopoulos et al,[32] 2013	19	Prospective	37	FDG-PET/CT provides relevant additional information for patients with colorectal carcinoma and liver metastases
Chua et al,[25] 2007	131 (75 with colorectal liver metastases)	Retrospective	25	FDG-PET/CT performed better in detecting both colorectal and noncolorectal liver metastases and frequently altered patient management
Lake et al,[42] 2014	133	—	20	FDG-PET CT in this setting may prevent futile operations, guide the resection of local regional nodal disease, and downstage many patients thought to have extrahepatic disease on conventional imaging

metastases and in 10 patients (20%) clinical management based on conventional imaging was changed as a result of FDG-PET findings. Sorensen and colleagues[39] showed in a prospective study that in 54 patients with CRC liver metastases an additional FDG-PET scan changed the treatment plan in 19% of the cases. In a study by Engledow and colleagues[40] 64 patients with CRC liver metastases were included and all underwent FDG-PET/CT and conventional imaging. FDG-PET/CT caused a change of management in 22 patients (34%), upstaging in 20, and downstaging in 2 patients. Joyce and colleagues[41] prospectively included 64 patients referred with potentially resectable liver metastases based on conventional imaging. All patients received FDG-PET and a change in clinical management occurred in 17 patients (24%). Lake and colleagues[42] showed that, out of 133 patients with colorectal liver metastases, FDG-PET/CT had a major impact on staging of extrahepatic disease in 20% of the patients compared with the initial CT.

In conclusion, most studies claim that FDG-PET or FDG-PET/CT can have an additional benefit when selecting patients with CRC for hepatic metastasectomy. However, there are a few studies that suggest that FDG-PET/CT may not have such a large impact on surgical management as others have reported.[19,30] Timing of FDG-PET/CT is crucial because chemotherapy negatively influences sensitivity. Studies indicate a high sensitivity and specificity of FDG-PET/CT for patients with colorectal liver metastases on a patient basis. On a lesion basis, FDG-PET/CT is less sensitive and less specific (Maffione and colleagues[23]).

Can a Preoperative Fluorodeoxyglucose-PET/Computed Tomography Scan Improve Overall Survival in Patients with Resectable Liver Metastases?

In a study by Yip and colleagues[43] the survival outcomes of patients with colorectal liver metastases were evaluated. The overall survival rates of 3 groups of patients were compared. The first group was a palliative group with occult extrahepatic disease found by FDG-PET/CT (n = 80). The second group was the group of patients with extensive multisite disease recognized on conventional imaging or disease progression during chemotherapy (n = 161). The third group of patients was the group of patients with resected hepatic disease (n = 291). The 5-year overall survival was significantly higher for the third group compared with the first and second groups (43%, 6.5%, and 6.1% respectively; P<.001). The investigators concluded that PET/CT seems to be effective in selecting patients with occult extrahepatic disease, which has poor survival outcomes. If this holds true, then the group of patients who received an FDG-PET/CT scan preoperatively should be a selected group of patients with better survival rates than patients who did not undergo an FDG-PET/CT scan preoperatively. This clinical question was investigated by Ayez and colleagues.[44] This study included 613 patients who all underwent resection of colorectal liver

metastases in the period between 2000 and 2009. The population was divided into 2 groups: the patients with an FDG-PET scan preoperatively (n = 206) and patients without an FDG-PET scan preoperatively (n = 407). No statistical difference was seen in median disease-free survival and overall survival between the groups. In the study by Wiering and colleagues,[35] overall survival and disease-free survival at 3 years did not differ between the group selected for hepatic surgery by conventional imaging and the group selected for additional FDG-PET imaging. These findings indicate that, despite less surgery in the patients staged with FDG-PET/CT, survival is not negatively influenced. In the study by Fernandez and colleagues,[45] the 5-year overall survival for patients with colorectal liver metastases after hepatic resection was 58% in a cohort of 100 patients. This survival was better than the 5-year overall survival of 6070 patients in 19 previously established studies in patients without preoperative FDG-PET. Riedl and colleagues[46] correlated the standardized uptake values (SUVs) of patients with hepatic metastases from CRC with overall survival and showed that survival was significantly longer for patients with a low SUV than for patients with a high SUV.

SUSPECTED RECURRENCE OF DISEASE

In approximately one-third of patients with CRC, recurrence occurs within the first 2 years after surgery and the most frequent site of recurrence is the area of surgery. Several studies have shown that FDG-PET is sensitive and specific in detecting recurrence in patients with colorectal carcinoma and can significantly affect patient management.[47–49] **Fig. 2** shows an example of a patient with rectal cancer with recurrent disease detected on FDG-PET/CT.

Our search included 1 randomized controlled trial by Sobhani and colleagues[50] They included 130 patients with CRC who had undergone curative therapy and who were randomly assigned to undergo either conventional follow-up or follow-up with FDG-PET. No difference in recurrence rate was found between the groups; however, recurrences were detected after a shorter period of time in the FDG-PET group. In the FDG-PET group, recurrences were also more frequently cured by surgery compared with the conventional group. Scott and colleagues[51] showed in a multicenter prospective trial that, in 93 patients with recurrent disease, FDG-PET/CT detected additional lesions in 45 patients (48.4%). FDG-PET/CT changed management plans in 61 patients (65.6%). In 13 patients (13%) a change was made from curative

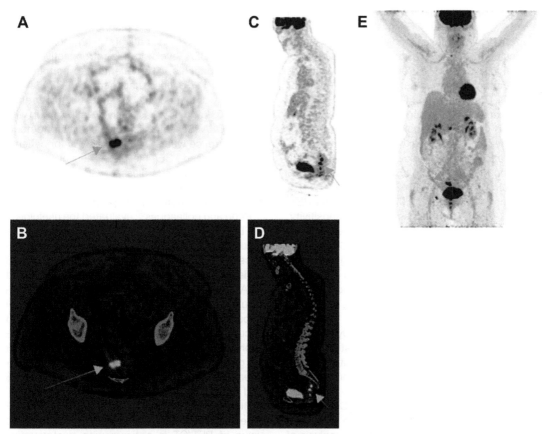

Fig. 2. Patient with increasing carcinoembryonic antigen levels, suspected of recurrent rectal cancer. FDG-PET transverse (*A*) and sagittal (*C*) sections and maximal intensity projection (*E*). Fused FDG-PET/CT transverse (*B*) and sagittal (*D*) sections. The arrows indicate local recurrence of the rectum carcinoma.

to palliative treatment after FDG-PET/CT and in 14 patients (15%) a change was made from palliative to curative treatment. During follow-up (1 year), progressive disease was detected in 60.5% of patients with additional lesions on FDG-PET/CT and in 36.2% of the patients with no additional lesions detected by FDG-PET/CT ($P = .04$). Shamim and colleagues[52] analyzed a retrospective cohort of 32 patients with recurrent CRC who received chemotherapy, of whom 20 were nonresponders and 12 were responders. All patients received FDG-PET/CT at baseline and after chemotherapy. Among nonresponders there was a significant increase in mean maximal standardized uptake value (SUV_{max}) after follow-up (baseline 8.1 ± 5.2 and follow-up 14.1 ± 9.0), and among responders there was a significant decrease in mean SUV_{max} (baseline 11.8 ± 10.1 and follow-up 3.7 ± 4.1).

In a meta-analysis up to 2011, Maas and colleagues[53] investigated which whole-body imaging modality had the highest accuracy for detecting local and distant CRC recurrence in patients with clinically or biochemically suspected recurrence.

They included 14 studies showing that FDG-PET and FDG-PET/CT were more accurate that CT with areas under the curves of 0.94 (0.90–0.97) for PET, 0.94 (0.87–0.98) for PET/CT, and 0.83 (0.72–0.90) for CT.

DETECTING RECURRENCE WITH FLUORODEOXYGLUCOSE-PET/COMPUTED TOMOGRAPHY IN PATIENTS WITH INCREASED CARCINOEMBRYONIC ANTIGEN LEVELS

Serial blood monitoring of carcinoembryonic antigen (CEA) levels is the most frequently used method to detect asymptomatic recurrences. It is estimated that, in 90% of patients with increased CEA levels after surgery, tumor has recurred.[54] However, serum CEA levels do not provide any information regarding the sites of recurrence. It can be a challenge when a patient has increased CEA levels but no apparent relapse can be localized.

In 2013, Lu and colleagues[55] conducted a systematic review and meta-analysis to assess the diagnostic performance of FDG-PET or PET/CT in patients with increased CEA levels and suspected recurrent disease. Eleven studies with 510 patients were included, of which 10 studies had a retrospective design and 1 study a prospective design. Diagnostic performance was calculated separately for FDG-PET (7 studies) and FDG-PET/CT (4 studies). In the detection of recurrence of patients with increased CEA levels, pooled estimates of sensitivity, specificity, and positive and negative likelihood ratios were respectively 90.3% (95% confidence interval [CI], 85.5%–94.0%), 80.0% (95% CI, 67.0%–89.6%), 2.88 (95% CI, 1.37–6.07), and 0.12 (95% CI, 0.07–0.20) for FDG-PET. For FDG-PET/CT, pooled estimates of sensitivity, specificity, and positive and negative likelihood ratios were respectively 94.1% (95% CI, 89.4%–97.1%), 77.2% (95% CI, 66.4%–85.9%), 4.7 (95% CI, 0.82–12.12), and 0.06 (95% CI, 0.03 and 0.13).

Giacomobono and colleagues[56] showed that quantitative assessment by SUV_{max} may be helpful in patients presenting with increased CEA levels. In this retrospective study a worse overall survival was observed in patients with SUV_{max} greater than 5.7 compared with patients with SUV_{max} of less than 5.7 (median survival, 16 vs 31 months; $P = .002$).

Studies have shown that FDG-PET/CT is superior to CT in detecting recurrent disease in patients with increased CEA levels. In the meta-analysis of Lu and colleagues,[55] studies revealed enough information to perform a pooled estimation of sensitivity and specificity for diagnostic CT scan, which revealed a sensitivity and specificity of 51.3% and 90.2%, respectively. Ozkan and colleagues[57] showed in a retrospective study with 69 patients a sensitivity of 97% and a specificity of 61% for FDG-PET/CT, and a sensitivity of 51% and specificity of 61% for contrast-enhanced CT.

Panagioditis and colleagues[58] conducted a prospective study in which the role of FDG-PET/CT was investigated in the diagnosis of recurrent CRC in patients with increased tumor marker levels (CEA and/or cancer antigen (CA) 19-9) and negative contrast-enhanced CT scans. A total of 43 patients (of whom 22 were ultimately diagnosed with recurrent disease) were included in this study and FDG-PET/CT had a sensitivity of 97% (95% CI, 0.82–0.99) and a specificity of 80% (95% CI, 0.44–0.96).

DETECTING RECURRENCE OF COLORECTAL CANCER IN PATIENTS WITH NORMAL LEVELS OF CARCINOEMBRYONIC ANTIGEN

More recently there have been studies indicating that PET/CT may be useful in detecting recurrence in patients with normal CEA levels. Sanli and colleagues[59] compared the diagnostic performance of FDG-PET/CT in patients with normal and increased CEA levels. In this retrospective study with 235 patients, 118 patients had normal CEA levels and 117 patients had increased CEA levels. Sensitivity and specificity for detecting recurrence were 100% and 84% respectively in the group with normal CEA. Sensitivity and specificity for detecting recurrence was 97.1% and 84.6% for patients with increased CEA levels. The investigators concluded that, regardless of CEA levels, FDG-PET/CT can detect recurrence. There have been several other studies that support this.

Peng and colleagues[60] evaluated the usefulness of FDG-PET/CT in the early detection of resectable recurrences of CRC and the impact on clinical disease management. In this retrospective study, 128 patients were included, of whom 49 had increased CEA levels (group 1) and 79 had clinically suspicious recurrences but no increase in CEA level (group 2). The overall sensitivity, specificity, and accuracy were 98.4%, 89.2%, and 93.8% respectively for group 1% and 100%, 88.9%, and 95.9% for group 2. FDG-PET/CT changed clinical management in 63.6% of the patients in group 1% and 39.2% of the patients in group 2.

Bu and colleagues[61] retrospectively investigated the association between the diagnostic value of PET/CT in patients with postoperative recurrence and metastasis of CRC, and the different levels of CEA. In total, 105 patients were included, of whom 87 had recurrence and metastatic CRC. Of the 68 patients in the CEA-positive group, FDG-PET/CT correctly diagnosed recurrence and metastases in 58 cases (85.3%). Of the 37 patients in the CEA-negative group, recurrence and metastasis was correctly diagnosed in 28 cases (75.7%). No statistical difference ($P<.221$) was found between the groups for monitoring the detection rates for recurrence and metastasis.

Zhang and colleagues[62] evaluated the diagnostic performance of FDG-PET/CT in surveillance of postoperative patients with CRC compared with contrast-enhanced CT and assessed the role of FDG-PET/CT in patients with different CEA concentrations. This retrospective study included 106 patients. FDG-PET/CT had a sensitivity, specificity, and accuracy of respectively 95.2%, 82.6%, and 92.5%. CT showed a sensitivity, specificity, and accuracy of 80.7%, 73.9%, and 79.3%. The sensitivity and accuracy were significantly higher for FDG-PET/CT compared with CT ($P = .004$ and $P = .013$). No statistical difference was found between patients with normal and increased CEA levels.

ASSESSMENT OF TREATMENT RESPONSE
Colorectal Cancer

Follow-up of patients to measure the effect of treatment is usually based on conventional imaging and is usually based on the Response Evaluation Criteria in Solid Tumors (RECIST), measuring changes in the diameter of the lesions. However, RECIST has limitations, because a decrease in tumor size does not always correspond with an improvement in prognosis. Because FDG-PET/CT focuses on metabolic changes, it may be able to measure tumor response before anatomic changes occur. In a systematic review up to 2009, de Geus-Oei and colleagues[63] showed that FDG-PET has a high predictive value in the therapeutic management of CRC. De Geus-Oei and colleagues[64] showed in a prospective study that FDG-PET can be used for chemotherapy response evaluation in a clinical setting. Fifty patients with advanced CRC underwent FDG-PET before and after 2 months from the start of chemotherapy. Nineteen patients received FDG-PET after the start of treatment. This study showed a significant predictive value of FDG-PET on overall and progression-free survival at broad ranges of Δ metabolic rate of glucose and ΔSUV. Hendlisz and colleagues[65] evaluated 41 patients with metastatic CRC and found that metabolic responding patients (23 patients) had a significantly longer overall survival compared with metabolic nonresponding patients (hazard ratio, 0.28; 95% CI, 0.10–0.76). However, the difference in progression-free survival was not statistically significant (hazard ratio, 0.57; 95% CI, 0.27–1.21) between the groups. In a prospective study by Mertens and colleagues,[66] 18 patients with CRC and potentially resectable liver metastases were included, of whom 16 underwent hepatic metastasectomy. An FDG-PET/CT scan was performed before treatment and after 5 cycles of chemotherapy (oxaliplatin plus 5-fluorouracil and leucovorin [FOLFOX]/irinotecan plus 5-fluorouracil and leucovorin [FOLFIRI]) and bevacizumab. Eight patients showed a partial response, 9 patients showed stable disease, and 1 patient showed progressive disease, according to RECIST. Results showed that follow-up SUV_{max}, standardized added metabolic activity (SAM), and ΔSAM were significant prognostic factors for progression-free survival and overall survival. Patients with SUV_{max} greater than 2.85 showed a median progression free survival 10.4 months, compared to 14.7 months in the group of patients with SUV_{max} less than 2.85. Patients with SUV_{max} greater than 2.85 showed a median overall survival of 32 months compared to a

median overall survival that had not yet been reached in the group of patients with SUX_{max} less than 2.85. The group of patients with high follow-up SAM and low ΔSAM had a median progression-free survival and overall survival of 9.4 months and 32 months, respectively. The group of patients with low follow-up SAM and high ΔSAM had a median progression-free survival and overall survival of 14.7 months ($P = .002$) and a median overall survival that had not been reached ($P = .002$). Baseline SUV_{max} and the SAM were not correlated with progression-free and overall survival. Lau and colleagues[67] showed that, in patients undergoing resection of colorectal liver metastases, FDG-PET is predictive of prognosis by assessing tumor metabolic response. They showed in a population of 80 patients that FDG-PET parameters after chemotherapy were predictive of overall survival and recurrence-free survival. Overall survival was 86% at 3 years for patients with metabolic response and 38% for patients with nonmetabolic response ($P = .003$). Baseline FDG-PET parameters were not predictive of prognosis and also RECIST did not predict outcome. A similar study by Small and colleagues[68] included 54 patients with colorectal liver metastases, who all received neoadjuvant chemotherapy followed by hepatic surgery. Response to chemotherapy on both CT and PET/CT were predictive of time to recurrence. However, for overall survival, only response to chemotherapy on CT (according to RECIST) was predictive.

In the last few years, some studies have used the PET Response Criteria in Solid tumors (PERCIST) to measure FDG-PET response to treatment.[69] In a study by Skougaard and colleagues,[70] 61 patients with metastatic CRC who were treated with cetuximab and irinotecan were included. Response evaluation was performed by CT using RECIST criteria and by FDG-PET/CT using PERCIST criteria. There was a poor morphologic and metabolic agreement, mainly because a large proportion of the patients who had stable disease on CT turned out to have partial metabolic response on FDG-PET/CT. Although the study was not powered to draw firm conclusions about survival outcome, the hazard ratio of both RECIST criteria and PERCIST criteria correlated with overall survival. Our search included a randomized control trial by Bystrom and colleagues,[71] who evaluated the value of FDG-PET in the response to palliative chemotherapy and prediction of long-term outcome in patients with metastatic CRC.[71] Note that patients were randomized in 2 different chemotherapy groups and that there was no randomization in diagnostic modality. Fifty-one patients were randomly assigned to receive irinotecan with either the Nordic bolus 5-fluorouracil (n = 27) and folinic acid schedule or the Gramont schedule (Leucovorin and 5-Flourouracil [Lv5FU2]-irinotecan) (n = 28). No differences in PET response and outcomes could be found between the treatment groups, so they were analyzed together. Each patient underwent an FDG-PET scan 1 to 14 days before start of treatment and immediately before the third cycle of chemotherapy. A strong correlation was found between metabolic response (changes in SUV) and objective response ($r = 0.57$; $P = .00001$), with a sensitivity of 77% and a specificity of 76%. However, no significant correlation was detected between metabolic response and time to progression ($P = .5$) or overall survival ($P =.1$).

Our conclusion is that most studies show that, by measuring metabolic response, FDG-PET/CT (or FDG-PET) can be of value to estimate prognosis in patients receiving treatment of advanced or metastatic CRC. Baseline parameters measured by FDG-PET/CT do not seem to show predictive value.

RECTAL CANCER

For patients with rectal cancer located within the mesorectal fascia, radical surgery of the mesorectum is the standard of treatment. In patients with locally advanced rectal cancer (LARC), treatment with surgery is often not sufficient because they are at the highest risk for failure of local treatment. For these patients neoadjuvant chemoradiation therapy can be successful.[72] To determine the effect of preoperative therapy remains a challenge for conventional imaging methods, because they are limited in differentiating between therapy-induced anatomic alterations (like fibrosis, necrosis, or inflammation tissue) and tumor foci.[73] Studies have shown that FDG-PET was better in predicting therapy outcomes than CT and MR imaging.[74,75] De Geus-Oei and colleagues[63] showed in a review that, in patients with primary rectal cancer, FDG-PET could predict outcome after neoadjuvant chemotherapy and local treatment. More recent studies using FDG-PET/CT confirm this.[76] In a prospective study by Calvo and colleagues,[76] 38 patients with LARC were included. SUV_{max} parameters were significantly correlated with disease-free survival and overall survival. In a retrospective study with 70 patients with LARC, Shanmugan and colleagues[77] showed that FDG-PET/CT can predict response to chemoradiation therapy. A posttherapy SUV less than 4 and a decrease of SUV of greater than 63%

were predictive of overall survival and recurrence-free survival.

Most of the studies mentioned earlier investigate tumor response by FDG-PET/CT by measuring metabolic response before and after neoadjuvant chemotherapy. It can be important to predict the effect of preoperative therapy in an even earlier stage because it may be helpful in determining long-term prognosis, it could optimize surgical approach, and it might improve quality of life by avoiding unnecessary surgery in patients who are not likely to benefit from an operation. Also, determining failure of therapy in an early stage may change chemotherapy management by switching to or adding a second agent. Furthermore, if it can be determined earlier that radiotherapy is ineffective, patients could be spared weeks of unnecessary radiotherapy. Several studies have investigated tumor response during preoperative therapy in patients with LARC. Janssen and colleagues[78] showed that, in patients with rectal cancer referred for preoperative chemoradiation, significant reductions in SUV_{max} were found after the first week of treatment ($P<.001$). Hatt and colleagues[79] investigated various FDG-PET parameters at baseline, after 1 week, and after 2 weeks of chemoradiation. Total lesion glycolysis, SUV_{max}, and mean SUV (SUV_{mean}) were predictive of tumor response after 2 weeks. No FDG-PET parameter was predictive after 1 week of chemoradiation therapy. At baseline only SUV_{mean} was predictive of tumor response. However, this finding is not confirmed by other studies. In a recent meta-analysis by Maffione and colleagues,[80] 10 studies with, in total, 302 patients were included to investigate the predictive value of FDG-PET/CT in early response of patients with LARC receiving neoadjuvant chemoradiation. In the total cohort, FDG-PET/CT showed good predictive value with a sensitivity and specificity of 79% and 78%, respectively.

However, not all studies support the use of FDG-PET in patients with LARC after neoadjuvant chemotherapy. In a prospective study by Ruby and colleagues[81] with 127 patients with LARC receiving neoadjuvant chemoradiation, no prognostic information was found by FDG-PET/CT. Another prospective study[82] from the same group showed that, in 121 patients, FDG-PET/CT was not able to distinguish between pathologic complete response and pathologic incomplete response. The investigators concluded that FDG-PET should not be used to predict response in this category of patients.

In a more recent meta-analysis by Li and colleagues,[83] 31 studies (2004–2013) on FDG-PET/CT predicting pathologic response to preoperative chemoradiotherapy were reviewed. The investigators suggested that, among 4 parameters (response index, posttreatment SUV_{max} [SUV_{max}-post], total lesion glycolysis before and after chemotherapy, and visual response), the SUV_{max}-post was the optimal parameter to measure tumor regression grade in patients wit preoperative rectal cancer. Results regarding the optimal scan time point were inconclusive, although there was a trend in favor of conducting the posttreatment FDG-PET/CT scan during therapy. In a meta-analysis by Zhang and colleagues,[84] subgroup analysis showed a higher sensitivity and specificity for patients who received FDG-PET/CT during the chemoradiation therapy (sensitivity 86% and specificity 80%) than for patients who received FDG-PET/CT after chemoradiation therapy (sensitivity 78% and specificity 62%).

An important limitation of these studies is that no universal method is used to quantify tumor response. Examples used in studies are tumor regression grade,[85] total lesion glycolysis,[75] and pathologic complete response.[77] Another limitation of FDG-PET/CT is that chemoradiation can induce significant accumulation of inflammation cells, such as macrophages, neutrophils, fibroblasts, and granulation tissue. These cells have a high glucose metabolism, and thus a high FDG uptake, which might cause misclassification of patients as nonresponders.

In summary, FDG-PET/CT seems a good (early) predictor of outcome in patients with LARC receiving neoadjuvant chemoradiation. More studies are required to investigate the optimal point of time during or after the neoadjuvant treatment for patients to undergo an FDG-PET/CT to evaluate treatment response.

SUMMARY

Studies show that FDG-PET/CT can have a significant clinical impact in patients with CRC in various stages of the disease. In patients with suspected recurrent disease and patients with liver metastases who might be eligible for surgery, FDG-PET/CT has clinically relevant advantages compared with conventional imaging. Also, FDG-PET/CT can be a useful modality to monitor treatment response. The value of FDG-PET/CT for primary staging in patients with colorectal carcinoma is limited, but studies show that there may be added value in patients with more advanced disease. The evidence is based mostly on retrospective and prospective cohort studies, because few randomized controlled trials have been conducted. More randomized controlled trials would give more weight to the evidence discussed in this article.

REFERENCES

1. Ferlay J, Steliarova-Foucher E, Lortet-Tieulent J, et al. Cancer incidence and mortality patterns in Europe: estimates for 40 countries in 2012. Eur J Cancer 2013;49(6):1374–403.
2. Furukawa H, Ikuma H, Seki A, et al. Positron emission tomography scanning is not superior to whole body multidetector helical computed tomography in the preoperative staging of colorectal cancer. Gut 2006;55(7):1007–11.
3. Petersen RK, Hess S, Alavi A, et al. Clinical impact of FDG-PET/CT on colorectal cancer staging and treatment strategy. Am J Nucl Med Mol Imaging 2014; 4(5):471–82.
4. Cipe G, Ergul N, Hasbahceci M, et al. Routine use of positron-emission tomography/computed tomography for staging of primary colorectal cancer: does it affect clinical management? World J Surg Oncol 2013;11:49.
5. Lee JH, Lee MR. Positron emission tomography/computed tomography in the staging of colon cancer. Ann Coloproctol 2014;30(1):23–7.
6. Park IJ, Kim HC, Yu CS, et al. Efficacy of PET/CT in the accurate evaluation of primary colorectal carcinoma. Eur J Surg Oncol 2006;32(9):941–7.
7. Kantorova I, Lipska L, Belohlavek O, et al. Routine (18)F-FDG PET preoperative staging of colorectal cancer: comparison with conventional staging and its impact on treatment decision making. J Nucl Med 2003;44(11):1784–8.
8. Veit-Haibach P, Kuehle CA, Beyer T, et al. Diagnostic accuracy of colorectal cancer staging with whole-body PET/CT colonography. JAMA 2006;296(21): 2590–600.
9. Llamas-Elvira JM, Rodriguez-Fernandez A, Gutierrez-Sainz J, et al. Fluorine-18 fluorodeoxyglucose PET in the preoperative staging of colorectal cancer. Eur J Nucl Med Mol Imaging 2007; 34(6):859–67.
10. Engelmann BE, Loft A, Kjaer A, et al. Positron emission tomography/computed tomography for optimized colon cancer staging and follow up. Scand J Gastroenterol 2014;49(2):191–201.
11. Davey K, Heriot AG, Mackay J, et al. The impact of 18-fluorodeoxyglucose positron emission tomography-computed tomography on the staging and management of primary rectal cancer. Dis Colon Rectum 2008;51(7):997–1003.
12. Gearhart SL, Frassica D, Rosen R, et al. Improved staging with pretreatment positron emission tomography/computed tomography in low rectal cancer. Ann Surg Oncol 2006;13(3):397–404.
13. Ozis SE, Soydal C, Akyol C, et al. The role of 18F-fluorodeoxyglucose positron emission tomography/computed tomography in the primary staging of rectal cancer. World J Surg Oncol 2014;12:26.

14. Eglinton T, Luck A, Bartholomeusz D, et al. Positron-emission tomography/computed tomography (PET/CT) in the initial staging of primary rectal cancer. Colorectal Dis 2010;12(7):667–73.

15. Bassi MC, Turri L, Sacchetti G, et al. FDG-PET/CT imaging for staging and target volume delineation in preoperative conformal radiotherapy of rectal cancer. Int J Radiat Oncol Biol Phys 2008;70(5):1423–6.

16. Heriot AG, Hicks RJ, Drummond EG, et al. Does positron emission tomography change management in primary rectal cancer? A prospective assessment. Dis Colon Rectum 2004;47(4):451–8.

17. Stangl R, Altendorf-Hofmann A, Charnley RM, et al. Factors influencing the natural history of colorectal liver metastases. Lancet 1994;343(8910):1405–10.

18. Ruers TJ, Wiering B, van der Sijp JR, et al. Improved selection of patients for hepatic surgery of colorectal liver metastases with (18)F-FDG PET: a randomized study. J Nucl Med 2009;50(7):1036–41.

19. Moulton CA, Gu CS, Law CH, et al. Effect of PET before liver resection on surgical management for colorectal adenocarcinoma metastases: a randomized clinical trial. JAMA 2014;311(18):1863–9.

20. Akhurst T, Kates TJ, Mazumdar M, et al. Recent chemotherapy reduces the sensitivity of [18F]fluorodeoxyglucose positron emission tomography in the detection of colorectal metastases. J Clin Oncol 2005;23(34):8713–6.

21. Lee M, Yeum TS, Kim JW, et al. Recent chemotherapy reduces the maximum-standardized uptake value of 18F-fluoro-deoxyglucose positron emission tomography in colorectal cancer. Gut Liver 2014; 8(3):254–64.

22. Glazer ES, Beaty K, Abdalla EK, et al. Effectiveness of positron emission tomography for predicting chemotherapy response in colorectal cancer liver metastases. Arch Surg 2010;145(4):340–5 [discussion: 345].

23. Maffione AM, Lopci E, Bluemel C, et al. Diagnostic accuracy and impact on management of (18)F-FDG PET and PET/CT in colorectal liver metastasis: a meta-analysis and systematic review. Eur J Nucl Med Mol Imaging 2015;42(1):152–63 [Systematic reviews and meta-analysis].

24. Akiyoshi T, Oya M, Fujimoto Y, et al. Comparison of preoperative whole-body positron emission tomography with MDCT in patients with primary colorectal cancer. Colorectal Dis 2009;11(5):464–9.

25. Chua SC, Groves AM, Kayani I, et al. The impact of 18F-FDG PET/CT in patients with liver metastases. Eur J Nucl Med Mol Imaging 2007;34(12):1906–14.

26. Selzner M, Hany TF, Wildbrett P, et al. Does the novel PET/CT imaging modality impact on the treatment of patients with metastatic colorectal cancer of the liver? Ann Surg 2004;240(6):1027–34 [discussion: 1035–6].

27. Seo HJ, Kim MJ, Lee JD, et al. Gadoxetate disodium-enhanced magnetic resonance imaging versus contrast-enhanced 18F-fluorodeoxyglucose positron emission tomography/computed tomography for the detection of colorectal liver metastases. Invest Radiol 2011;46(9):548–55.

28. Cantwell CP, Setty BN, Holalkere N, et al. Liver lesion detection and characterization in patients with colorectal cancer: a comparison of low radiation dose non-enhanced PET/CT, contrast-enhanced PET/CT, and liver MRI. J Comput Assist Tomogr 2008;32(5):738–44.

29. Carnaghi C, Tronconi MC, Rimassa L, et al. Utility of 18F-FDG PET and contrast-enhanced CT scan in the assessment of residual liver metastasis from colorectal cancer following adjuvant chemotherapy. Nucl Med Rev Cent East Eur 2007;10(1):12–5.

30. Ramos E, Valls C, Martinez L, et al. Preoperative staging of patients with liver metastases of colorectal carcinoma. Does PET/CT really add something to multidetector CT? Ann Surg Oncol 2011; 18(9):2654–61.

31. Rojas Llimpe FL, Di Fabio F, Ercolani G, et al. Imaging in resectable colorectal liver metastasis patients with or without preoperative chemotherapy: results of the PROMETEO-01 study. Br J Cancer 2014;111(4): 667–73.

32. Georgakopoulos A, Pianou N, Kelekis N, et al. Impact of 18F-FDG PET/CT on therapeutic decisions in patients with colorectal cancer and liver metastases. Clin Imaging 2013;37(3):536–41.

33. Briggs RH, Chowdhury FU, Lodge JP, et al. Clinical impact of FDG PET-CT in patients with potentially operable metastatic colorectal cancer. Clin Radiol 2011;66(12):1167–74.

34. McLeish AR, Lee ST, Byrne AJ, et al. Impact of (1)(8)F-FDG-PET in decision making for liver metastectomy of colorectal cancer. ANZ J Surg 2012;82(1–2):30–5.

35. Wiering B, Krabbe PF, Dekker HM, et al. The role of FDG-PET in the selection of patients with colorectal liver metastases. Ann Surg Oncol 2007;14(2):771–9.

36. Teague BD, Morrison CP, Court FG, et al. Role of FDG-PET in surgical management of patients with colorectal liver metastases. ANZ J Surg 2004; 74(8):646–52.

37. Arulampalam TH, Costa DC, Loizidou M, et al. Positron emission tomography and colorectal cancer. Br J Surg 2001;88(2):176–89.

38. Ruers TJ, Langenhoff BS, Neeleman N, et al. Value of positron emission tomography with [F-18] fluorodeoxyglucose in patients with colorectal liver metastases: a prospective study. J Clin Oncol 2002;20(2):388–95.

39. Sorensen M, Mortensen FV, Hoyer M, et al, Liver tumour board at Aarhus University Hospital. FDG-PET improves management of patients with colorectal liver metastases allocated for local treatment: a consecutive prospective study. Scand J Surg 2007;96(3):209–13.

40. Engledow AH, Skipworth JR, Pakzad F, et al. The role of 18FDG PET/CT in the management of colorectal liver metastases. HPB (Oxford) 2012;14(1):20–5.

41. Joyce DL, Wahl RL, Patel PV, et al. Preoperative positron emission tomography to evaluate potentially resectable hepatic colorectal metastases. Arch Surg 2006;141(12):1220–6 [discussion: 1227].

42. Lake ES, Wadhwani S, Subar D, et al. The influence of FDG PET-CT on the detection of extrahepatic disease in patients being considered for resection of colorectal liver metastasis. Ann R Coll Surg Engl 2014;96(3):211–5.

43. Yip VS, Poston GJ, Fenwick SW, et al. FDG-PET-CT is effective in selecting patients with poor long term survivals for colorectal liver metastases. Eur J Surg Oncol 2014;40(8):995–9.

44. Ayez N, de Ridder J, Wiering B, et al. Preoperative FDG-PET-scan in patients with resectable colorectal liver metastases does not improve overall survival: a retrospective analyses stratified by clinical risk score. Dig Surg 2013;30(4–6):451–8.

45. Fernandez FG, Drebin JA, Linehan DC, et al. Five-year survival after resection of hepatic metastases from colorectal cancer in patients screened by positron emission tomography with F-18 fluorodeoxyglucose (FDG-PET). Ann Surg 2004;240(3):438–47 [discussion: 447–50].

46. Riedl CC, Akhurst T, Larson S, et al. 18F-FDG PET scanning correlates with tissue markers of poor prognosis and predicts mortality for patients after liver resection for colorectal metastases. J Nucl Med 2007;48(5):771–5.

47. Desai DC, Zervos EE, Arnold MW, et al. Positron emission tomography affects surgical management in recurrent colorectal cancer patients. Ann Surg Oncol 2003;10(1):59–64.

48. Watson AJ, Lolohea S, Robertson GM, et al. The role of positron emission tomography in the management of recurrent colorectal cancer: a review. Dis Colon Rectum 2007;50(1):102–14 [Systematic reviews and meta-analysis].

49. Even-Sapir E, Parag Y, Lerman H, et al. Detection of recurrence in patients with rectal cancer: PET/CT after abdominoperineal or anterior resection. Radiology 2004;232(3):815–22.

50. Sobhani I, Tiret E, Lebtahi R, et al. Early detection of recurrence by 18FDG-PET in the follow-up of patients with colorectal cancer. Br J Cancer 2008;98(5):875–80.

51. Scott AM, Gunawardana DH, Kelley B, et al. PET changes management and improves prognostic stratification in patients with recurrent colorectal cancer: results of a multicenter prospective study. J Nucl Med 2008;49(9):1451–7.

52. Shamim SA, Kumar R, Halanaik D, et al. Role of FDG-PET/CT in detection of recurrent disease in colorectal cancer. Nucl Med Commun 2010;31(6):590–6.

53. Maas M, Rutten IJ, Nelemans PJ, et al. What is the most accurate whole-body imaging modality for assessment of local and distant recurrent disease in colorectal cancer? A meta-analysis: imaging for recurrent colorectal cancer. Eur J Nucl Med Mol Imaging 2011;38(8):1560–71 [Systematic reviews and meta-analysis].

54. Moertel CG, Fleming TR, Macdonald JS, et al. An evaluation of the carcinoembryonic antigen (CEA) test for monitoring patients with resected colon cancer. JAMA 1993;270(8):943–7.

55. Lu YY, Chen JH, Chien CR, et al. Use of FDG-PET or PET/CT to detect recurrent colorectal cancer in patients with elevated CEA: a systematic review and meta-analysis. Int J Colorectal Dis 2013;28(8):1039–47 [Systematic reviews and meta-analysis].

56. Giacomobono S, Gallicchio R, Capacchione D, et al. F-18 FDG PET/CT in the assessment of patients with unexplained CEA rise after surgical curative resection for colorectal cancer. Int J Colorectal Dis 2013;28(12):1699–705.

57. Ozkan E, Soydal C, Araz M, et al. The role of 18F-FDG PET/CT in detecting colorectal cancer recurrence in patients with elevated CEA levels. Nucl Med Commun 2012;33(4):395–402.

58. Panagiotidis E, Datseris IE, Rondogianni P, et al. Does CEA and CA 19-9 combined increase the likelihood of 18F-FDG in detecting recurrence in colorectal patients with negative CeCT? Nucl Med Commun 2014;35(6):598–605.

59. Sanli Y, Kuyumcu S, Ozkan ZG, et al. The utility of FDG-PET/CT as an effective tool for detecting recurrent colorectal cancer regardless of serum CEA levels. Ann Nucl Med 2012;26(7):551–8.

60. Peng NJ, Hu C, King TM, et al. Detection of resectable recurrences in colorectal cancer patients with 2-[18F]fluoro-2-deoxy-D-glucose-positron emission tomography/computed tomography. Cancer Biother Radiopharm 2013;28(6):479–87.

61. Bu W, Wei R, Li J, et al. Association between carcinoembryonic antigen levels and the applied value of F-fluorodeoxyglucose positron emission tomography/computed tomography in post-operative recurrent and metastatic colorectal cancer. Oncol Lett 2014;8(6):2649–53.

62. Zhang Y, Feng B, Zhang G-L, et al. Value of 8F-FDG PET-CT in surveillance of postoperative colorectal cancer patients with various carcinoembryonic antigen concentrations. World J Gastroenterol 2014;20(21):6608–14.

63. de Geus-Oei LF, Vriens D, van Laarhoven HW, et al. Monitoring and predicting response to therapy with 18F-FDG PET in colorectal cancer: a systematic review. J Nucl Med 2009;50(Suppl 1):43S–54S [Systematic reviews and meta-analysis].

64. de Geus-Oei LF, van Laarhoven HW, Visser EP, et al. Chemotherapy response evaluation with FDG-PET in patients with colorectal cancer. Ann Oncol 2008; 19(2):348–52.

65. Hendlisz A, Golfinopoulos V, Garcia C, et al. Serial FDG-PET/CT for early outcome prediction in patients with metastatic colorectal cancer undergoing chemotherapy. Ann Oncol 2012;23(7):1687–93.

66. Mertens J, De Bruyne S, Van Damme N, et al. Standardized added metabolic activity (SAM) IN (1)(8)F-FDG PET assessment of treatment response in colorectal liver metastases. Eur J Nucl Med Mol Imaging 2013;40(8):1214–22.

67. Lau LF, Williams DS, Lee ST, et al. Metabolic response to preoperative chemotherapy predicts prognosis for patients undergoing surgical resection of colorectal cancer metastatic to the liver. Ann Surg Oncol 2014;21(7):2420–8.

68. Small RM, Lubezky N, Shmueli E, et al. Response to chemotherapy predicts survival following resection of hepatic colo-rectal metastases in patients treated with neoadjuvant therapy. J Surg Oncol 2009;99(2): 93–8.

69. Wahl RL, Jacene H, Kasamon Y, et al. From RECIST to PERCIST: evolving considerations for PET response criteria in solid tumors. J Nucl Med 2009; 50(Suppl 1):122S–50S.

70. Skougaard K, Johannesen HH, Nielsen D, et al. CT versus FDG-PET/CT response evaluation in patients with metastatic colorectal cancer treated with irinotecan and cetuximab. Cancer Med 2014;3(5): 1294–301.

71. Bystrom P, Berglund A, Garske U, et al. Early prediction of response to first-line chemotherapy by sequential [18F]-2-fluoro-2-deoxy-D-glucose positron emission tomography in patients with advanced colorectal cancer. Ann Oncol 2009;20(6):1057–61.

72. de Wilt JH, Vermaas M, Ferenschild FT, et al. Management of locally advanced primary and recurrent rectal cancer. Clin Colon Rectal Surg 2007;20(3): 255–63.

73. Vliegen RF, Beets GL, Lammering G, et al. Mesorectal fascia invasion after neoadjuvant chemotherapy and radiation therapy for locally advanced rectal cancer: accuracy of MR imaging for prediction. Radiology 2008;246(2):454–62.

74. Denecke T, Rau B, Hoffmann KT, et al. Comparison of CT, MRI and FDG-PET in response prediction of patients with locally advanced rectal cancer after multimodal preoperative therapy: is there a benefit in using functional imaging? Eur Radiol 2005;15(8): 1658–66.

75. Guillem JG, Moore HG, Akhurst T, et al. Sequential preoperative fluorodeoxyglucose-positron emission tomography assessment of response to preoperative chemoradiation: a means for determining longterm outcomes of rectal cancer. J Am Coll Surg 2004;199(1):1–7.

76. Calvo FA, Sole CV, de la Mata D, et al. (1)(8)F-FDG PET/CT-based treatment response evaluation in locally advanced rectal cancer: a prospective validation of long-term outcomes. Eur J Nucl Med Mol Imaging 2013;40(5):657–67.

77. Shanmugan S, Arrangoiz R, Nitzkorski JR, et al. Predicting pathological response to neoadjuvant chemoradiotherapy in locally advanced rectal cancer using 18FDG-PET/CT. Ann Surg Oncol 2012;19(7): 2178–85.

78. Janssen MH, Ollers MC, van Stiphout RG, et al. Evaluation of early metabolic responses in rectal cancer during combined radiochemotherapy or radiotherapy alone: sequential FDG-PET-CT findings. Radiother Oncol 2010;94(2):151–5.

79. Hatt M, van Stiphout R, le Pogam A, et al. Early prediction of pathological response in locally advanced rectal cancer based on sequential 18F-FDG PET. Acta Oncol 2013;52(3):619–26.

80. Maffione AM, Chondrogiannis S, Capirci C, et al. Early prediction of response by (1)(8)F-FDG PET/CT during preoperative therapy in locally advanced rectal cancer: a systematic review. Eur J Surg Oncol 2014;40(10):1186–94 [Systematic reviews and meta-analysis].

81. Ruby JA, Leibold T, Akhurst TJ, et al. FDG-PET assessment of rectal cancer response to neoadjuvant chemoradiotherapy is not associated with long-term prognosis: a prospective evaluation. Dis Colon Rectum 2012;55(4):378–86.

82. Guillem JG, Ruby JA, Leibold T, et al. Neither FDG-PET Nor CT can distinguish between a pathological complete response and an incomplete response after neoadjuvant chemoradiation in locally advanced rectal cancer: a prospective study. Ann Surg 2013; 258(2):289–95.

83. Li C, Lan X, Yuan H, et al. 18F-FDG PET predicts pathological response to preoperative chemoradiotherapy in patients with primary rectal cancer: a meta-analysis. Ann Nucl Med 2014;28(5):436–46.

84. Zhang C, Tong J, Sun X, et al. 18F-FDG-PET evaluation of treatment response to neo-adjuvant therapy in patients with locally advanced rectal cancer: a meta-analysis. Int J Cancer 2012;131(11):2604–11 [Systematic reviews and meta-analysis].

85. Janssen MH, Ollers MC, van Stiphout RG, et al. PET-based treatment response evaluation in rectal cancer: prediction and validation. Int J Radiat Oncol Biol Phys 2012;82(2):871–6.

86. Arulampalam TH, Francis DL, Visvikis D, et al. FDG-PET for the pre-operative evaluation of colorectal liver metastases. Eur J Surg Oncol 2004;30(3): 286–91.

PET/Computed Tomography in Renal, Bladder, and Testicular Cancer

Kirsten Bouchelouche, MD, DMSc[a],*, Peter L. Choyke, MD[b]

KEYWORDS

- PET/CT • Renal cancer • Bladder cancer • Testicular cancer

KEY POINTS

- PET/computed tomography (CT) with F-18 fluorodeoxyglucose (FDG) may be used in selected high-risk renal cancer patients and when conventional imaging is negative or if there is a potential tumor thrombus.
- In metastatic renal cancer, FDG PET/CT is used to monitor targeted molecular therapies.
- FDG PET/CT is used for staging and restaging in muscle-invasive bladder cancer, and may add important prognostic information.
- FDG PET/CT may be used for staging, restaging, and follow-up of testicular cancer, and for the evaluation of residual tumors in patients with seminoma.

INTRODUCTION

PET/computed tomography (CT) has become one of the most important imaging modalities for patients with cancer and PET/CT with F-18 fluoro-deoxyglucose (FDG) has become ubiquitous as a tool for staging and follow-up of many cancer patients. In urology, FDG is the most common PET radiotracer used in renal, bladder, and testicular cancers, but its role is hampered by physiologic excretion of FDG through the urinary system masking FDG uptake in primary renal and bladder carcinomas. Thus, new PET agents have been introduced and tested in both malignancies. In this review, we focus on the role of PET/CT in staging, detection of recurrent and metastatic disease, response assessment, and prognosis in renal, bladder, and testicular cancers.

USE OF PET IN RENAL CELL CARCINOMA
Overview of Renal Cell Carcinoma

Renal cell carcinoma (RCC) represents approximately 3% of human cancers. With the advent of widespread cross-sectional imaging, the detection of small renal cancers has increased, and the majority of these are well-differentiated and are cured by operative resection.[1] Nonetheless, renal cancer remains a significant cause of cancer death owing to the variable aggressiveness of some tumors. Renal cancers are categorized as clear cell (60%–80%), papillary (10%), chromophobe–oncocytic (5%), and other tumors such as sarcomatoid, squamous cell, and leiomyosarcoma. Accompanying the increase in small RCCs, there has been an increase in the diagnosis of small benign tumors, such as oncocytomas and

The authors have nothing to disclose.
[a] Department of Nuclear Medicine & PET Centre, Aarhus University Hospital, Skejby, Brendstrupgaardsvej 100, Aarhus DK-8200, Denmark; [b] Molecular Imaging Program, Building 10, Room B3B6B9F, Center for Cancer Research, National Cancer Institute (NCI), Bethesda, MD, USA
* Corresponding author.
E-mail address: kirsbouc@rm.dk

PET Clin 10 (2015) 361–374
http://dx.doi.org/10.1016/j.cpet.2015.03.002
1556-8598/15/$ – see front matter Published by Elsevier Inc

angiomylipomas, that can mimic RCC.[1] Because RCCs can be highly lethal, it is important to identify, characterize, and stage them and then to monitor them during treatment. A decade ago, PET played almost no role in RCC. In recent years, a fuller understanding of the role of PET in the management of RCC has been realized.

Renal cancers can be stratified as localized, locally advanced, or metastatic. Herein, we consider the role of FDG PET in each of these settings. In the final section, we consider other PET agents that have been proposed to evaluate RCC.

Primary Renal Cell Carcinoma

Traditionally, FDG PET has played a minor role in the diagnosis of RCC. Contrast-enhanced CT and MRI have proven effective at detecting solid renal masses suspicious for RCC. However, both modalities are nonspecific and cannot distinguish benign and malignant lesions. For many small lesions that are indeterminate, a biopsy is recommended to rule out benign disease before intervention, although this recommendation is often not followed.[1] It would be tempting to use FDG PET in this setting; however, PET/CT has a sensitivity of only approximately 60% for RCC, although it is 90% specific for malignancy.[2] Thus, a negative FDG PET is not helpful clinically. This is in part owing to the lower metabolic status of many RCCs, but also because FDG PET is primarily excreted through the kidneys, making RCCs isointense with renal parenchyma.[3] If they were located elsewhere in the body, where the background was lower, they might be considered positive, but in the kidney they are often difficult to detect. The uptake of FDG in renal tumors depends on size.[3] FDG is exquisitely sensitive for type II papillary renal cancers (**Figs. 1** and **2**), especially when found in conjunction with the hereditary leiomyoma RCC

syndrome.[3] Sarcomatoid tumors are also reliably PET avid.[3] However, in general, FDG has modest uptake and can also be taken up in benign renal tumors.[3] Thus, FDG PET has played a minor role in primary RCC evaluation. Moreover, FDG has proven insensitive in cystic renal masses owing to the low burden of solid tissue in such lesions.[4] Interestingly C-11 acetate has been reported to be useful in this setting, having a 100% positive predictive value (PPV), although a sensitivity of only 50%. C-11 acetate is excreted via the pancreas and, therefore, avoids the confusion of renal parenchymal enhancement found with FDG. In any case, C-11 acetate is limited to masses of greater than 1.5 cm in diameter[4] and has the unavoidable disadvantage of a short half-life ($t\sqrt{2}$ = 20 minutes), limiting the study to sites with cyclotrons and radiochemistry. Occasionally, an FDG PET scan performed for another malignancy reveals a lesion within the kidney. It is uncertain whether this lesion represents a metastasis or another primary tumor.[5] Unfortunately, uptake in the lesion is not specific in this regard, and a biopsy is usually performed to clarify this dilemma. Thus, FDG PET plays a minor role in the diagnosis of primary RCC. Diagnosis is generally made on CT and/or MRI and, if questions arise, a biopsy is usually recommended. FDG plays an important role in particular subtypes of renal cancer, such as type II papillary and sarcomatoid.

Staging of Renal Cell Carcinoma

FDG PET also plays a relatively minor role in the initial staging of RCC. The majority of cancers discovered on CT or MRI is small and localized with a low risk of metastases; therefore, additional studies are unwarranted. Higher risk, larger tumors are more FDG PET avid. For local staging, FDG PET has been found useful in determining whether

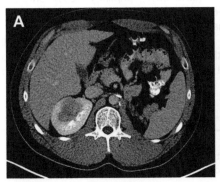
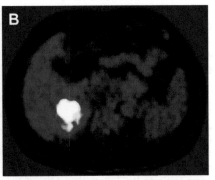
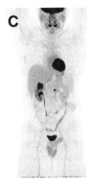

Fig. 1. Solitary renal cancer in the right upper pole. This patient had a type II papillary renal cancer in the right kidney (*A*) and was considered high risk for metastatic disease. The F-18 fluorodeoxyglucose PET/CT demonstrates increased activity in the upper pole of the kidney corresponding the mass on CT (*B*) and no evidence of metastatic disease elsewhere (*C*).

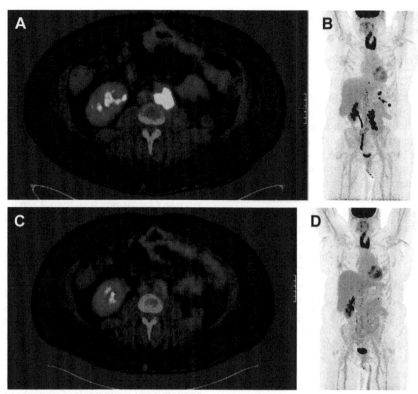

Fig. 2. Patient with aggressive type II papillary renal cancer associated with hereditary leiomyoma renal cell carcinoma syndrome, which has recurred after left nephrectomy. PET/CT with F18-fluorodeoxyglucose demonstrates intense uptake in the left paraaortic adenopathy on transverse PET/CT (*A*) and coronal projection image (*B*). After therapy with a combination of targeted therapies, the activity and size of the adenopathy have decreased dramatically (*C, D*). The patient has maintained a good response for 2 years.

thrombus in the renal vein and inferior vena cava is malignant or "bland,"[6] a distinction that is considered important by some surgeons.[7] In general CT, MRI, and bone scan in symptomatic patients are considered sufficient staging studies to clear a patient for surgery. Occasionally, when an isolated potential metastasis is detected, FDG PET can be used to confirm metabolic activity, thereby confirming the diagnosis of metastatic disease (**Fig. 3**). However, in general FDG PET is not used widely for RCC staging. Surveillance imaging after surgery is also discouraged, because there is no level 1 evidence that early intervention improves survival.[8] American Urologic Association guidelines suggest that more advanced initial tumors may warrant increased surveillance and

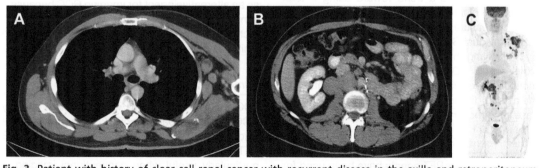

Fig. 3. Patient with history of clear cell renal cancer with recurrent disease in the axilla and retroperitoneum. Transverse CT scan shows several abnormal nodes in the left axilla (*A*). Retroperitoneal adenopathy is also seen (*B*). Coronal PET demonstrates extensive uptake in the axilla and shoulder muscles as well as retroperitoneal adenopathy (*C*).

FDG PET could play a role here, although this has not been studied.[8]

Metastatic Renal Cell Carcinoma

FDG PET in RCC is most often used in patients with metastatic disease who are on novel, targeted therapies. Renal cancer is not responsive to conventional chemotherapy and, thus, this therapy is rarely, if ever, used. A variety of targeted therapies, which include tyrosine kinase inhibitors (such as sorafinib and sunitinib) that have antiangiogenic mechanisms and mammalian target of rapamycin inhibitors (such as everolimus) have demonstrated efficacy and small but important improvements in overall survival (OS). These targeted agents do not behave generally in the same manner as conventional cytotoxic agents. Although tumor size measurements, embodied in the RECIST criteria, have proven adequate for monitoring chemotherapy, for other cancers with modern targeted therapies, there is often little change in the size of the lesions and some metastases even increase even while the drug is prolonging survival.[9] Thus, FDG PET activity could play a role in monitoring the effectiveness of targeted therapies with tyrosine kinase inhibitors.

Ferda and colleagues[10] demonstrated that the initial uptake of lesions correlated with prognosis, with patients whose renal tumors exhibit a maximum standardized uptake values (SUV_{max}) of greater than 10 having significantly worse survival than those with SUV_{max} less than 10. Decreases in FDG uptake also correlated with outcome[9–11] and were independent of where the lesion was located (eg, bone, lung, node). More dramatic decreases in SUV_{max} correlated with better progression-free survival and OS.[2] The advantage of FDG PET over conventional modalities is most apparent in bone and musculoskeletal metastases, which are difficult to assess on CT and MRI because the bone damage continues to be seen even when the lesion is responding. There is a trend toward using a total metabolic volume or total lesion glycolysis as an overall measure of disease burden,[12,13] rather than individual SUV_{max} scores. This is calculated by multiplying the SUV_{max} and the number of lesions. Thus, FDG PET is used increasingly to monitor the efficacy of treatment of patients with metastatic disease who are receiving tyrosine kinase inhibitors and other targeted therapies.

Other Agents for Renal Cell Carcinoma

A number of other PET agents have been used for renal cancer. Sodium fluoride PET has not been reported commonly in RCC, but recent reports suggest it will be more sensitive than conventional bone scans, much as it in other malignancies. This is true even for predominantly lytic renal cancer bone metastases.[14]

More than 95% of clear cell renal cancers express carbonic anhydrase IX on their cell membrane. An antibody, cG250, was developed as a potential therapeutic agent, but results of early trials showed modest or no benefit.[15] However, it was thought that labeling the antibody with I-124 could produce an effective imaging agent for clear cell carcinoma.[15] The REDECT trial of I-124 girentuximab (cG250) showed an 86% sensitivity and 86% specificity for clear cell carcinoma.[15] The agent was not as useful for lesions less than 2 cm in diameter or in non–clear cell renal cancers. The advantages of this agent are that it is specific for clear cell carcinoma and has a sensitivity comparable with biopsy,[15] but the disadvantage is that less common, but nevertheless aggressive, cancers may be negative. It may play a role in patients too ill to undergo biopsy or in those patients for whom adequate conventional studies cannot be obtained. However, the study requires 3 to 7 days because of the long clearance time of the antibody and this may make it impractical.[6] Moreover, it is unclear whether the niche applications of this agent would make it economically sustainable. Suggestions have been made to exchange the I-124 with Zr-89, which may result in better imaging, but this does not clarify the actual clinical role of this agent.[6,16]

F-18 Fluoromisonidazole has also been suggested as an imaging agent for RCC based on the level of hypoxia in many renal tumors; however, this agent has not been studied extensively and early reports show only modest uptake in RCCs. It was not predictive of response to therapy.[17] Interestingly, initial studies show a decrease in hypoxia after initiating tyrosine kinase inhibitor, therapy likely owing to "vascular normalization", followed by an increase in hypoxia as antiangiogenic effects begin to predominate.[17]

As mentioned, C-11 acetate has been proposed as an alternative agent for imaging RCC because it is not excreted through the kidney. However, the technical limitations of this agent are likely to inhibit its widespread use.

Summary

FDG PET/CT is not used widely in most primary RCCs, although particular RCC subtypes are quite avid for the agent. In high-risk, larger patients FDG PET may be useful in preoperative staging and is particularly useful when conventional imaging is negative or there is a potential tumor thrombus. In metastatic RCC, FDG PET/CT is used increasingly to monitor targeted molecular therapies such as tyrosine kinase inhibitors. Sodium fluoride PET seems to be a useful method in detecting subtle bone metastases, but it has not yet replaced conventional bone scan. Several other PET agents targeting carbonic anhydrase IX, hypoxia, and fatty acid synthesis have been proposed and tested but none are in widespread use.

USE OF PET IN BLADDER CANCER
Overview of Bladder Cancer

Bladder carcinoma (BC) is the ninth most common cancer worldwide and the most frequent type of cancer of the urinary tract.[18] Painless hematuria is the most common presenting complaint.[19] More than 90% of BCs are urothelial (transitional cell) carcinomas, 5% are squamous cell carcinomas, and less than 2% are adenocarcinomas.[19] At presentation, approximately 30% of patients have muscle-invasive BC.[18] Muscle-invasive BC is an aggressive epithelial tumor with a high rate of early systemic dissemination. The common sites of metastatic disease include liver, lung, bone, and adrenal glands. The standard method of diagnosing BC continues to be based on direct visualization of the bladder with cystoscopy and subsequent biopsy/resection. The optimal management of these patients depends on accurate staging and detection of metastatic disease. Generally, muscle-invasive bladder-confined BC is treated with radical cystectomy with pelvic lymph node dissection (PLND), whereas metastatic disease is treated with cisplatin-based combination chemotherapy.[19] The extent of extravesical involvement determines whether the patient is a candidate for neoadjuvant chemotherapy before definitive treatment.

Primary Bladder Cancer

Both CT and MRI are used widely for imaging of primary BC. For local tumor assessment, MRI is reported to be more accurate than CT.[18] MRI is superior to CT for determining depth of bladder wall infiltration.[20] Both CT and MRI have limited capability for detecting microscopic invasion of the perivesical fat, but they may be used to find T3b disease or higher with good diagnostic accuracy.[21] The role of FDG PET/CT in the detection of localized BC is limited because of the difficulty in differentiating radiotracer activity excreted into the urine from tumor activity in the bladder. Several methods have been proposed to overcome radioactivity interference in urine, such as FDG wash out, early images, late images after voiding, dual phase imaging, catheterization, bladder irrigation, and forced diuresis.[22–29] A recent metaanalysis evaluated the diagnostic accuracy of FDG PET/CT for detecting bladder lesions.[30] Six studies met the inclusion criteria. The pooled sensitivity and specificity of PET or PET/CT for the detection of BC was 80.0% and 84.0%, respectively. When compared with results of MRI and CT published in other studies, FDG PET/CT showed no superiority in detecting local bladder lesions.[30]

Staging

Assessment of lymph node (LN) metastases based solely on size is limited by the inability of both CT and MRI to identify metastases in normal-sized or minimally enlarged nodes. Thus, the sensitivity for detection of LN metastases is low for both imaging modalities.[20] Specificity is also low because nodal enlargement may be owing to benign disease. Given the ability of PET to detect metabolic activity, investigators have begun exploring the use of PET in staging BC (**Figs. 4** and **5**).[29,31–36] A recent metaanalysis of FDG PET/CT for the staging and restaging of BC found that the pooled sensitivity was 82%, the pooled specificity was 89%, and the global accuracy was 92%.[37] FDG PET/CT detects more malignant disease than conventional CT/MRI in 20% to 40% of patients,[32,33]

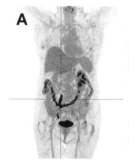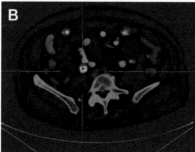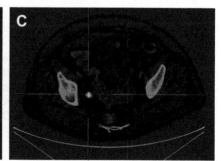

Fig. 4. Patient with newly diagnosed muscle-invasive bladder cancer. Tumor in the bladder wall could not be visualized with F-18 fluorodeoxyglucose (FDG) PET owing to FDG activity in the urine. However, unexpected focal increased FDG activity in the right ureter was seen (A, B), which was owing to malignancy. A lymph node metastasis was also seen in the right side of pelvis (C).

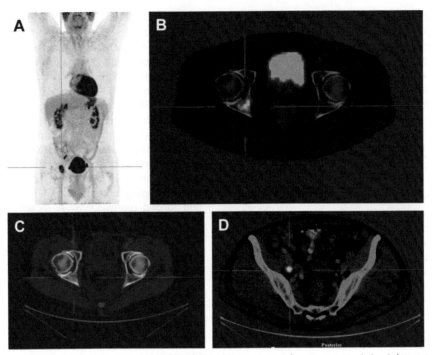

Fig. 5. Patient with newly diagnosed muscle-invasive bladder cancer. A bone metastasis in right acetabulum can be seen on F-18 fluorodeoxyglucose PET/CT (*A, B*), but with only minimal changes on CT (*C*). A lymph node metastasis is seen in the right side of the pelvis (*D*).

and FDG PET/CT may change the clinical management in up to 68% of the patients.[32] Upstaging is more frequent than downstaging.[33] For diagnosing LN-positive disease, Swinnen and colleagues[34] reported the accuracy, the sensitivity, and the specificity of 84%, 46%, and 97% for FDG PET/CT, respectively. When analyzing the results of CT alone, there was an accuracy of 80%, sensitivity of 46%, and specificity of 92%. The study found no advantage for combined FDG PET/CT over CT alone for LN staging of invasive BC. FDG PET/CT has also been compared with MRI for LN staging in patients with BC (n = 18).[31] The specificities for detection of LN metastases for MRI and FDG PET/CT were 80% and 93.33%, respectively. The negative predictive values (NPV) were 80% and 87.5% for MRI and FDG PET/CT, respectively. The differences in specificity and NPV were not significant. However, the trend of the data indicates an advantage of FDG PET/CT over MRI.[31] Larger prospective studies are needed to further elucidate the clinical role of FDG PET/CT in LN staging of BC.

Restaging

The overall prognosis for recurrent BC is poor. However, additional salvage and/or palliative therapies are prompted when disease is discovered.

Accurate restaging is, therefore, important before additional costly and toxic therapies are considered. There are few data available regarding the utility of FDG PET/CT in assessing for recurrence and metastatic disease in patients who have previously undergone treatment for their primary BC.[27,28,38] Jadvar and colleagues[38] retrospectively assessed the diagnostic ability of FDG PET or PET/CT in recurrent and metastatic BC. In the study, all 35 patients were treated previously for their primary disease. The metastatic sites detected in the study included mediastinum, lung, and bone. FDG PET/CT affected the clinical management in 17% of patients, by prompting either additional therapy or a wait-and-watch strategy. The few studies indicate that FDG PET may be useful for the detection of recurrent tumor in the pelvis, differentiation between local recurrent disease versus postoperative or postirradiation fibrosis/necrosis, and for the detection of distant metastases.

Response to Therapy

In muscle-invasive BC neoadjuvant chemotherapy is an established standard treatment that improves the OS of patients with BC.[39] However, the nonresponse rate is relative high. Monitoring the LN response to neoadjuvant chemotherapy may enable patient selection for surgery. Evaluation of the LN response with conventional imaging modalities is usually difficult and inaccurate. This is mainly owing to difficulty with identifying viable tumor in residual (necrotic) masses and small tumor deposits in LNs of normal size. Recently, FDG PET/CT was used for monitoring the response of pelvic LN metastasis to neoadjuvant chemotherapy for BC (n = 19).[40] Metabolic response was assessed according to EORTC (European Organization for Research and Treatment of Cancer) recommendations based on the change in FDG uptake on FDG PET/CT. Radiologic response was assessed on CT according to RECIST (Response Evaluation Criteria in Solid Tumors). All patients underwent PLND with histopathologic evaluation of LNs. PET/CT and CT correctly distinguished responders (95%) from nonresponders (79%) and complete responders (68%) from patients with residual disease (63%). Although no definitive conclusions can be drawn from these preliminary data, PET/CT seemed to be feasible for evaluating the LN response to neoadjuvant chemotherapy. However, this has to be confirmed in large clinical trials.

Prognostic Value

Only 2 studies have focused on the prognostic value of FDG PET/CT. Kibel and colleagues[41] reported sensitivity, specificity, PPV, and NPV of 70%, 94%, 78%, and 91%, respectively, for FDG PET/CT in 42 patients with BC. Median follow-up was 14.9 months. FDG PET/CT detected occult metastatic disease in 17% (7/42) of the patients with negative conventional preoperative evaluations. Recurrence free survival, OS, and disease-free survival were all significantly poorer in the patients with positive FDG PET/CT than in those with negative FDG-PET/CT. In the study, FDG PET/CT was strongly correlated with survival. Recently, Mertens and colleagues[42] also investigated the association between extravesical FDG-avid lesions on PET/CT and mortality in patients with muscle-invasive BC. Of the 211 patients included in the study, 98 (46.4%) had 1 or more extravesical lesions on PET/CT, and 113 (53.5%) had a negative PET/CT. Conventional CT revealed extravesical lesions in 51 patients (24.4%). Median follow-up was 18 months. Patients with a positive PET/CT had a significantly shorter OS and disease-free survival (median OS, 14 vs 50 months [P = .001]; disease-free survival, 16 vs 50 months [P<.001]). On multivariable analysis, the presence of extravesical lesions on PET/CT was an independent prognostic indicator of mortality. This association was not significant for conventional CT. The results indicate that the presence of extravesical

FDG-avid lesions on PET/CT might be considered an independent indicator of mortality.

Other Agents for Bladder Cancer

Investigators have attempted to improve the sensitivity of PET by using tracers that are not excreted in the urine like FDG. Tracers like C-11 choline, C-11 acetate, and C-11 methionine have been used for that purpose. Furthermore, sodium fluoride has been used for detection of bone metastasis.

Choline

Few data are available on the role of C-11 choline PET/CT in BC.[43–49] The sensitivity for detection of LN metastasis is relative low.[46,48,49] Recently, Brunocilla and colleagues[48] investigated the diagnostic accuracy of choline PET/CT in preoperative LN staging of BC suitable for radical cystectomy and extended PLND. Overall, 844 LNs were evaluated, and 38 (4.5%) showed metastatic involvement. On a patient-based analysis, choline PET/CT showed a sensitivity of 42% and specificity of 84%, whereas CT showed a sensitivity of 14% and specificity of 89%. On an LN-based analysis, choline PET/CT showed a sensitivity of 10% and specificity of 64%, whereas CT showed a sensitivity of 2% and specificity of 63%. In contrast, in another study (n = 44) choline PET/CT was not able to improve diagnostic efficacy in preoperative LN staging compared with CT.[43] C-11 choline PET may be more useful for restaging of BC suspected of relapse, especially for LN evaluation and distant metastases.[44] Recently, the prognostic value of choline PET/CT in the preoperative staging of muscle-invasive BC was investigated.[45] In this prospective study, 44 patients with localized BC were staged with choline PET/CT before radical cystectomy with PLND. The results of imaging were correlated with OS and cancer specific death (CSD). There was no difference in OS and CSD between the patient groups when stratified for organ confined versus non–organ-confined disease or LN involvement defined by either choline PET/CT or CT. The authors concluded that neither CT nor choline PET/CT was able to sufficiently predict OS or CSD in BC patients treated with radical cystectomy. However, a major limitation of the study is the relatively small number of patients included.

Methionine

C-11 methionine uptake in tissue is an indication of amino acid transport and metabolism, which is often increased in malignant tumors. In a small study, methionine was superior to FDG; however, tumor was identified with a sensitivity of

78% (18/23) only with methionine PET.[50] Methionine uptake was correlated with tumor grade. However, methionine did not improve staging of BC. In another study, methionine PET was used for the evaluation of therapy response in 44 patients with varying stages of BC treated with chemotherapy.[51] The diagnostic accuracy of PET was poor and the technique could not monitor the therapeutic effect of neoadjuvant chemotherapy, producing results that correlated with therapy outcome.

Acetate

Another tracer with little or no urinary excretion is C-11 acetate. A small study (n = 16) prospectively evaluated MRI, acetate PET/CT, and CT for staging of BC.[52] MRI, acetate PET/CT, and CT demonstrated similar levels of accuracy. For all modalities, a history of intravesical and/or systemic chemotherapy affected staging accuracy. In another small study (n = 14), acetate PET/CT was compared with choline PET/CT in BC.[53] Acetate and choline scans were performed within 1 week. The 2 tracers demonstrated equivalent results in the preoperative evaluation.

Sodium fluoride

Lytic bone metastases of BC may be better detected using sodium fluoride PET scans compared with conventional technetium 99mTc-methylene diphosphonate (MDP) bone scan. Recently, sodium fluoride PET was compared with MDP bone scan in the detection of skeletal metastases in BC.[54] In this prospective study, 48 patients with BC underwent PET and bone scan within 48 hours. Skeletal metastases diagnosed on each of these techniques was compared against a final diagnosis based on CT, MRI, skeletal survey, clinical follow-up, and histologic correlation. The sensitivity, specificity, positive PPV, NPV, and accuracy of MDP planar bone scan were 82.35%, 64.51%, 56%, 86.95%, and 70.83%; of MDP single photon emission CT/CT were 88.23%, 74.19%, 65.21%, 92%, and 79.16%; and of fluoride PET/CT were 100%, 87.09%, 80.95%, 100%, and 91.66%, respectively. In the study, fluoride PET/CT was superior to both MDP planar bone scan and MDP single photon emission CT/CT. Fluoride PET/CT identified bony metastases and changed the management in 17 of 48 patients (35%).

Summary

FDG PET/CT is not used for the evaluation of primary tumor in the bladder because of urinary excretion of FDG. Several methods have been proposed to overcome interference from radioactivity in urine. However, FDG PET/CT is increasingly used for staging and restaging in muscle-invasive BC, and FDG PET/CT may add important prognostic information. Tracers with no or little urinary excretion have been proposed and tested in BC, but are not recommended in international guidelines.

USE OF PET IN TESTICULAR CANCER
Overview of Testicular Cancer

Testicular cancer represents between 1% and 1.5% of male cancers and 5% of urologic tumors, with 3 to 10 new cases occurring per 100,000 males per year.[55] Over the last 30 years, the incidence of testicular cancer has increased.[56] Only 1% to 2% is bilateral at diagnosis. The histologic type varies, although there is a clear predominance (90%–95%) of germ cell tumors (GCT).[55] Testicular cancers are classified as seminomas, which account for approximately 40% of GCT or nonseminomatous GSTs (NSGCT), which account for approximately 60%.[57] The clinical management of testicular GCT depends on the pathology, staging, and prognostic stratification.[58] Testicular tumors show excellent cure rates.[57] This is mainly owing to careful staging at the time of diagnosis, adequate early treatment based on chemotherapeutic combinations with or without radiotherapy and surgery, and very strict follow-up and salvage therapies. Testicular cancer typically spreads by the lymphatic route through channels along testicular vessels to the retroperitoneum.[59] Hematogenous spread is predominantly to the lungs. Testicular cancer normally appears as a painless, unilateral scrotal mass.[57] In approximately 20% of cases, the first symptom is scrotal pain. Orchidectomy and pathologic examination of the testis are necessary to confirm the diagnosis and to define the local extension.[55] Serum tumor markers (alpha fetoprotein, human chorionic gonadotropin, and lactate dehydrogenase) are prognostic factors and contribute to diagnosis and staging.[55] Imaging plays an important role in the clinical management of testicular cancer. In this section, we give an overview of PET/CT in testicular cancer.

Primary Testicular Cancer

Currently, diagnostic ultrasound (US) serves to confirm the presence of a testicular mass and to explore the contralateral testis.[60] The sensitivity of US to detect testicular tumor is almost 100%, and it has an important role in determining whether a mass is intratesticular or extratesticular.[60] MRI offers greater sensitivity and specificity than US for diagnosing tumors.[60,61] MRI of scrotum has a sensitivity of 100% and a specificity of 95% to 100%,[62] but its high cost does not justify its clinical use. FDG PET/CT does not have a role in the primary evaluation of a scrotal mass.

Staging

To determine the presence of metastatic disease, the LN pathway must be screened and the presence of visceral metastases must be determined.[55] Retroperitoneal and mediastinal LNs are most often assessed by CT. The supraclavicular nodes can be assessed by physical examination. CT has a sensitivity of 70% to 80% in determining the state of the retroperitoneal LN, and MRI produce similar results to CT.[55] However, MRI is not recommended for routine imaging in staging of testicular cancer because of the high cost and limited access to MRI, although MRI may be useful when CT and US are inconclusive, when the patients has an allergy to CT contrast media, or in cases where the radiation dose should be reduced. FDG PET is a potentially useful diagnostic tool for initial staging in patients with GCT. Studies have suggested improved diagnostic accuracy of FDG PET compared with CT imaging in a range of settings.[63–66] In 1 study, 70% of patients with normal-sized nodes who subsequently developed relapse could be identified at presentation by the use of PET.[64] Recently, Ambrosini and colleagues[67] performed a retrospective study in 51 seminoma and 70 NSGCT. FDG demonstrated good sensitivity and specificity for seminoma lesions (92% and 84%, respectively), but its sensitivity was lower for NSGCT (sensitivity and specificity were 77% and 95%, respectively). The FDG scan influenced the clinical management of 92% (47/51) seminomas, and 84% (59/70) NSGCT. Sharma and colleagues[68] demonstrated high diagnostic accuracy of FDG PET/CT for restaging both seminomatous and nonseminomatous malignant GCTs in a large patient population (n = 92). FDG PET/CT showed sensitivity, specificity, PPV, NPV, and accuracy of 94.2%, 75.0%, 83.0%, 90.9%, and 85.8% overall; 90.0%, 74.0%, 72.0%, 90.9%, and 80.8% in seminomatous GCT; and 96.8%, 76.9%, 91.1%, 90.9%, and 91.1% in nonseminomatous GCT, respectively.[68] The difference in PET/CT accuracy for seminomatous and nonseminomatous GCTs was not significant. The results support the potential usefulness of FDG PET/CT for the assessment of patients with GCT.

Residual Disease

In patients with metastatic seminoma, postchemotherapy residual masses are present in 55% to 80%. In lesions greater than 3 cm, viable tumor is expected in 11% to 37% of cases. Surgery is

technically demanding owing to fibrosis and it is often incomplete and associated with increased morbidity. Thus, it is important to discriminate between residual tumor and fibrosis or necrosis. CT and MRI cannot predict adequately the histology of residual masses.[69] For many years, FDG PET has been considered as the gold standard for discriminating between residual tumors and necrosis or fibrosis (Fig. 6). Several prospective and retrospective studies evaluated the diagnostic performance of FDG-PET or PET/CT in the postchemotherapy management of patients with GCT.[65,67,70–79] Recently, Treglia and colleagues[80] published a metaanalysis about the diagnostic performance of FDG PET and PET/CT in the postchemotherapy management of patients with seminoma. Nine studies including 375 scans were included. The pooled analysis demonstrated a sensitivity of 78%, a specificity of 86%, PPV of 58%, NPV of 94%, and accuracy of 84%. A better diagnostic accuracy of FDG PET or PET/CT in evaluating residual or recurrent lesions greater than 3 cm compared with those less than 3 cm was found. However, possible sources of false-negative and false-positive results for postchemotherapy residual or recurrent seminoma on FDG PET or PET/CT should be kept in mind. False-negative findings may be owing to small lesions (with size below the resolution of the method) or with low proliferative activity (and consequently low FDG uptake). False-positive results may be owing to inflammatory lesions. The results of the metaanalysis support the role of FDG PET or PET/CT in the postchemotherapy management of patients with seminoma. Bachner and colleagues[70] performed a retrospective validation of the large SEMPET trial published in 2004.[74] A total of 11 centers participated and a total of 127 FDG PET studies were evaluated. The authors compared PET scans carried out before and after a cutoff level of 6 weeks after the end of the last chemotherapy cycle. PET sensitivity, specificity, NPV, and PPV were 50%, 77%, 91%, and 25%, respectively, before the cutoff and 82%, 90%, 95%, and 69% after the cutoff. PET accuracy significantly improved from 73% before to 88% after the cutoff (P = .032).

The presence of vital carcinoma and mature teratoma is common (55%) in residual masses in patients with NSGCT. In patients with metastatic NSGCT, residual masses after cisplatin-based combination chemotherapy consist of necrosis in 40%, persisting vital carcinoma in 20%, and mature teratoma in 40% of patients.[81] Oechsle and colleagues[77] conducted a large, prospective, multicenter study to evaluate the accuracy of FDG PET in NSGCT for the prediction of histology

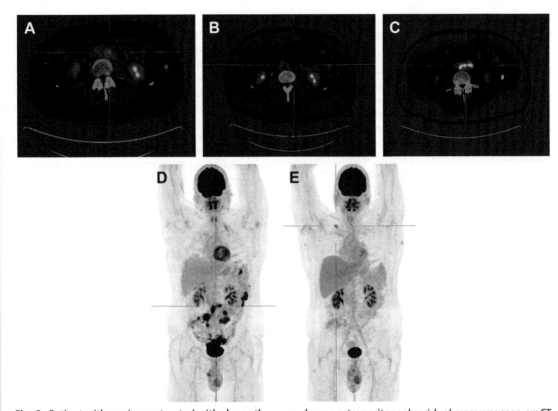

Fig. 6. Patient with seminoma treated with chemotherapy, where a retroperitoneal residual mass was seen on CT. F-18 fluorodeoxyglucose (FDG) PET/CT demonstrated moderate activity in a small area of the known residual mass (*A*). After a new cycle of chemotherapy, FDG PET/CT showed complete regression of FDG activity in the residual mass (*B*). However, control FDG PET/CT 3 months later demonstrated relapse in the retroperitoneal mass (*C*) and multiple peritoneal metastases (*D*). After 1 more cycle of chemotherapy, FDG PET/CT demonstrated complete regression (*E*). Only few benign inflammatory elements in cutis were seen.

compared with CT and serum tumor markers. A total of 121 patients with stage IIC or III NSGCT scheduled for secondary resection after cisplatin-based chemotherapy were included. FDG PET was performed after completion of chemotherapy. Prediction of tumor viability with FDG PET was correct in 56%, which did not reach the expected clinically relevant level of 70%, and was not better than the accuracy of CT (55%) or serum tumor markers (56%). Sensitivity and specificity of FDG PET were 70% and 48%, respectively. PPV were not different (55%, 61%, and 59% for CT, STM and PET, respectively). Judging only vital carcinoma as true malignant finding, the NPV increased to 83% for FDG PET. The results indicate that, in NSGCT, FDG-PET is less helpful in predicting histology in residual masses after chemotherapy than in patients with pure seminomatous GCT. Whether NSGCT has lower FDG uptake than seminoma remains to be evaluated further in the future in prospective, large-scale studies.

Other Agents for Testicular Cancer

Until recently, FDG has been the only radiotracer used for PET imaging of GCT. Increased uptake of FDG is regarded as an indicator of viable tumor. However, FDG uptake is not specific for tumor; inflammatory and granulomatous tissues also show FDG accumulation. The role of FDG PET in staging nonseminomatous GCT residues is limited because FDG PET cannot differentiate mature teratoma from necrosis and fibrosis. The thymidine analog F-18-fluorothymidine (FLT) is a cell proliferation marker. Recently, a small study (n = 11) investigated the addition of FLT PET to FDG PET for early response monitoring and prediction of the histology of residual tumor masses in patients with metastatic GCT.[82] The authors concluded that, despite the lower incidence of false-positive results with FLT PET than with FDG PET, PET-negative residual masses after chemotherapy of metastatic nonseminomatous GCT still require resection, because the low NPV of FDG

PET cannot be improved by application of the pro-liferation marker FLT.[82]

Summary

FDG PET/CT has no role in primary evaluation of a scrotal mass, but can be used for staging in GCT. However, FDG PET is not yet included in the international guidelines for staging of testicular cancer. For detection of residual disease, FDG PET/CT is an accurate diagnostic method in the postchemotherapy management of patients with seminoma.

REFERENCES

1. Sahni VA, Silverman SG. Imaging management of incidentally detected small renal masses. Semin Intervent Radiol 2014;31:9.

2. Caldarella C, Muoio B, Isgro MA, et al. The role of fluorine-18-fluorodeoxyglucose positron emission tomography in evaluating the response to tyrosine-kinase inhibitors in patients with metastatic primary renal cell carcinoma. Radiol Oncol 2014;48:219.

3. Makis W, Ciarallo A, Rakheja R, et al. Spectrum of malignant renal and urinary bladder tumors on 18F-FDG PET/CT: a pictorial essay. Clin Imaging 2012;36:660.

4. Oyama N, Ito H, Takahara N, et al. Diagnosis of complex renal cystic masses and solid renal lesions using PET imaging: comparison of 11C-acetate and 18F-FDG PET imaging. Clin Nucl Med 2014; 39:e208.

5. Aras M, Dede F, Ones T, et al. Is the value of FDG PET/CT in evaluating renal metastasis underestimated? A case report and review of the literature. Mol Imaging Radionucl Ther 2013;22:109.

6. Czarnecka AM, Kornakiewicz A, Kukwa W, et al. Frontiers in clinical and molecular diagnostics and staging of metastatic clear cell renal cell carcinoma. Future Oncol 2014;10:1095.

7. Ravina M, Hess S, Chauhan MS, et al. Tumor thrombus: ancillary findings on FDG PET/CT in an oncologic population. Clin Nucl Med 2014;39:767.

8. Smaldone MC, Uzzo RG. Balancing process and risk: standardizing posttreatment surveillance for renal cell carcinoma. J Urol 2013;190:417.

9. Chen JL, Appelbaum DE, Kocherginsky M, et al. FDG-PET as a predictive biomarker for therapy with everolimus in metastatic renal cell cancer. Cancer Med 2013;2:545.

10. Ferda J, Ferdova E, Hora M, et al. 18F-FDG-PET/CT in potentially advanced renal cell carcinoma: a role in treatment decisions and prognosis estimation. Anticancer Res 2013;33:2665.

11. Kakizoe M, Yao M, Tateishi U, et al. The early response of renal cell carcinoma to tyrosine kinase inhibitors evaluated by FDG PET/CT was not influenced by metastatic organ. BMC Cancer 2014;14:390.

12. Farnebo J, Gryback P, Harmenberg U, et al. Volumetric FDG-PET predicts overall and progression-free survival after 14 days of targeted therapy in metastatic renal cell carcinoma. BMC Cancer 2014;14:408.

13. Yoon HJ, Paeng JC, Kwak C, et al. Prognostic implication of extrarenal metabolic tumor burden in advanced renal cell carcinoma treated with targeted therapy after nephrectomy. Ann Nucl Med 2013;27:748.

14. Fuccio C, Spinapolice EG, Cavalli C, et al. 18F-Fluoride PET/CT in the detection of bone metastases in clear cell renal cell carcinoma: discordance with bone scintigraphy. Eur J Nucl Med Mol Imaging 1930;40:2013.

15. Divgi CR, Uzzo RG, Gatsonis C, et al. Positron emission tomography/computed tomography identification of clear cell renal cell carcinoma: results from the REDECT trial. J Clin Oncol 2013;31:187.

16. Cheal SM, Punzalan B, Doran MG, et al. Pairwise comparison of 89Zr- and 124I-labeled cG250 based on positron emission tomography imaging and nonlinear immunokinetic modeling: in vivo carbonic anhydrase IX receptor binding and internalization in mouse xenografts of clear-cell renal cell carcinoma. Eur J Nucl Med Mol Imaging 2014;41:985.

17. Ammari S, Thiam R, Cuenod CA, et al. Radiological evaluation of response to treatment: application to metastatic renal cancers receiving anti-angiogenic treatment. Diagn Interv Imaging 2014;95:527.

18. Witjes JA, Comperat E, Cowan NC, et al. EAU guidelines on muscle-invasive and metastatic bladder cancer: summary of the 2013 guidelines. Eur Urol 2014;65:778.

19. Kaufman DS, Shipley WU, Feldman AS. Bladder cancer. Lancet 2009;374:239.

20. Bouchelouche K, Turkbey B, Choyke PL. PET/CT and MRI in bladder cancer. J Cancer Sci Ther 2012;S14(1):7692.

21. Rajesh A, Sokhi HK, Fung R, et al. Bladder cancer: evaluation of staging accuracy using dynamic MRI. Clin Radiol 2011;66:1140.

22. Mertens LS, Fioole-Bruining A, Vegt E, et al. Detecting primary bladder cancer using delayed (18)F-2-fluoro-2-deoxy-D-glucose-positron emission tomography/computed tomography imaging after forced diuresis. Indian J Nucl Med 2012;27:145.

23. Mertens LS, Bruin NM, Vegt E, et al. Catheter-assisted 18F-FDG-PET/CT imaging of primary bladder cancer: a prospective study. Nucl Med Commun 2012;33:1195.

24. Chondrogiannis S, Marzola MC, Colletti PM, et al. Proposal of a new acquisition protocol for bladder cancer visualization with 18F-FDG PET/CT. Clin Nucl Med 2015;40(1):e78–80.

25. Yildirim-Poyraz N, Ozdemir E, Uzun B, et al. Dual phase 18F-fluorodeoxyglucose positron emission tomography/computed tomography with forced diuresis in diagnostic imaging evaluation of bladder cancer. Rev Esp Med Nucl Imagen Mol 2013;32:214.

26. Yang Z, Cheng J, Pan L, et al. Is whole-body fluorine-18 fluorodeoxyglucose PET/CT plus additional pelvic images (oral hydration-voiding-refilling) useful for detecting recurrent bladder cancer? Ann Nucl Med 2012;26:571.

27. Anjos DA, Etchebehere EC, Ramos CD, et al. 18F-FDG PET/CT delayed images after diuretic for restaging invasive bladder cancer. J Nucl Med 2007; 48:764.

28. Harkirat S, Anand S, Jacob M. Forced diuresis and dual-phase F-fluorodeoxyglucose-PET/CT scan for restaging of urinary bladder cancers. Indian J Radiol Imaging 2010;20:13.

29. Kosuda S, Kison PV, Greenough R, et al. Preliminary assessment of fluorine-18 fluorodeoxyglucose positron emission tomography in patients with bladder cancer. Eur J Nucl Med 1997;24:615.

30. Wang N, Jiang P, Lu Y. Is fluorine-18 fluorodeoxyglucose positron emission tomography useful for detecting bladder lesions? A meta-analysis of the literature. Urol Int 2014;92:143.

31. Jensen TK, Holt P, Gerke O, et al. Preoperative lymph-node staging of invasive urothelial bladder cancer with 18F-fluorodeoxyglucose positron emission tomography/computed axial tomography and magnetic resonance imaging: correlation with histopathology. Scand J Urol Nephrol 2011;45:122.

32. Apolo AB, Riches J, Schoder H, et al. Clinical value of fluorine-18 2-fluoro-2-deoxy-D-glucose positron emission tomography/computed tomography in bladder cancer. J Clin Oncol 2010;28:3973.

33. Mertens LS, Fioole-Bruining A, Vegt E, et al. Impact of (18) F-fluorodeoxyglucose (FDG)-positron-emission tomography/computed tomography (PET/CT) on management of patients with carcinoma invading bladder muscle. BJU Int 2013;112:729.

34. Swinnen G, Maes A, Pottel H, et al. FDG-PET/CT for the preoperative lymph node staging of invasive bladder cancer. Eur Urol 2010;57:641.

35. Bachor R, Kotzerke J, Reske SN, et al. Lymph node staging of bladder neck carcinoma with positron emission tomography. Urologe A 1999;38:46 [in German].

36. Drieskens O, Oyen R, Van PH, et al. FDG-PET for preoperative staging of bladder cancer. Eur J Nucl Med Mol Imaging 2005;32:1412.

37. Lu YY, Chen JH, Liang JA, et al. Clinical value of FDG PET or PET/CT in urinary bladder cancer: a systemic review and meta-analysis. Eur J Radiol 2012; 81:2411.

38. Jadvar H, Quan V, Henderson RW, et al. [F-18]-Fluorodeoxyglucose PET and PET-CT in diagnostic imaging evaluation of locally recurrent and metastatic bladder transitional cell carcinoma. Int J Clin Oncol 2008;13:42.

39. Meeks JJ, Bellmunt J, Bochner BH, et al. A systematic review of neoadjuvant and adjuvant chemotherapy for muscle-invasive bladder cancer. Eur Urol 2012;62:523.

40. Mertens LS, Fioole-Bruining A, van Rhijn BW, et al. FDG-positron emission tomography/computerized tomography for monitoring the response of pelvic lymph node metastasis to neoadjuvant chemotherapy for bladder cancer. J Urol 2013;189:1687.

41. Kibel AS, Dehdashti F, Katz MD, et al. Prospective study of [18F]fluorodeoxyglucose positron emission tomography/computed tomography for staging of muscle-invasive bladder carcinoma. J Clin Oncol 2009;27:4314.

42. Mertens LS, Mir MC, Scott AM, et al. 18F-fluorodeoxyglucose–positron emission tomography/computed tomography aids staging and predicts mortality in patients with muscle-invasive bladder cancer. Urology 2014;83:393.

43. Maurer T, Souvatzoglou M, Kubler H, et al. Diagnostic efficacy of [11C]choline positron emission tomography/computed tomography compared with conventional computed tomography in lymph node staging of patients with bladder cancer prior to radical cystectomy. Eur Urol 2012;61:1031.

44. Graziani T, Ceci F, Lopes FL, et al. 11C-Choline PET/CT for restaging of bladder Cancer. Clin Nucl Med 2015;40(1):e1–5.

45. Maurer T, Horn T, Souvatzoglou M, et al. Prognostic value of C-choline PET/CT and CT for predicting survival of bladder Cancer patients treated with radical cystectomy. Urol Int 2014;93:207.

46. Picchio M, Treiber U, Beer AJ, et al. Value of 11C-choline PET and contrast-enhanced CT for staging of bladder cancer: correlation with histopathologic findings. J Nucl Med 2006;47:938.

47. Gofrit ON, Mishani E, Orevi M, et al. Contribution of 11C-choline positron emission tomography/computerized tomography to preoperative staging of advanced transitional cell carcinoma. J Urol 2006; 176:940.

48. Brunocilla E, Ceci F, Schiavina R, et al. Diagnostic accuracy of (11)C-choline PET/CT in preoperative lymph node staging of bladder cancer: a systematic comparison with contrast-enhanced CT and histologic findings. Clin Nucl Med 2014;39:e308.

49. de Jong IJ, Pruim J, Elsinga PH, et al. Visualisation of bladder cancer using (11)C-choline PET: first clinical experience. Eur J Nucl Med Mol Imaging 2002; 29:1283.

50. Ahlstrom H, Malmstrom PU, Letocha H, et al. Positron emission tomography in the diagnosis and staging of urinary bladder cancer. Acta Radiol 1996;37:180.

51. Letocha H, Ahlstrom H, Malmstrom PU, et al. Positron emission tomography with L-methyl-11C-methionine in the monitoring of therapy response in muscle-invasive transitional cell carcinoma of the urinary bladder. Br J Urol 1994;74:767.

52. Vargas HA, Akin O, Schoder H, et al. Prospective evaluation of MRI, (1)(1)C-acetate PET/CT and contrast-enhanced CT for staging of bladder cancer. Eur J Radiol 2012;81:4131.

53. Orevi M, Klein M, Mishani E, et al. 11C-acetate PET/CT in bladder urothelial carcinoma: intraindividual comparison with 11C-choline. Clin Nucl Med 2012;37:e67.

54. Chakraborty D, Bhattacharya A, Mete UK, et al. Comparison of 18F fluoride PET/CT and 99mTc-MDP bone scan in the detection of skeletal metastases in urinary bladder carcinoma. Clin Nucl Med 2013;38:616.

55. Albers P, Albrecht W, Algaba F, et al. EAU guidelines on testicular cancer. Update 2011. European Association of Urology. Actas Urol Esp 2012;36:127 [in Spanish].

56. Manecksha RP, Fitzpatrick JM. Epidemiology of testicular cancer. BJU Int 2009;104:1329.

57. Horwich A, Shipley J, Huddart R. Testicular germ-cell cancer. Lancet 2006;367:754.

58. Flechon A, Rivoire M, Droz JP. Management of advanced germ-cell tumors of the testis. Nat Clin Pract Urol 2008;5:262.

59. Jana S, Blaufox MD. Nuclear medicine studies of the prostate, testes, and bladder. Semin Nucl Med 2006;36:51.

60. Kim W, Rosen MA, Langer JE, et al. US MR imaging correlation in pathologic conditions of the scrotum. Radiographics 2007;27:1239.

61. Cassidy FH, Ishioka KM, McMahon CJ, et al. MR imaging of scrotal tumors and pseudotumors. Radiographics 2010;30:665.

62. Johnson JO, Mattrey RF, Phillipson J. Differentiation of seminomatous from nonseminomatous testicular tumors with MR imaging. AJR Am J Roentgenol 1990;154:539.

63. Hain SF, O'Doherty MJ, Timothy AR, et al. Fluorodeoxyglucose PET in the initial staging of germ cell tumours. Eur J Nucl Med 2000;27:590.

64. Lassen U, Daugaard G, Eigtved A, et al. Whole-body FDG-PET in patients with stage I non-seminomatous germ cell tumours. Eur J Nucl Med Mol Imaging 2003;30:396.

65. Hain SF, O'Doherty MJ, Timothy AR, et al. Fluorodeoxyglucose positron emission tomography in the evaluation of germ cell tumours at relapse. Br J Cancer 2000;83:863.

66. Cremerius U, Wildberger JE, Borchers H, et al. Does positron emission tomography using 18-fluoro-2-deoxyglucose improve clinical staging of testicular cancer?—Results of a study in 50 patients. Urology 1999;54:900.

67. Ambrosini V, Zucchini G, Nicolini S, et al. 18F-FDG PET/CT impact on testicular tumours clinical management. Eur J Nucl Med Mol Imaging 2014;41:668.

68. Sharma P, Jain TK, Parida GK, et al. Diagnostic accuracy of integrated (18)F-FDG PET/CT for restaging patients with malignant germ cell tumours. Br J Radiol 2014;87:20140263.

69. Stomper PC, Kalish LA, Garnick MB, et al. CT and pathologic predictive features of residual mass histologic findings after chemotherapy for nonseminomatous germ cell tumors: can residual malignancy or teratoma be excluded? Radiology 1991;180:711.

70. Bachner M, Loriot Y, Gross-Goupil M, et al. 2-18fluoro-deoxy-D-glucose positron emission tomography (FDG-PET) for postchemotherapy seminoma residual lesions: a retrospective validation of the SEMPET trial. Ann Oncol 2012;23:59.

71. Siekiera J, Malkowski B, Jozwicki W, et al. Can we rely on PET in the follow-up of advanced seminoma patients? Urol Int 2012;88:405.

72. Hinz S, Schrader M, Kempkensteffen C, et al. The role of positron emission tomography in the evaluation of residual masses after chemotherapy for advanced stage seminoma. J Urol 2008;179:936.

73. Lewis DA, Tann M, Kesler K, et al. Positron emission tomography scans in postchemotherapy seminoma patients with residual masses: a retrospective review from Indiana University Hospital. J Clin Oncol 2006;24:e54.

74. De Santis M, Becherer A, Bokemeyer C, et al. 2-18fluoro-deoxy-D-glucose positron emission tomography is a reliable predictor for viable tumor in postchemotherapy seminoma: an update of the prospective multicentric SEMPET trial. J Clin Oncol 2004;22:1034.

75. Spermon JR, De Geus-Oei LF, Kiemeney LA, et al. The role of (18)fluoro-2-deoxyglucose positron emission tomography in initial staging and re-staging after chemotherapy for testicular germ cell tumours. BJU Int 2002;89:549.

76. Ganjoo KN, Chan RJ, Sharma M, et al. Positron emission tomography scans in the evaluation of postchemotherapy residual masses in patients with seminoma. J Clin Oncol 1999;17:3457.

77. Oechsle K, Hartmann M, Brenner W, et al. [18F]Fluorodeoxyglucose positron emission tomography in nonseminomatous germ cell tumors after chemotherapy: the German multicenter positron emission tomography study group. J Clin Oncol 2008;26:5930.

78. Becherer A, De Santis M, Karanikas G, et al. FDG PET is superior to CT in the prediction of viable tumour in post-chemotherapy seminoma residuals. Eur J Radiol 2005;54:284.

79. De Santis M, Bokemeyer C, Becherer A, et al. Predictive impact of 2-18fluoro-2-deoxy-D-glucose positron emission tomography for residual

postchemotherapy masses in patients with bulky seminoma. J Clin Oncol 2001;19:3740.

80. Treglia G, Sadeghi R, Annunziata S, et al. Diagnostic performance of fluorine-18-fluorodeoxyglucose positron emission tomography in the postchemotherapy management of patients with seminoma: systematic review and meta-analysis. Biomed Res Int 2014;2014:852681.

81. Hartmann JT, Schmoll HJ, Kuczyk MA, et al. Post-chemotherapy resections of residual masses from metastatic non-seminomatous testicular germ cell tumors. Ann Oncol 1997;8:531.

82. Pfannenberg C, Aschoff P, Dittmann H, et al. PET/CT with 18F-FLT: does it improve the therapeutic management of metastatic germ cell tumors? J Nucl Med 2010;51:845.

Value of FDG PET/CT in Patient Management and Outcome of Skeletal and Soft Tissue Sarcomas

Sara Sheikhbahaei, MD, MPH[a], Charles Marcus, MD[a],
Nima Hafezi-Nejad, MD, MPH[a], Mehdi Taghipour, MD[a],
Rathan M. Subramaniam, MD, PhD, MPH[a,b,c,*]

KEYWORDS

- Fluorodeoxyglucose • PET • Computed tomography • Patient management • Skeletal sarcoma
- Soft tissue sarcoma

KEY POINTS

- Fluorodeoxyglucose (FDG)-PET/computed tomography (CT) helps to ensure accurate histopathologic examination by guiding biopsy toward the most biologically significant regions in large and heterogeneous sarcomas: metabolic biopsy.
- To evaluate therapy response in osteosarcoma, Ewing sarcoma, and gastrointestinal stromal tumors, quantitative FDG-PET imaging markers such as maximum standardized uptake value or visual interpretation are more accurate than traditional size-based response criteria, because the tumor may not always change in size in response to therapy.
- FDG-PET/CT has a promising role in surveillance and detection of local recurrences in patients with sarcomas, because the conventional imaging may not distinguish between posttherapeutic changes/fibrosis from disease relapse and may show artifacts hindering accurate tumor visualization.

INTRODUCTION

Bone and soft tissue sarcomas are a heterogeneous group of relatively rare tumors.[1,2] The incidence of bone and soft tissue tumors has increased during the last 35 years. In the United States, approximately 3000 new bone sarcomas and 12,000 new soft tissue sarcomas were expected to be diagnosed in 2014.[3] The 5-year survival rate for all types of bone and soft tissue sarcomas is about 65%.[3] The survival depends on several factors, including the subtype of cancer, presence of metastasis, location, and the grade of tumor.[4] With the development of new anticancer drugs, identifying patients who might benefit from alternative treatment strategies early in the course of treatment is crucial.[1,5]

Fluorodeoxyglucose (FDG)-PET/computed tomography (CT) is a new imaging modality, which combines anatomic localization by CT with functional PET imaging and which has a promising role in the management of many solid tumors.[6–18] It has been

Disclosure: Dr Subramaniam – Phillips Health Care Molecular Imaging board meeting; Bayer Health care – clinical trial.
[a] Russell H Morgan Department of Radiology and Radiological Sciences, Johns Hopkins School of Medicine, JHOC 3230, 601 North Caroline Street, Baltimore, MD 21287, USA; [b] Department of Oncology, Johns Hopkins School of Medicine, 401 North Broadway, Baltimore, MD 21231, USA; [c] Department of Health Policy and Management, Johns Hopkins Bloomberg School of Public Health, 624 North Broadway, Baltimore, MD 21205, USA
* Corresponding author. Russell H Morgan Department of Radiology and Radiological Sciences, Johns Hopkins Medical Institutions, 601 North Caroline Street/JHOC 3235, Baltimore, MD 21287.
E-mail address: rsubram4@jhmi.edu

PET Clin 10 (2015) 375–393
http://dx.doi.org/10.1016/j.cpet.2015.03.003
1556-8598/15/$ – see front matter © 2015 Elsevier Inc. All rights reserved.

increasingly used in the evaluation of bone and soft tissue sarcomas,[1,4,5,19–22] and its impact on the management of these tumors is discussed in the following sections.

Tumor Staging and Grading

A prospective multicenter trial of patients with bone and soft tissue sarcoma[23] suggested that FDG-PET could provide important additional information in initial tumor staging and have an impact on therapy planning. A previous meta-analysis[24] reported pooled sensitivity and specificity (95% confidence interval [CI]) of 91% (89%–93%) and 85% (82%–88%) for FDG-PET/CT in the detection of bone and soft tissue sarcomas, respectively. Compared with conventional imaging modalities (ultrasonography, CT, magnetic resonance [MR] imaging), FDG-PET/CT is equally effective in identifying primary tumors (100%) and is superior in the identification of metastatic lymph nodes (25% vs 95%) and bone metastasis (57% vs 90%).[23] However, the specificity of FDG-PET/CT in staging of bone and soft tissue lesions is not higher than conventional imaging, because both benign and malignant lesions may show abnormal metabolic activity in PET.[22]

In bone and soft tissue sarcoma, histologic grading is considered an important prognostic factor.[21] The value of FDG-PET/CT in grading of sarcomas is not to replace the existing gold standard of histopathology but to improve the preoperative prognostic assessment and guide further management.[1,20] FDG-PET has been reported to provide useful information about sarcoma grade, even when the cell type is unknown.[4,21] A study of 89 patients with bone and soft tissue sarcoma showed that the standardized uptake value (SUV) of FDG-PET was strongly associated with the histologic grading, cellularity, mitotic activity, and P53 expression.[25] Although an increase in maximum SUV (SUV_{max}) was observed in higher grade of sarcomas, there remains a significant overlap between SUV values. FDG uptake does not reliably discriminate grades II versus III and benign versus grade I sarcomas. Therefore, PET/CT scans need to be interpreted in the overall clinical context for each individual patient.[25] Besides, identifying regions with the highest SUV_{max} could assist in a more accurate sampling of large and heterogeneous sarcomas.[5,21]

Monitoring of Treatment Response

One of the advantages of FDG-PET/CT in evaluation of patients with sarcomas is its ability to assess therapeutic response early during treatment.[1,5,19,21,26] Posttreatment changes measured by FDG avidity of the tumor are considered an indicator of the efficacy of the regimen.[1,5] Because the biochemical changes in a tumor usually occur before the morphologic changes, using a functional imaging modality can enable clinicians to evaluate the therapeutic effectiveness earlier than conventional anatomic imaging.[5,20] Besides, quantitative FDG-PET has been shown to be significantly more accurate than traditional tumor response criteria (size based),[27] such as RECIST (Response Evaluation Criteria in Solid Tumors) in sarcomas, because sarcomas, including gastrointestinal stromal tumors (GISTs), may not necessarily change in size in response to therapy.[27–29] Thus, use of early interim FDG-PET/CT allows a noninvasive assessment of histologic response to treatment in bone and soft tissue tumors.[22]

Follow-up and Recurrence Detection

Follow-up of patients with sarcomas could help to detect local or distant recurrences in a timely manner, allowing prompt initiation of further treatment.[5,20,22] In addition, synchronous cancers may arise in survivors of bone sarcomas, either related to or independent of irradiation.[30] FDG-PET imaging can be useful for follow-up of patients after sarcoma treatment and has been found to have a profound effect on patient prognosis.[1,5,21,31,32] Anatomic imaging alone had not been accurate enough for surveillance of bone and soft tissue tumors, because of posttreatment changes, including anatomic distortion, disruption of normal tissue planes, and metal artifacts.[4,21,22]

Survival and Prognostic Stratification

Studies of various cancers[6] have widely shown that quantitative metabolic parameters derived from FDG-PET/CT have value in predicting disease progression and survival. The usefulness of metabolic FDG-PET/CT parameters identified at staging or later during follow-up in outcome prediction was also studied in patients with bone and soft tissue tumors.[5,21,22,31–33] Several studies of bone and soft tissue sarcomas[31,34] consistently indicated that the presence and volume of necrosis and the baseline SUV_{max} are strong independent adverse prognostic factors for clinical outcome. Recent studies also showed that the percentage reduction of pretherapy to posttherapy SUV_{max} is significantly associated with patient outcome. Thus, midtherapy PET to evaluate the interim treatment response could strengthen the outcome prediction in patients with sarcomas.[32,35] Besides, volume-based PET measurements (eg, metabolic tumor volume [MTV] and total lesion glycolysis) represent total tumor uptake and thus may provide superior prognostic information to

SUV_{max}.[33] However, there is no consensus in the advantage of volumetric PET parameters over SUV_{max} in soft tissue tumors.[33,34] This situation might be a result of small sample size, the inclusion of different subtypes of soft tissue tumors in each study, or adoption of different methods for delineation of PET parameters.[34]

The remainder of this article reviews the value of FDG-PET/CT imaging in the management of common bone and soft tissue sarcomas including osteosarcoma (OS), Ewing sarcoma (ES), chondrosarcoma (CS), rhabdomyosarcoma (RS), liposarcoma (LS), malignant fibrous histiocytoma (MFH), and GIST.

OSTEOSARCOMA

OS is the most common bone malignancy in children and adolescents.[4,36] It is also considered the second most common bone cancer in adults, accounting for approximately 28% of adult primary bone cancers.[4,36] OS is classified into several subtypes based on the location within the bone, cell type, tumor grade, and so forth. The subtypes vary in clinical presentation and features, radiographic appearance, and prognosis. Conventional central intramedullary OS is the most common subtype of OS and accounts for nearly 75% of cases; it usually presents with an immature cloudlike bone formation in the metaphyses of long bones.[4,36] The diagnosis of OS is based on a combination of histopathologic and imaging features. Plain radiographs remain the preferred initial imaging test for the diagnosis of OS followed by MR imaging.[36]

PET/CT imaging provides detailed information on tumor staging, treatment monitoring, and follow-up of OS.[4,20,25,37–39] Tumor staging and histologic grading have an important role in treatment planning and prognosis.[38,40] The area of the tumor with the highest degree of anaplasia and mitotic rate is used to determine the histologic grading. The accuracy of tumor grading may suffer from sampling error, because there is marked heterogeneity in biological activity within the tumors, particularly in large masses.[21] Some studies[25,37] have proposed that FDG-PET/CT-guided biopsy helps to ensure accurate grading and prognostication. Other studies[41,42] have shown that the SUV_{max} is correlated with the histopathologic tumor characteristics and can differentiate between high-grade and low-grade OS,[37,39,41] serving as a surrogate marker of tumor grading. Recommended treatment of localized OS ranges from surgery in low-grade tumors to a combination of neoadjuvant chemotherapy or radiation therapy followed by surgery in high-grade tumors.[36,43]

Although the definitive marker for evaluating therapeutic response is determined by the histopathologic analysis, it can be performed only after surgical resection of tumor.[39] In histopathologic analysis, the tumor is considered to have a good treatment response if the degree of necrosis is higher than 90% after preoperative chemotherapy.[25,33,44] FDG-PET/CT has a promising role in evaluating treatment response, as a noninvasive alternative.[39] Several studies[21,45,46] have suggested that preoperative FDG-PET/CT could significantly determine the treatment response to neoadjuvant therapy and prognosis and that it is useful in tailoring surgery or further treatment options. These studies[21,41,47] suggest incorporating FDG-PET metabolic parameters in survival-predicting models for OS. A meta-analysis of 8 studies comprising 178 patients[39] evaluated the predictive value of posttreatment SUV to tumor necrosis rates in patients with OS treated with neoadjuvant chemotherapy. These investigators suggested that posttreatment SUV of 2.5 or less is valuable for predicting the histologic response to chemotherapy with a sensitivity and specificity of 0.73 (0.54–0.87) and 0.86 (0.51–0.97), respectively. Recent studies emphasized that combined metabolic and volumetric PET/CT parameters can independently predict histologic response after neoadjuvant chemotherapy in OS.[47,48] Further, Byun and colleagues[40] suggested that the addition of baseline MTV to histologic response predicts survival more accurately than histologic response alone. These investigators reported that the 5-year metastasis-free survival rates in patients with baseline MTV of 105 (mL) or less and good histologic response were 100% compared with 38% in those with MTV greater than 105 and poor histologic response. In another study, Bajpai and colleagues[47] suggested that an initial tumor size of less than 300 mL on PET was independently associated with good histologic response (odds ratio = 17.6) and could predict histologic response better when combined with the SUV ratio before and after treatment (histologic response proportions of 83% in combined model vs 37% with MTV alone). Moreover, FDG-PET/CT has also been reported to be a useful imaging modality in the detection of recurrence and follow-up of patients with OS after tumor resection.[4,22,37,49] Studies[38,46–57] describing the performance of FDG-PET in the therapeutic response and surveillance of OS are summarized in **Table 1**.

A recent study[57] including 20 patients with pediatric OS (101 lesions) showed that follow-up FDG-PET/CT provided a diagnostic benefit in 17.4% of examinations and was superior to conventional imaging (CT and MR imaging) modalities in the detection of bone lesions and complementary to CT in characterizing lung nodules. Overall, the performance of FDG-PET is superior to CT and MR imaging in the detection of local recurrences in OS, because the latter could not differentiate between posttherapeutic tissue changes or fibrosis from local relapse.[4] Besides, in patients with metallic implants after a limb-sparing procedure, imaging artifacts often hamper MR imaging or CT findings.[22] However, PET imaging performed more than 6 months after surgery is useful in identifying residual or recurrent tumor from postsurgical healing (**Figs. 1 and 2**).[22,49]

EWING SARCOMA

ES family tumors (ESFT) are the second most common primary malignant bone tumor in children and adolescents.[58] ES also represents approximately 6% of all primary malignant bone tumors in adults.[3] ESFT include ES, peripheral primitive neuroectodermal tumor, and Askin tumor (tumor of the chest wall).[43] ESFT are high-grade, small, blue, round-cell tumors, which can arise both from bone and soft tissues. These tumors occur about 9 times more commonly in whites than in African Americans.[43,58]

Initial presentation and tumor staging are currently the most important clinical prognostic factors for survival in ESFT.[59] The survival of patients depends highly on the presence or absence of metastasis. The 5-year survival rate of patients with localized ES is about 70% compared with 25% to 30% in those with metastasis.[3] Tumor size, primary site (distal extremities) and site of metastasis (lung/pleural) are all important prognostic factors.[43,58–60] Staging must be oriented to accurately detect lung, bone, and bone marrow metastases.[43] **Table 2** summarized studies evaluating the diagnostic performance of staging/restaging FDG-PET in patients with ES.[57,61–67]

FDG-PET/CT scan is considered a useful tool in the diagnosis of ESFT.[57–59,63,67] A meta-analysis of 5 selected studies reported a pooled sensitivity and specificity (95% CI) of 96% (91%–99%) and 92% (87%–96%), respectively, for FDG-PET/CT in staging and restaging patients with ESFT.[58] In a recent study, Quartuccio and colleagues[57] compared the diagnostic accuracy of PET/CT and conventional imaging (CT, MR imaging, bone scanning) in the staging and follow-up of pediatric skeletal ES, The study included a total of 311 lesions. In the per scan comparison, the diagnostic benefit of FDG-PET/CT was 27.8% in initial staging and 9.1% in the follow-up. FDG-PET/CT provided a diagnostic benefit in 21 of 44 (47.7%)

patients with ES at least once during clinical management.[57]

Advances in therapeutic approaches and the use of multimodal therapeutic regimens have increased the cure rate of ESFT to more than 50%.[60,67] The accurate staging of ESFT could also improve the treatment planning and target volume definition.[60] The detection of occult metastases by FDG-PET/CT may change treatment decisions.[23] Generally, a tumor assessment must be performed after neoadjuvant chemotherapy to tailor subsequent treatment. Patients may further be considered for preoperative radiotherapy, limb salvage surgery, or amputation. Dynamic MR imaging can also assess the response to chemotherapy.[60] FDG-PET/CT has been shown to provide additional information regarding the biological activity of tumors and is useful in the preoperative staging and assessment of therapeutic response after neoadjuvant chemotherapy (**Fig. 3**).[60]

Moreover, FDG-PET/CT has shown high diagnostic accuracy for recurrence detection in the follow-up of patients with ESFT when disease recurrence is suspected (clinically or by imaging) or during routine follow-up.[67] In a study of 53 patients (71 scans),[67] FDG-PET/CT showed a sensitivity of 95% and a specificity of 87% in detecting recurrence in patients with skeletal ES. Another study[63] reported that FDG-PET/CT is more accurate than PET alone in the follow-up of ES. FDG-PET/CT is also sensitive in the detection of osseous metastases and recurrent bone lesions compared with other conventional imaging, such as MR imaging or bone scintigraphy (**Fig. 4**).[60,68] Nevertheless, FDG-PET/CT is shown to have a lower sensitivity in staging small lesions, particularly pulmonary metastases, compared with spiral CT.[23,57,69] Early detection of lung metastasis in ES could substantially improve survival, because of the possibility of curative treatment.

CHONDROSARCOMA

CS accounts for more than 40% of primary bone cancers in adults.[3] Most CS are locally aggressive, nonmetastatic, and low-grade tumors.[43]

FDG-PET was proposed as a promising modality for additional assessment when a diagnosis of CS was suspected.[70] Brenner and colleagues[71] developed an SUV cutoff for prediction of relapse in patients with CS. In their report, selecting patients with SUV values greater than 4 had a sensitivity and specificity of 90% and76%, respectively.[71] These investigators further investigated the role of PET in the grading of CS. Moreover, they suggested that the use of PET could enhance

Table 1
Summary of studies describing value of FDG-PET in the therapeutic response and surveillance of OS

PET Performed After Preoperative NAC

Author, Year	Design	No. of Patients (GR/PR)	Treatment	Modality	PET Variable (Cut Point)	Sensitivity (%)	Specificity (%)	PPV (%)	NPV (%)	DA (%)
Hawkins et al,[50] 2002	—	14 (5/9)[a]	NAC + surgery	PET	SUV_{max} 2 (2)	60	92.3	75	85.7	—
Ye et al,[51] 2008	P	15 (8/7)	2 cycles of NAC + surgery	PET	SUV_{max} 2/SUV_{max} 1 (0.5)	63	71	71	63	—
Cheon et al,[46] 2009	P	70 (33/37)	2 cycles of NAC + surgery	PET	SUV_{max} 2 (5)	—	—	78	93	84
Hamada et al,[52] 2009	R	11 (5/6)	NAC + surgery	PET	SUV_{max} 2 (2.5)	100	100	100	100	—
Denecke et al,[53] 2010	P	11 (5/6)	NAC + surgery	PET	SUV_{max} 2 (2.8)	80	100	100	86	91
Bajpai et al,[47] 2011	P	31 (10/21)	3 cycles of NAC + surgery	PET/CT	SUV_{max} 2 (3.3)	80	76.2	61.5	88.9	—
Gaston et al,[54] 2011	R	19 (10/9)	NAC + surgery	PET	SUV_{max} 2 (2.5)	100	60	100	69	—
Im et al,[48] 2012[a]	P	14 (5/9)[a]	2 cycles of NAC + surgery	PET/CT	SUV_{max} 2 (3)	100	88.9	83.3	100	92.9
Kong et al,[38] 2013	P	26 (13/13)	2 cycles of NAC + surgery	PET/CT	SUV_{max} 2 (5)	61.5	92.3	88.9	70.6	76.9
Byun et al,[55] 2014	P	30 (13/17)	2 cycles of NAC + surgery	PET	SUV_{max} 2 (5)	58.8	92.3	90.9	63.2	73.3

PET Performed After Completion of Surgery/as a Follow-up

Author, Year	Design	No. of Patients (No. of Scans Included), Analysis	Treatment	Modality (Interpretation)	Reference Standard	Sensitivity (%)	Specificity (%)	PPV (%)	NPV (%)	DA (%)
Byun et al,[56] 2013	R	206 (833), scan level	Surgery + chemotherapy	PET/CT (visual)	Pathology, clinical, and imaging FU ≥6 mo	94.5	98.1	77.6	99.6	97.8
Chang et al,[49] 2014	R	109 (355), patient level	NAC + limb salvage surgery	PET/CT (SUV_{max} 4.6)	Pathology, imaging FU ≥6 mo	88.9	76	25	98.7	77.1
Quartuccio et al,[57] 2015	R	20 (75), scan level			Note: The overall concordance between FDG-PET/CT and conventional imaging (CT, MR imaging, bone scan) was 82.4%. FDG-PET/CT provided diagnostic benefit of 17.4%, showing fewer false-positive lesions (6.7%, 5/75) and more true-positive lesions (10.7%, 8/75).					

Histologic response evaluated according to the degree of tumor necrosis as good (≥90%), and poor (<90%) response.
Abbreviations: DA, diagnostic accuracy; FU, follow-up; GR, good histologic response; NAC, neoadjuvant chemotherapy; No, number; NPV, negative predictive value; P, prospective; PPV, positive predictive value; PR, poor histologic response; R, retrospective; SUV_{max} 1, SUV_{max} before NAC; SUV_{max} 2, SUV_{max} after NAC.
[a] Patients with sarcomas other than OS were excluded from the study.

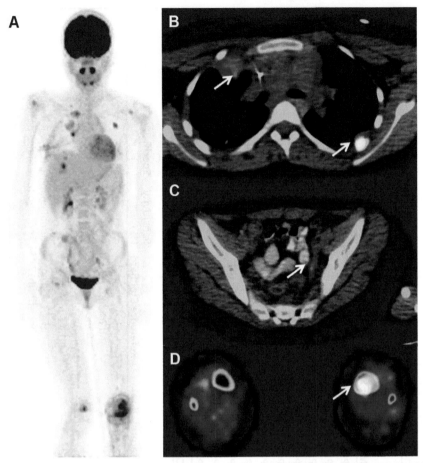

Fig. 1. Osteosarcoma (OS): anterior maximum intensity projection (*A*) and axial fused PET/CT (*B–D*) images of a 15-year-old girl with OS of the left tibia, status post limb salvage radical resection and chemotherapy. She presented a year after completion of treatment with progressive right-sided chest pain. The restaging FDG-PET/CT study showed multiple foci of increased FDG uptake involving pleural-based nodules/masses (*B, white arrow*), pelvic nodes (*C, white arrow*), and the left proximal tibia (*D, white arrow*), consistent with metastatic disease.

the outcome prediction, especially when being accompanied by histopathologic grading.[71] Feldman and colleagues[72] used whole-body FDG-PET in the evaluation of cartilage neoplasms. They suggested an SUV cutoff value of 2 to differentiate benign from malignant cartilage neoplasms. Despite a limited number of patients, these investigators proposed whole-body FDG-PET as a valuable adjunct modality in identifying the differential diagnosis of CS.[72] In their later studies, they expanded their SUV cutoff of 2 to be used in differentiating benign from malignant osteochondroma as well.[73] The idea that PET may have potential benefits in differentiating benign versus malignant osteochondroma was confirmed by other investigators as well.[74]

Newer studies have evaluated the role of PET in correlation with treatment measures in CS. Stacchiotti and colleagues[75,76] investigated the role of PET in the evaluation of response to sunitinib in

CS. Although the number of patients included in the study was small (n = 10), response evaluation was assessable.[75,76] PET has the potential to be used in evaluating the treatment response after radiotherapy[77] and antioxidant therapies.[78] Hybrid PET-MR imaging may elucidate additional valuable information about degree of differentiation, morphologic mapping, and even histopathology of CS.[79]

RHABDOMYOSARCOMA

RS constitutes more than half of soft tissue sarcomas in children. It is one of the musculoskeletal sarcomas that was the target for various types of PET studies.[80] The role of PET in the diagnosis, staging, outcome prediction, and monitoring of disease remission and recurrence in patients with RS is reviewed.[81,82]

Several studies have evaluated the role of PET in the diagnosis and staging of RS.[2] PET findings can

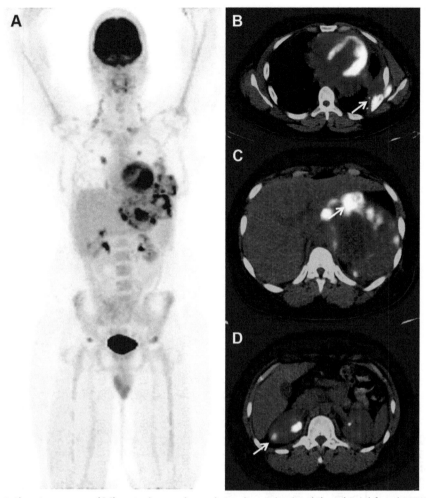

Fig. 2. Metastatic osteosarcoma (OS): anterior maximum intensity projection (*A*) and axial fused PET/CT (*B–D*) images of a 21-year-old man with a history of left distal tibial OS, post amputation and multiple courses of chemotherapy. The restaging FDG-PET/CT study performed 1 year after treatment completion showed multiple foci of increased FDG uptake involving the lung (*B*), soft tissue of the abdomen (*C*), and right kidney (*D*) (*white arrows*), consistent with widespread metastatic disease.

be correlated with that of MR imaging and CT, at staging, evaluation of treatment response, and identifying metastases (**Fig. 5**).[2] In a study of 35 patients with RS,[83] PET/CT could correctly diagnose the overall TNM stage in 86% of patients compared with 54% for conventional imaging (bone scintigraphy, chest radiograph, CT or MR imaging) (*P*<.01). PET/CT shows higher accuracies for nodal staging (97% vs 87%) and identifying metastasis (89% vs 63%), compared with the conventional imaging. This finding is also true in the restaging of RS, wherein PET information can change the treatment options.[83,84] However, there is no consensus regarding the routine use of PET in addition to CT for the staging of soft tissue sarcomas, including RS.[85] Formerly, it was considered that PET did not have a significant impact on the management plan, and the routine use of

PET in addition to CT for initial staging or metastasis detection may provide only a small additional benefit.[82,85] Nevertheless, a new systematic review has concluded that PET may improve accuracy of tumor detection and staging in childhood RS.[86]

Earlier PET studies reported a favorable accuracy for PET in detecting RS recurrence.[87] Further studies[88] showed a promising role for PET in detection of recurrence, especially in patients treated with radiotherapy. Although PET has the advantage of being used for monitoring disease outcome in childhood RS,[89] it may assist in the detection of local recurrence.[90] Despite the ability of PET to improve accuracy at initial staging, treatment monitoring, and follow-up, there is a need for more, larger studies to draw meaningful clinical comparisons.[91,92]

Table 2
Diagnostic performance of staging/restaging FDG-PET in patients with ES

Author, Year	Design	Disease (No. of Patients)	No. of Scans Included	Modality	Target	Sensitivity (%)	Specificity (%)	PPV (%)	NPV (%)	DA (%)	Reference Standard
Franzius et al,[61] 2000	R	ES (38)	66	PET	Staging/restaging	100 (82–100)	96 (85–99)	91 (72–98)	100 (92–100)	97 (90–100)	Pathology, anatomic imaging, clinical FU 20 mo
Gyorke et al,[62] 2006	R	ES (10), PNET (13)	33	PET	Staging/restaging	96 (87–100)	92 (84–97)	—	—	91 (76–98)	Pathology, imaging, clinical FU 6 mo
Gerth et al,[63] 2007	R	ES (53)	163	PET	Staging/FU	96 (87–100)	92 (84–97)	89 (78–96)	97 (91–100)	94 (91–100)	Pathology, imaging, clinical FU
Kleis et al,[64] 2008	R	ES (9), OS (1)	83	PET/CT	Staging/FU	85 (73–96)	59 (44–74)	—	—	—	Pathology, clinical and imaging FU ≥6 mo
Charest et al,[65] 2009	R	ES (22)	22	PET/CT	Staging/restaging	100 (74–100)	100 (69–100)	—	—	—	Pathology
Mody et al,[66] 2010	R	ES (11), PNET (5)	27	PET/CT	Staging/restaging	87 (60–98)	83 (52–98)	—	—	—	Pathology, imaging, clinical FU ≥12 mo
Sharma et al,[67] 2013	R	Skeletal ES (53)	71	PET/CT	FU	95 (83–99)	87 (70–96)	90 (77–97)	93 (77–99)	91.5	Pathology, clinical/imaging FU ≥6 mo
Quartuccio et al,[57] 2015	R	ES (44)[a]	346	PET/CT	Staging/FU	90.3	77.8	69.9	93.3	82	Pathology, FU ≥6 mo

Diagnostic accuracy data reported as % (95% CI) were possible.
Abbreviations: DA, diagnostic accuracy; FU, follow-up; NPV, negative predictive value; P, prospective; PNET, primitive neurectodermal tumors; PPV, positive predictive value; R, retrospective.
[a] Lesion-based analysis reported.

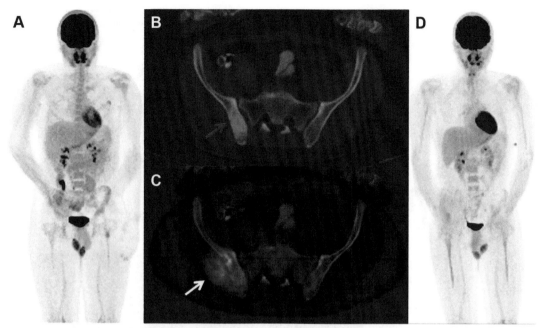

Fig. 3. Ewing sarcoma (ES): anterior maximum intensity projection (*A*), axial CT (*B*), and fused PET/CT (*C*) images of a 15-year-old boy, recently diagnosed with ES. The staging FDG-PET/CT study shows an FDG-avid (SUV$_{max}$ 2.90) (*red arrow*) sclerotic lesion (*white arrow*) in the right posterior iliac bone extending into the gluteal soft tissue, consistent with the patient's known primary ES. He underwent chemoradiation. The restaging FDG-PET/CT (*D*) study 6 months after completion of treatment shows no definite evidence of metabolically active FDG-avid disease, consistent with complete treatment response.

LIPOSARCOMA

LS is considered one of the most common soft tissue sarcomas in adults.[3] Earlier studies suggested the glucose utilization rate, assessed by PET, as a marker of differentiation of LS.[44,93] FDG-PET can successfully differentiate between low-grade and high-grade LS.[44] FDG uptake cutoffs were shown to be able to determine the histopathologic grade of the tumor in LS.[44] Because glucose utilization can be measured in PET, it can potentially determine the therapy response and tissue necrosis as well.[94] PET can significantly differentiate remnant tumor from necrosis and dead tissue after radiotherapy.[95] Moreover, PET may diagnose local recurrence and the malignancy grade of recurrent LS.[96] Accurate identification of disease recurrence is vital in patients with LS, because it has been predicted that the recurrence rate in LS can be as high as 93% after surgery.[96]

PET was shown to accurately diagnose LS (**Fig. 6**).[2,97] PET, in addition to CT or MR imaging for anatomic localization, is a useful modality at initial diagnosis, assessing treatment response and metastatic involvement.[2] In myxoid LS, there is a high incidence of metastasis, and with the heterogeneous histologic features of the tumor, the combined approach (FDG-PET/CT and MR

imaging) may yield more accurate staging.[98] Despite reports that indicate a high diagnostic accuracy for PET in LS, use of PET is not recommended as a routine investigation.[82,85] Critics argue that the routine use of PET in the initial evaluation of LS adds little to conventional imaging and is not likely to change the treatment options.[85] Nevertheless, recent studies have focused on selected use of PET in grading, staging, and metastasis workup of patients with LS.[99,100] PET may be useful in the classification of these lesions even before histologic grading.[101] PET evaluation of FDG kinetics is proposed to unveil the diagnosis, histologic grading, and prognosis of soft tissue sarcomas, such as LS.[102] In addition to the staging and grading, PET is suggested as a prognosis assessment tool in the evaluation of patients with LS.[103] Specifically, an SUV$_{max}$ greater than 3.6 was suggested as a significant indicator of higher recurrence and metastasis as well as lower disease-free survival.[103]

MALIGNANT FIBROUS HISTIOCYTOMA

MFH is considered the most frequent type of soft tissue sarcoma in adults, with the highest incidence in the fifth to seventh decades of

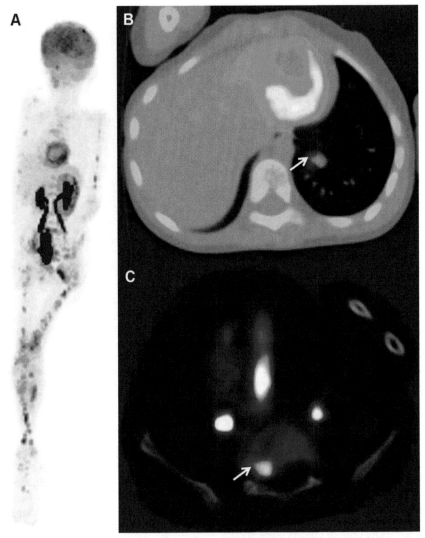

Fig. 4. Ewing sarcoma (ES): anterior maximum intensity projection (*A*) and axial fused PET/CT (*B, C*) images of a 7-year-old boy with stage IV ES of the left proximal tibia. He underwent chemotherapy. The restaging FDG-PET/CT study performed 6 months after completion of treatment shows innumerable foci of increased FDG activity throughout the axial and appendicular skeleton, vertebra (*C*), and left lung nodule (*B*) (*white arrows*), consistent with widespread metastatic disease.

life.[4,104] The most common location of primary MFH is in the extremities (70%), especially the lower extremities, followed by the retroperitoneum (16%).[104,105] Several studies of patients with soft tissue sarcomas (including MFH)[4,25] have shown that FDG-PET/CT has a high diagnostic accuracy at initial assessment, grading, detection of recurrence, and prognostication. Because the incidence of MFH is low, there is no study evaluating the efficacy of FDG-PET/CT in MFH exclusively. However, several case reports have observed high FDG uptake in MFH and shown that FDG-PET/CT correctly detects primary MFH, even in uncommon locations including the superior mediastinum (SUV_{max} = 17.4),[104] kidneys (SUV_{max} = 6.8),[105] stomach (SUV_{max} = 24.6),[106] prostate (SUV = 46.8),[107] lung (SUV_{max} = 12.1),[108] and maxillary sinus (SUV_{max} = 16.9),[109] as well as metastatic lesions in lung and bilateral adrenal glands.[110]

GASTROINTESTINAL STROMAL TUMORS

GISTs are the most common mesenchymal neoplasm of the gastrointestinal tract, accounting for approximately 5% of all sarcomas.[29,58] They are most frequently encountered in the stomach and proximal small bowel but can occur anywhere

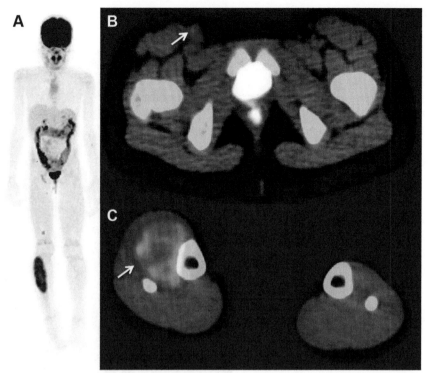

Fig. 5. Rhabdomyosarcoma (RS): anterior maximum intensity projection (*A*) and axial fused PET/CT (*B*, *C*) images of a 7-year-old girl with right calf alveolar RS, who underwent a staging FDG-PET/CT study. The PET/CT study showed FDG activity (SUV$_{max}$ 6.68) corresponding to the primary right leg RS with metabolically active right popliteal (*C*) and inguinal lymphadenopathy (*B*) (*white arrows*).

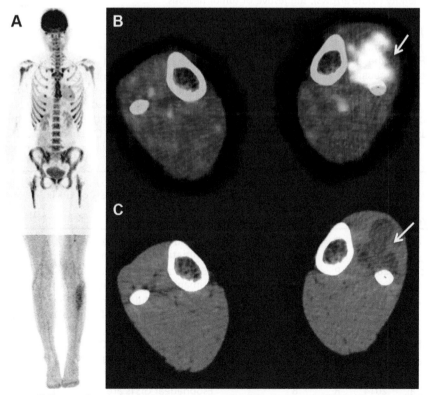

Fig. 6. Liposarcoma (LS): anterior maximum intensity projection (*A*), axial fused PET/CT (*B*), and axial CT (*C*) images of an 18-year-old woman with LS who underwent a staging FDG-PET/CT study. The study showed an intensely FDG-avid (SUV$_{max}$ 8.6) mass in the left anterolateral calf (*white arrows*), consistent with the newly diagnosed LS.

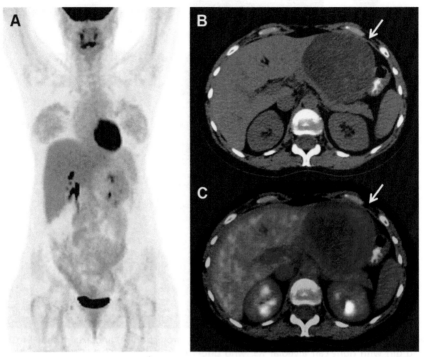

Fig. 7. Gastrointestinal stromal tumor (GIST): anterior maximum intensity projection (*A*), axial fused PET/CT (*B*), and axial CT (*C*) images of a 42-year-old woman with a recent diagnosis of a GIST involving the stomach. The study showed a 10-cm mass along the lesser curvature of the stomach with mild FDG uptake (SUV_{max} 1.7) and central hypodensity (*white arrows*), suggestive of tumor necrosis.

along the digestive tract or in the mesentery and retroperitoneum (**Fig. 7**).[3,111,112]

Use of PET in the evaluation of GIST had a remarkably successful history, especially compared with other soft tissue sarcomas.[29,112] PET has a comparable accuracy in contrast with endoscopic ultrasonography and endoscopic biopsy in gastric GIST[113] and is particularly indicated in indeterminate CT or MR imaging findings. There is a direct association between FDG-PET SUV values and the malignant potential of a gastric GIST (**Table 3**).[114–119] Cutoffs of 2.2, 4.2, and 6.5 were supposed to classify patients with gastric GIST as very low, low, intermediate, and high risk, respectively.[113]

On the other hand, unlike conventional imaging modalities such as CT scans, FDG-PET can detect increased metabolic activity in most GISTs and

Table 3
Summary of studies describing value of FDG-PET in the primary diagnosis of GISTs

Author, Year	Design	No. of Patients	Comments
Gayed et al,[114] 2004	R	54	PET and CT are comparable in staging GISTs before initiation of therapy
Kaneta et al,[115] 2009	P	41	PET has an incremental value over conventional imaging for the diagnostic of patients with GISTs
Otomi et al,[116] 2010	R	20	PET/CT is useful for primary examinations of GIST and the degree of FDG uptake is a useful indicator of risk category
Koch et al,[117] 2013	R	8	Anorectal GISTs are FDG avid ($SUV_{max} = 11$)
Yoshikawa et al,[118] 2013	R	10	PET/CT easily can predict the malignant potential of GIST ($SUV_{max} >4.3–6.3$)
Winant et al,[119] 2014	R	8	Esophageal GISTs are unusual but were markedly FDG avid on PET ($SUV_{max} >16$)

Abbreviations: P, prospective; R, retrospective.

Table 4
Summary of studies describing value of FDG-PET in therapy assessment of GISTs

Author, Year	Design	Number of Patients	Time of Posttherapy Scan	Comments
Van Oosterom et al,[123] 2001	P	17	1 and 4 wk	14 of 17 patients showed pretreatment uptake of FDG and could be assessed for PET response. 3 progressions, 10 complete response and 1 stable disease, which corresponded with CT
Demetri et al,[121] 2002	P	64	1, 3, and 6 mo	PET is useful for monitoring the therapeutic effect of imatinib in patients with GIST
Antoch et al,[124] 2004	R	20	1, 3, and 6 mo	PET/CT can provide additional information in GIST tumor response when compared with PET and CT alone
Choi et al,[125] 2004	R	36	2 mo	PET is sensitive and specific for evaluating GIST tumor response but cannot be used in patients with no FDG uptake in primary tumor scan
Gayed et al,[114] 2004	R	49	2 mo	PET is superior to CT in predicting early response to therapy
Jager et al,[126] 2004	P	16	1 wk	FDG uptake changes after 1 wk of treatment were of greater magnitude than tumor volume changes on CT at 8 wk
Goerres et al,[127] 2005	P	34	3 mo	Patients without FDG uptake after the start of treatment had a better prognosis than patients with residual activity
Goldstein et al,[128] 2005	—	18	2 mo	PET is a useful modality to monitor treatment response to Imatinib in patients with malignant GIST
Holdsworth et al,[129] 2007	P	63	1 mo	The change in PET SUV$_{max}$ was predictive of prolonged treatment success in patients with GIST
Demetri et al,[130] 2009	P	97	1 wk	PET showed decreased tumor glycolytic activity after 1 wk of starting sunitinib in patients with GIST who had failure response to imatinib
Prior et al,[131] 2009	P	23	4 wk	Week 4 FDG-PET is useful for early assessment of treatment response and for the prediction of clinical outcome
Maurel et al,[132] 2010	P	26	2 mo	Patients having disease control assessed by PET had longer overall survival than those patients who were classified as progressive disease
Fuster et al,[122] 2011	P	21	2 mo	PET is useful in assessing response of GIST refractory to imatinib
Stroobants et al,[133] 2012	P	21	1 wk	11 complete response, 2 partial response, 8 stable or progression. PET response was associated with a longer progression-free survival

also the subsequent functional changes that occur after the initiation of treatment.[29,111,112,120] Hybrid modalities such as FDG-PET/CT can be more accurate in the identification of these tumors and can play a complementary role in their evaluation.[29]

PET has specific value in posttreatment monitoring of patients with GIST (Table 4).[114,121–133] Recent studies[134–137] have focused on the use of PET as a sensitive modality in the posttreatment evaluation of many newly introduced drugs, including imatinib, panobinostat, cediranib, and retaspimycin.[134–138] Moreover, PET has an essential role in determining treatment in patients with GIST before surgery.[139] The role of PET in the detection of viable tissue after treatment and its power in clarifying the extent of the disease are the main advantages of PET assessments in GIST.[140,141] Despite the clinically promising accuracy of PET in the evaluation of GIST, it may not have similar high sensitivities in the detection of smaller lesions.[29] False-negative PET results in GIST tumors are a new entity that has attracted attention in recent studies.[142] For example, non–contrast-enhanced ultrasonography has been proposed as an alternative for GIST metastases that are negative in PET and CT.[143] In case of recurrence, PET/CT can be a feasible, reliable, and accurate method of restaging, even in the absence of a staging study.[144] However, in patients with GIST who undergo complete tumor resection (R0) with low likelihood of disease spread, PET may not be a sufficient tool for the diagnosis of clinically occult metastasis.[145] In similar clinical settings, individualized protocol studies along with concurrent interpretation using PET and CT assessments play a remarkable role in the posttreatment evaluation of GIST.[140]

SUMMARY

FDG-PET/CT has been increasingly used in bone and soft tissue sarcomas and provides advantages in the initial tumor staging, tumor grading, therapy assessment, and recurrence detection in these tumors. FDG-PET/CT metabolic parameters are reliable predictors of survival in sarcomas and could be implemented in risk stratification models along with other prognostic factors in these patients.

REFERENCES

1. Kasper B, Hohenberger P, Strauss LG, et al. The use of fluorine-18 fluorodeoxyglycose-positron emission tomography for treatment monitoring in patients with soft tissue sarcomas. Hell J Nucl Med 2010;13:40–4.

2. Tewfik JN, Greene GS. Fluorine-18-deoxyglucose-positron emission tomography imaging with magnetic resonance and computed tomographic correlation in the evaluation of bone and soft-tissue sarcomas: a pictorial essay. Curr Probl Diagn Radiol 2008;37:178–88.

3. Available at: http://www.cancer.gov. Accessed April 2015.

4. Choi YY, Kim JY, Yang SO. PET/CT in benign and malignant musculoskeletal tumors and tumor-like conditions. Semin Musculoskelet Radiol 2014;18:133–48.

5. Quak E, van de Luijtgaarden AC, de Geus-Oei LF, et al. Clinical applications of positron emission tomography in sarcoma management. Expert Rev Anticancer Ther 2011;11:195–204.

6. Paidpally V, Chirindel A, Lam S, et al. FDG-PET/CT imaging biomarkers in head and neck squamous cell carcinoma. Imaging Med 2012;4:633–47.

7. Hadiprodjo D, Ryan T, Truong MT, et al. Parotid gland tumors: preliminary data for the value of FDG PET/CT diagnostic parameters. AJR Am J Roentgenol 2012;198:W185–90.

8. Agarwal A, Chirindel A, Shah BA, et al. Evolving role of FDG PET/CT in multiple myeloma imaging and management. AJR Am J Roentgenol 2013;200:884–90.

9. Jackson T, Chung MK, Mercier G, et al. FDG PET/CT interobserver agreement in head and neck cancer: FDG and CT measurements of the primary tumor site. Nucl Med Commun 2012;33:305–12.

10. Davison JM, Subramaniam RM, Surasi DS, et al. FDG PET/CT in patients with HIV. AJR Am J Roentgenol 2011;197:284–94.

11. Tahari AK, Alluri KC, Quon H, et al. FDG PET/CT imaging of oropharyngeal squamous cell carcinoma: characteristics of human papillomavirus-positive and -negative tumors. Clin Nucl Med 2014;39:225–31.

12. Shah B, Srivastava N, Hirsch AE, et al. Intra-reader reliability of FDG PET volumetric tumor parameters: effects of primary tumor size and segmentation methods. Ann Nucl Med 2012;26:707–14.

13. Paidpally V, Tahari AK, Lam S, et al. Addition of 18F-FDG PET/CT to clinical assessment predicts overall survival in HNSCC: a retrospective analysis with follow-up for 12 years. J Nucl Med 2013;54:2039–45.

14. Marcus C, Ciarallo A, Tahari AK, et al. Head and neck PET/CT: therapy response interpretation criteria (Hopkins criteria)–interreader reliability, accuracy, and survival outcomes. J Nucl Med 2014;55:1411–6.

15. Antoniou AJ, Marcus C, Tahari AK, et al. Follow-up or surveillance 18F-FDG PET/CT and survival outcome in lung cancer patients. J Nucl Med 2014;55:1062–8.

16. Sridhar P, Mercier G, Tan J, et al. FDG PET metabolic tumor volume segmentation and pathologic volume of primary human solid tumors. AJR Am J Roentgenol 2014;202:1114–9.

17. Marcus C, Paidpally V, Antoniou A, et al. 18F-FDG PET/CT and lung cancer: value of fourth and subsequent posttherapy follow-up scans for patient management. J Nucl Med 2015;56:204–8.

18. Karantanis D, Kalkanis D, Czernin J, et al. Perceived misinterpretation rates in oncologic 18F-FDG PET/CT studies: a survey of referring physicians. J Nucl Med 2014;55:1925–9.

19. Costelloe CM, Chuang HH, Madewell JE. FDG PET/CT of primary bone tumors. AJR Am J Roentgenol 2014;202:W521–31.

20. Schuetze SM. Utility of positron emission tomography in sarcomas. Curr Opin Oncol 2006;18:369–73.

21. Benz MR, Tchekmedyian N, Eilber FC, et al. Utilization of positron emission tomography in the management of patients with sarcoma. Curr Opin Oncol 2009;21:345–51.

22. Garner HW, Kransdorf MJ, Peterson JJ. Posttherapy imaging of musculoskeletal neoplasms. Radiol Clin North Am 2011;49:1307–23, vii.

23. Volker T, Denecke T, Steffen I, et al. Positron emission tomography for staging of pediatric sarcoma patients: results of a prospective multicenter trial. J Clin Oncol 2007;25:5435–41.

24. Bastiaannet E, Groen H, Jager PL, et al. The value of FDG-PET in the detection, grading and response to therapy of soft tissue and bone sarcomas; a systematic review and meta-analysis. Cancer Treat Rev 2004;30:83–101.

25. Folpe AL, Lyles RH, Sprouse JT, et al. (F-18) Fluorodeoxyglucose positron emission tomography as a predictor of pathologic grade and other prognostic variables in bone and soft tissue sarcoma. Clin Cancer Res 2000;6:1279–87.

26. Peterson JJ. F-18 FDG-PET for detection of osseous metastatic disease and staging, restaging, and monitoring response to therapy of musculoskeletal tumors. Semin Musculoskelet Radiol 2007;11:246–60.

27. Evilevitch V, Weber WA, Tap WD, et al. Reduction of glucose metabolic activity is more accurate than change in size at predicting histopathologic response to neoadjuvant therapy in high-grade soft-tissue sarcomas. Clin Cancer Res 2008;14:715–20.

28. Jaffe CC. Response assessment in clinical trials: implications for sarcoma clinical trial design. Oncologist 2008;13:14–8.

29. Van den Abbeele AD. The lessons of GIST-PET and PET/CT: a new paradigm for imaging. Oncologist 2008;13:8–13.

30. Grimer R, Athanasou N, Gerrand C, et al. UK guidelines for the management of bone sarcomas. Sarcoma 2010;2010:317462.

31. Rakheja R, Makis W, Tulbah R, et al. Necrosis on FDG PET/CT correlates with prognosis and mortality in sarcomas. AJR Am J Roentgenol 2013;201:170–7.

32. Eary JF, Conrad EU, O'Sullivan J, et al. Sarcoma mid-therapy [F-18]fluorodeoxyglucose positron emission tomography (FDG PET) and patient outcome. J Bone Joint Surg Am 2014;96:152–8.

33. Choi ES, Ha SG, Kim HS, et al. Total lesion glycolysis by 18F-FDG PET/CT is a reliable predictor of prognosis in soft-tissue sarcoma. Eur J Nucl Med Mol Imaging 2013;40:1836–42.

34. Hong SP, Lee SE, Choi YL, et al. Prognostic value of 18F-FDG PET/CT in patients with soft tissue sarcoma: comparisons between metabolic parameters. Skeletal Radiol 2014;43:641–8.

35. Schuetze SM, Rubin BP, Vernon C, et al. Use of positron emission tomography in localized extremity soft tissue sarcoma treated with neoadjuvant chemotherapy. Cancer 2005;103:339–48.

36. Fox MG, Trotta BM. Osteosarcoma: review of the various types with emphasis on recent advancements in imaging. Semin Musculoskelet Radiol 2013;17:123–36.

37. Brenner W, Bohuslavizki KH, Eary JF. PET imaging of osteosarcoma. J Nucl Med 2003;44:930–42.

38. Kong CB, Byun BH, Lim I, et al. (1)(8)F-FDG PET SUVmax as an indicator of histopathologic response after neoadjuvant chemotherapy in extremity osteosarcoma. Eur J Nucl Med Mol Imaging 2013;40:728–36.

39. Hongtao L, Hui Z, Bingshun W, et al. 18F-FDG positron emission tomography for the assessment of histological response to neoadjuvant chemotherapy in osteosarcomas: a meta-analysis. Surg Oncol 2012;21:e165–70.

40. Byun BH, Kong CB, Park J, et al. Initial metabolic tumor volume measured by 18F-FDG PET/CT can predict the outcome of osteosarcoma of the extremities. J Nucl Med 2013;54:1725–32.

41. Rakheja R, Makis W, Skamene S, et al. Correlating metabolic activity on 18F-FDG PET/CT with histopathologic characteristics of osseous and soft-tissue sarcomas: a retrospective review of 136 patients. AJR Am J Roentgenol 2012;198:1409–16.

42. Schulte M, Brecht-Krauss D, Heymer B, et al. Grading of tumors and tumorlike lesions of bone: evaluation by FDG PET. J Nucl Med 2000;41:1695–701.

43. ESMO/European Sarcoma Network Working Group. Bone sarcomas: ESMO clinical practice guidelines for diagnosis, treatment and follow-up. Ann Oncol 2014;25(Suppl 3):iii113–23.

44. Adler LP, Blair HF, Williams RP, et al. Grading liposarcomas with PET using [18F]FDG. J Comput Assist Tomogr 1990;14:960–2.

45. Nair N, Ali A, Green AA, et al. Response of osteosarcoma to chemotherapy. Evaluation with F-18 FDG-PET scans. Clin Positron Imaging 2000;3:79–83.

46. Cheon GJ, Kim MS, Lee JA, et al. Prediction model of chemotherapy response in osteosarcoma by 18F-FDG PET and MRI. J Nucl Med 2009;50: 1435–40.

47. Bajpai J, Kumar R, Sreenivas V, et al. Prediction of chemotherapy response by PET-CT in osteosarcoma: correlation with histologic necrosis. J Pediatr Hematol Oncol 2011;33:e271–8.

48. Im HJ, Kim TS, Park SY, et al. Prediction of tumour necrosis fractions using metabolic and volumetric 18F-FDG PET/CT indices, after one course and at the completion of neoadjuvant chemotherapy, in children and young adults with osteosarcoma. Eur J Nucl Med Mol Imaging 2012;39:39–49.

49. Chang KJ, Kong CB, Cho WH, et al. Usefulness of increased F-FDG uptake for detecting local recurrence in patients with extremity osteosarcoma treated with surgical resection and endoprosthetic replacement. Skeletal Radiol 2014;44:529–37.

50. Hawkins DS, Rajendran JG, Conrad EU 3rd, et al. Evaluation of chemotherapy response in pediatric bone sarcomas by [F-18]-fluorodeoxy-D-glucose positron emission tomography. Cancer 2002;94: 3277–84.

51. Ye Z, Zhu J, Tian M, et al. Response of osteogenic sarcoma to neoadjuvant therapy: evaluated by 18F-FDG-PET. Ann Nucl Med 2008;22:475–80.

52. Hamada K, Tomita Y, Inoue A, et al. Evaluation of chemotherapy response in osteosarcoma with FDG-PET. Ann Nucl Med 2009;23:89–95.

53. Denecke T, Hundsdorfer P, Misch D, et al. Assessment of histological response of paediatric bone sarcomas using FDG PET in comparison to morphological volume measurement and standardized MRI parameters. Eur J Nucl Med Mol Imaging 2010;37:1842–53.

54. Gaston LL, Di Bella C, Slavin J, et al. 18F-FDG PET response to neoadjuvant chemotherapy for Ewing sarcoma and osteosarcoma are different. Skeletal Radiol 2011;40:1007–15.

55. Byun BH, Kong CB, Lim I, et al. Early response monitoring to neoadjuvant chemotherapy in osteosarcoma using sequential (1)(8)F-FDG PET/CT and MRI. Eur J Nucl Med Mol Imaging 2014;41: 1553–62.

56. Byun BH, Kong CB, Lim I, et al. Comparison of (18) F-FDG PET/CT and (99 m)Tc-MDP bone scintigraphy for detection of bone metastasis in osteosarcoma. Skeletal Radiol 2013;42:1673–81.

57. Quartuccio N, Fox J, Kuk D, et al. Pediatric bone sarcoma: diagnostic performance of (18)F-FDG PET/CT versus conventional imaging for initial staging and follow-up. AJR Am J Roentgenol 2015;204: 153–60.

58. Treglia G, Salsano M, Stefanelli A, et al. Diagnostic accuracy of (1)(8)F-FDG-PET and PET/CT in patients with Ewing sarcoma family tumours: a systematic review and a meta-analysis. Skeletal Radiol 2012;41:249–56.

59. Martin RC 2nd, Brennan MF. Adult soft tissue Ewing sarcoma or primitive neuroectodermal tumors: predictors of survival? Arch Surg 2003; 138:281–5.

60. Bernstein M, Kovar H, Paulussen M, et al. Ewing's sarcoma family of tumors: current management. Oncologist 2006;11:503–19.

61. Franzius C, Sciuk J, Daldrup-Link HE, et al. FDG-PET for detection of osseous metastases from malignant primary bone tumours: comparison with bone scintigraphy. Eur J Nucl Med 2000;27:1305–11.

62. Gyorke T, Zajic T, Lange A, et al. Impact of FDG PET for staging of Ewing sarcomas and primitive neuroectodermal tumours. Nucl Med Commun 2006;27:17–24.

63. Gerth HU, Juergens KU, Dirksen U, et al. Significant benefit of multimodal imaging: PET/CT compared with PET alone in staging and follow-up of patients with Ewing tumors. J Nucl Med 2007;48:1932–9.

64. Kleis M, Daldrup-Link H, Matthay K, et al. Diagnostic value of PET/CT for the staging and restaging of pediatric tumors. Eur J Nucl Med Mol Imaging 2009;36:23–36.

65. Charest M, Hickeson M, Lisbona R, et al. FDG PET/CT imaging in primary osseous and soft tissue sarcomas: a retrospective review of 212 cases. Eur J Nucl Med Mol Imaging 2009;36:1944–51.

66. Mody RJ, Bui C, Hutchinson RJ, et al. FDG PET imaging of childhood sarcomas. Pediatr Blood Cancer 2010;54:222–7.

67. Sharma P, Khangembam BC, Suman KC, et al. Diagnostic accuracy of 18F-FDG PET/CT for detecting recurrence in patients with primary skeletal Ewing sarcoma. Eur J Nucl Med Mol Imaging 2013; 40:1036–43.

68. Daldrup-Link HE, Franzius C, Link TM, et al. Whole-body MR imaging for detection of bone metastases in children and young adults: comparison with skeletal scintigraphy and FDG PET. AJR Am J Roentgenol 2001;177:229–36.

69. Franzius C, Daldrup-Link HE, Sciuk J, et al. FDG-PET for detection of pulmonary metastases from malignant primary bone tumors: comparison with spiral CT. Ann Oncol 2001;12:479–86.

70. Aoki J, Watanabe H, Shinozaki T, et al. FDG-PET in differential diagnosis and grading of chondrosarcomas. J Comput Assist Tomogr 1999;23:603–8.

71. Brenner W, Conrad EU, Eary JF. FDG PET imaging for grading and prediction of outcome in chondrosarcoma patients. Eur J Nucl Med Mol Imaging 2004;31:189–95.

72. Feldman F, Van Heertum R, Saxena C, et al. 18FDG-PET applications for cartilage neoplasms. Skeletal Radiol 2005;34:367–74.

73. Feldman F, Vanheertum R, Saxena C. 18Fluoro-deoxyglucose positron emission tomography evaluation of benign versus malignant osteochondromas: preliminary observations. J Comput Assist Tomogr 2006;30:858–64.

74. Purandare NC, Rangarajan V, Agarwal M, et al. Integrated PET/CT in evaluating sarcomatous transformation in osteochondromas. Clin Nucl Med 2009;34:350–4.

75. Stacchiotti S, Dagrada GP, Morosi C, et al. Extraskeletal myxoid chondrosarcoma: tumor response to sunitinib. Clin Sarcoma Res 2012;2:22.

76. Stacchiotti S, Pantaleo MA, Astolfi A, et al. Activity of sunitinib in extraskeletal myxoid chondrosarcoma. Eur J Cancer 2014;50:1657–64.

77. Bradshaw TJ, Yip S, Jallow N, et al. Spatiotemporal stability of Cu-ATSM and FLT positron emission tomography distributions during radiation therapy. Int J Radiat Oncol Biol Phys 2014;89:399–405.

78. Leung TK, Chen CH, Lai CH, et al. Bone and joint protection ability of ceramic material with biological effects. Chin J Physiol 2012;55:47–54.

79. Purohit BS, Dulguerov P, Burkhardt K, et al. Dedifferentiated laryngeal chondrosarcoma: combined morphologic and functional imaging with positron-emission tomography/magnetic resonance imaging. Laryngoscope 2014;124:E274–7.

80. Klem ML, Grewal RK, Wexler LH, et al. PET for staging in rhabdomyosarcoma: an evaluation of PET as an adjunct to current staging tools. J Pediatr Hematol Oncol 2007;29:9–14.

81. McLean TW, Buckley KS. Pediatric genitourinary tumors. Curr Opin Oncol 2010;22:268–73.

82. Roberge D, Vakilian S, Alabed YZ, et al. FDG PET/CT in initial staging of adult soft-tissue sarcoma. Sarcoma 2012;2012:960194.

83. Tateishi U, Hosono A, Makimoto A, et al. Comparative study of FDG PET/CT and conventional imaging in the staging of rhabdomyosarcoma. Ann Nucl Med 2009;23:155–61.

84. Suman KC, Sharma P, Singh H, et al. Primary rhabdomyosarcoma of pulmonary artery: 18F-FDG PET/CT for detecting recurrence in a rare tumor. Clin Nucl Med 2013;38:e155–6.

85. Roberge D, Hickeson M, Charest M, et al. Initial McGill experience with fluorodeoxyglucose PET/CT staging of soft-tissue sarcoma. Curr Oncol 2010;17:18–22.

86. Norman G, Fayter D, Lewis-Light K, et al. An emerging evidence base for PET-CT in the management of childhood rhabdomyosarcoma: systematic review. BMJ Open 2015;5:e006030.

87. De Wit M, Raabe A, Seegers B, et al. Time benefit in the assessment of recurrences following fractionated radiotherapy in an experimental tumour system using positron-emission tomography with 18F-fluorodeoxyglucose. Int J Radiat Biol 2004;80:529–39.

88. Raabe A, Buchert R, Seegers B, et al. Potential time benefit in the assessment of recurrent rat rhabdomyosarcoma using positron emission tomography (PET) with (18)fluorodeoxyglucose depends on therapy-specific growth delay. Strahlenther Onkol 2006;182:610–5.

89. Peng F, Rabkin G, Muzik O. Use of 2-deoxy-2-[F-18]-fluoro-D-glucose positron emission tomography to monitor therapeutic response by rhabdomyosarcoma in children: report of a retrospective case study. Clin Nucl Med 2006;31:394–7.

90. Arush MW, Israel O, Postovsky S, et al. Positron emission tomography/computed tomography with 18fluoro-deoxyglucose in the detection of local recurrence and distant metastases of pediatric sarcoma. Pediatr Blood Cancer 2007;49:901–5.

91. Rommel D, Abarca-Quinones J, Bol A, et al. Early monitoring of external radiation therapy by [18F]-fluoromethylcholine positron emission tomography and 3-T proton magnetic resonance spectroscopy: an experimental study in a rodent rhabdomyosarcoma model. Nucl Med Biol 2010;37:645–53.

92. Dharmarajan KV, Wexler LH, Gavane S, et al. Positron emission tomography (PET) evaluation after initial chemotherapy and radiation therapy predicts local control in rhabdomyosarcoma. Int J Radiat Oncol Biol Phys 2012;84:996–1002.

93. Kern KA, Brunetti A, Norton JA, et al. Metabolic imaging of human extremity musculoskeletal tumors by PET. J Nucl Med 1988;29:181–6.

94. Nieweg OE, Pruim J, Hoekstra HJ, et al. Positron emission tomography with fluorine-18-fluorodeoxyglucose for the evaluation of therapeutic isolated regional limb perfusion in a patient with soft-tissue sarcoma. J Nucl Med 1994;35:90–2.

95. Kosuda S, Wahl RL, Grossman HB. Demonstration of recurrent dedifferentiated liposarcoma of the spermatic cord by FDG-PET. Ann Nucl Med 1997;11:263–6.

96. Kole AC, Nieweg OE, van Ginkel RJ, et al. Detection of local recurrence of soft-tissue sarcoma with positron emission tomography using [18F]fluorodeoxyglucose. Ann Surg Oncol 1997;4:57–63.

97. Jadvar H, Fischman AJ. Evaluation of rare tumors with [F-18]fluorodeoxyglucose positron emission tomography. Clin Positron Imaging 1999;2:153–8.

98. Conill C, Setoain X, Colomo L, et al. Diagnostic efficacy of bone scintigraphy, magnetic resonance imaging, and positron emission tomography in bone metastases of myxoid liposarcoma. J Magn Reson Imaging 2008;27:625–8.

99. Kudo H, Inaoka T, Tokuyama W, et al. Round cell liposarcoma arising in the left foot: MRI and PET findings. Jpn J Radiol 2012;30:852–7.

100. Ozguven S, Aras M, Inanir S. Mesenteric metastases of purely myxoid liposarcoma: an unusual behavior of primary tumor depicted on fludeoxyglucose positron emission tomography/computerized tomography. Indian J Nucl Med 2015;30: 82–3.

101. Reddy MP, Sangster GP, Takalkar AM, et al. Accurate grading of 3 synchronous liposarcomas assessed by PET-CT in a single patient. Clin Nucl Med 2007;32:937–9.

102. Okazumi S, Dimitrakopoulou-Strauss A, Schwarzbach MH, et al. Quantitative, dynamic 18F-FDG-PET for the evaluation of soft tissue sarcomas: relation to differential diagnosis, tumor grading and prediction of prognosis. Hell J Nucl Med 2009;12:223–8.

103. Brenner W, Eary JF, Hwang W, et al. Risk assessment in liposarcoma patients based on FDG PET imaging. Eur J Nucl Med Mol Imaging 2006;33: 1290–5.

104. Choi BH, Yoon SH, Lee S, et al. Primary malignant fibrous histiocytoma in mediastinum: imaging with (18)F-FDG PET/CT. Nucl Med Mol Imaging 2012; 46:304–7.

105. Hwang SS, Park SY, Park YH. The CT and F-FDG PET/CT appearance of primary renal malignant fibrous histiocytoma. J Med Imaging Radiat Oncol 2010;54:365–7.

106. Zheng W, Chen J, Liu J, et al. FDG PET/CT findings of malignant fibrous histiocytoma of the stomach. Clin Nucl Med 2014. http://dx.doi.org/10.1097/rlu. 0000000000000610. [Epub ahead of print].

107. Dong A, Gong J, Wang Y, et al. MRI and FDG PET/CT findings of malignant fibrous histiocytoma of the prostate. Clin Nucl Med 2014;39:889–91.

108. Noh HW, Park KJ, Sun JS, et al. Primary pulmonary malignant fibrous histiocytoma mimics pulmonary artery aneurysm with partial thrombosis: various radiologic evaluations. Eur Radiol 2008;18:1653–7.

109. Ho L, Meka M, Gamble BK, et al. Left maxillary sinus malignant fibrous histiocytoma on FDG PET-CT. Clin Nucl Med 2009;34:967–8.

110. Kobayashi E, Kawai A, Seki K, et al. Bilateral adrenal gland metastasis from malignant fibrous histiocytoma: value of [F-18]FDG PET-CT for diagnosis of occult metastases. Ann Nucl Med 2006;20: 695–8.

111. Treglia G, Mirk P, Stefanelli A, et al. 18F-Fluorodeoxyglucose positron emission tomography in evaluating treatment response to imatinib or other drugs in gastrointestinal stromal tumors: a systematic review. Clin Imaging 2012;36:167–75.

112. King DM. The radiology of gastrointestinal stromal tumours (GIST). Cancer Imaging 2005;5:150–6.

113. Yamada M, Niwa Y, Matsuura T, et al. Gastric GIST malignancy evaluated by 18FDG-PET as compared with EUS-FNA and endoscopic biopsy. Scand J Gastroenterol 2007;42:633–41.

114. Gayed I, Vu T, Iyer R, et al. The role of 18F-FDG PET in staging and early prediction of response to therapy of recurrent gastrointestinal stromal tumors. J Nucl Med 2004;45:17–21.

115. Kaneta T, Takahashi S, Fukuda H, et al. Clinical significance of performing 18F-FDG PET on patients with gastrointestinal stromal tumors: a summary of a Japanese multicenter study. Ann Nucl Med 2009;23:459–64.

116. Otomi Y, Otsuka H, Morita N, et al. Relationship between FDG uptake and the pathological risk category in gastrointestinal stromal tumors. J Med Invest 2010;57:270–4.

117. Koch MR, Jagannathan JP, Shinagare AB, et al. Imaging features of primary anorectal gastrointestinal stromal tumors with clinical and pathologic correlation. Cancer Imaging 2013;12:557–65.

118. Yoshikawa K, Shimada M, Kurita N, et al. Efficacy of PET-CT for predicting the malignant potential of gastrointestinal stromal tumors. Surg Today 2013; 43:1162–7.

119. Winant AJ, Gollub MJ, Shia J, et al. Imaging and clinicopathologic features of esophageal gastrointestinal stromal tumors. AJR Am J Roentgenol 2014;203:306–14.

120. Evangelista L, Cervino AR, Gregianin M, et al. FDG-PET/CT visualises a case of primary hyperparathyroidism in patient with GIST. Minerva Endocrinol 2010;35:193–5.

121. Demetri GD, von Mehren M, Blanke CD, et al. Efficacy and safety of imatinib mesylate in advanced gastrointestinal stromal tumors. N Engl J Med 2002;347:472–80.

122. Fuster D, Ayuso JR, Poveda A, et al. Value of FDG-PET for monitoring treatment response in patients with advanced GIST refractory to high-dose imatinib. A multicenter GEIS study. Q J Nucl Med Mol Imaging 2011;55:680–7.

123. van Oosterom AT, Judson I, Verweij J, et al. Safety and efficacy of imatinib (STI571) in metastatic gastrointestinal stromal tumours: a phase I study. Lancet 2001;358:1421–3.

124. Antoch G, Kanja J, Bauer S, et al. Comparison of PET, CT, and dual-modality PET/CT imaging for monitoring of imatinib (STI571) therapy in patients with gastrointestinal stromal tumors. J Nucl Med 2004;45:357–65.

125. Choi H, Charnsangavej C, de Castro Faria S, et al. CT evaluation of the response of gastrointestinal stromal tumors after imatinib mesylate treatment: a quantitative analysis correlated with FDG PET findings. AJR Am J Roentgenol 2004;183: 1619–28.

126. Jager PL, Gietema JA, van der Graaf WT. Imatinib mesylate for the treatment of gastrointestinal stromal tumours: best monitored with FDG PET. Nucl Med Commun 2004;25:433–8.

127. Goerres GW, Stupp R, Barghouth G, et al. The value of PET, CT and in-line PET/CT in patients with gastrointestinal stromal tumours: long-term outcome of treatment with imatinib mesylate. Eur J Nucl Med Mol Imaging 2005;32:153–62.

128. Goldstein D, Tan BS, Rossleigh M, et al. Gastrointestinal stromal tumours: correlation of F-FDG gamma camera-based coincidence positron emission tomography with CT for the assessment of treatment response–an AGITG study. Oncology 2005;69:326–32.

129. Holdsworth CH, Badawi RD, Manola JB, et al. CT and PET: early prognostic indicators of response to imatinib mesylate in patients with gastrointestinal stromal tumor. AJR Am J Roentgenol 2007;189: W324–30.

130. Demetri GD, Heinrich MC, Fletcher JA, et al. Molecular target modulation, imaging, and clinical evaluation of gastrointestinal stromal tumor patients treated with sunitinib malate after imatinib failure. Clin Cancer Res 2009;15:5902–9.

131. Prior JO, Montemurro M, Orcurto MV, et al. Early prediction of response to sunitinib after imatinib failure by 18F-fluorodeoxyglucose positron emission tomography in patients with gastrointestinal stromal tumor. J Clin Oncol 2009;27:439–45.

132. Maurel J, Martins AS, Poveda A, et al. Imatinib plus low-dose doxorubicin in patients with advanced gastrointestinal stromal tumors refractory to high-dose imatinib: a phase I-II study by the Spanish group for research on sarcomas. Cancer 2010; 116:3692–701.

133. Stroobants S, Goeminne J, Seegers M, et al. 18FDG-Positron emission tomography for the early prediction of response in advanced soft tissue sarcoma treated with imatinib mesylate (Glivec). Eur J Cancer 2003;39:2012–20.

134. Gelibter A, Milella M, Ceribelli A, et al. PET scanning evaluation of response to imatinib mesylate therapy in gastrointestinal stromal tumor (GIST) patients. Anticancer Res 2004;24:3147–51.

135. Zaknun JJ, Kendler D, Moncayo R, et al. F-18 FDG PET for assessing tyrosine kinase-related signal transduction inhibition in a GIST c-kit-positive tumor patient by imatinib. Clin Nucl Med 2005;30:749–51.

136. Bauer S, Hilger RA, Muhlenberg T, et al. Phase I study of panobinostat and imatinib in patients with treatment-refractory metastatic gastrointestinal stromal tumors. Br J Cancer 2014;110:1155–62.

137. Judson I, Scurr M, Gardner K, et al. Phase II study of cediranib in patients with advanced gastrointestinal stromal tumors or soft-tissue sarcoma. Clin Cancer Res 2014;20:3603–12.

138. Wagner AJ, Chugh R, Rosen LS, et al. A phase I study of the HSP90 inhibitor retaspimycin hydrochloride (IPI-504) in patients with gastrointestinal stromal tumors or soft-tissue sarcomas. Clin Cancer Res 2013;19:6020–9.

139. Ronellenfitsch U, Wangler B, Niedermoser S, et al. Importance of PET for surgery of gastrointestinal stromal tumors. Chirurg 2014;85:493–9 [in German].

140. Valls-Ferrusola E, Garcia-Garzon JR, Ponce-Lopez A, et al. Patterns of extension of gastrointestinal stromal tumors (GIST) treated with imatinib (Gleevec(R)) by 18F-FDG PET/CT. Rev Esp Enferm Dig 2012;104:360–6.

141. Tokumoto N, Tanabe K, Misumi T, et al. The usefulness of preoperative 18FDG positron-emission tomography and computed tomography for predicting the malignant potential of gastrointestinal stromal tumors. Dig Surg 2014;31:79–86.

142. Williams A, Gutzeit A, Germer M, et al. PET-negative gastrointestinal stromal tumors. Case Rep Oncol 2013;6:508–13.

143. Dietrich C, Hartung E, Ignee A. The use of contrast-enhanced ultrasound in patients with GIST metastases that are negative in CT and PET. Ultraschall Med 2008;29:276–7.

144. Bertagna F, Bosio G, Orlando E, et al. Role of F-18-FDG-PET/CT in restaging of patients affected by gastrointestinal stromal tumours (GIST). Nucl Med Rev Cent East Eur 2010;13:76–80.

145. Hahn S, Bauer S, Heusner TA, et al. Postoperative FDG-PET/CT staging in GIST: is there a benefit following R0 resection? Eur J Radiol 2011;80: 670–4.

Fludeoxyglucose F 18 PET–Computed Tomography

Management Changes Effecting Patient Outcomes in Gynecologic Malignancies

Jacqueline C. Brunetti, MD[a,b],*

KEYWORDS

- [18]F FDG PET • PET-CT • Ovarian cancer • Cervical cancer • Endometrial cancer

KEY POINTS

- The treatment and follow-up of patients with cervical cancer is significantly affected by the use of F 18 fluorodeoxyglucose (^{18}F FDG) PET–computed tomography (CT) in initial staging, treatment planning, and monitoring therapy response.
- The prognostic information gleaned from primary lesion maximum standardized uptake value (SUVmax), metabolic tumor volume (MTV), and extent of para-aortic nodal metastatic disease may play a critical role in tailoring therapy based on patient tumor-specific factors rather than on International Federation of Gynecology and Obstetrics (FIGO) stage alone.
- [18]F FDG PET-CT imaging posttreatment provides accurate information regarding tumor response and valuable prognostic information that might direct more aggressive therapy or allow a more confident decision to choose palliation rather than cure.

INTRODUCTION

Overexpression of glucose transporter-1 (GLUT-1) in cancer cells resulting in increased transmembrane intracellular transport of glucose is the basis of deposition of ^{18}F FDG in primary and metastatic neoplastic lesions. The accuracy in tumor detection with ^{18}F FDG depends on the degree of GLUT-1 aberration, tumor size, cellular density, and mitotic rate. [18]F FDG PET-CT has been demonstrated to effect changes in patient management by improving detection of locoregional and distant metastases in tumors with increased glycolytic phenotype. Cervical, endometrial, and ovarian malignancies are such tumors. Although there are specific patterns on PET-CT that can favor a diagnosis of gynecologic malignancy, the value of this modality lies not in screening or initial diagnosis but in gains in accuracy in detection of metastatic disease and recurrent tumor. The possible roles imaging may play in influencing patient outcomes include facilitating early diagnosis, thus increasing likelihood of cure; improving accuracy in initial staging, thereby aiding optimal treatment choice; early detection of recurrent disease that allows initiation of potentially effective therapies; and diagnosis of widespread advanced disease that may lead to palliative rather than costly, futile treatment.

The author has nothing to disclose.
[a] Department of Radiology, Holy Name Medical Center, 718 Teaneck Road, Teaneck, NJ 07666, USA;
[b] Department of Radiology, Columbia University Medical Center, 622 W 168th Street, New York, NY 10032, USA
* Department of Radiology, Holy Name Medical Center, 718 Teaneck Road, Teaneck, NJ 07666.
E-mail address: brunetti@mail.holyname.org

PET Clin 10 (2015) 395–409
http://dx.doi.org/10.1016/j.cpet.2015.03.010
1556-8598/15/$ – see front matter © 2015 Elsevier Inc. All rights reserved.

This article reviews current accepted practice standards for patient management in endometrial, ovarian, and cervical cancer, with emphasis on therapeutic impact of ^{18}F FDG PET-CT in tumor staging, treatment monitoring, and detection of recurrent disease.

ENDOMETRIAL CANCER

Endometrial cancer is the most common gynecologic malignancy. For the year 2014, The National Cancer Institute projects 52,630 new diagnoses and 8590 deaths. Tumors are most frequent in the postmenopausal age group, although 20% to 25% may be detected before menopause. Postmenopausal vaginal bleeding is the most frequent presenting symptom and results in most patients being diagnosed at early stage. Risk factors include unopposed estrogen exposure, obesity, nulliparity, hereditary nonpolyposis colorectal cancer, tamoxifen therapy, diabetes, and high-fat diet. Two histologic classes have been identified. Type 1 cancers are hormonally driven, endometrioid cell type, arise in hyperplastic endometrium, present early with low grade, and have a low risk of recurrence. Type 2 tumors are of the less differentiated, clear-cell, or high-grade endometrioid type; present in atrophic endometrium; and are more frequently diagnosed at a later stage. Patients who present with type 2 lesions are at greater risk for recurrence. Endometrial cancer is surgically staged, and treatment is tailored to estimation of risk of recurrence based on histologic grade, degree of myometrial invasion, involvement of the cervix, lymphovascular invasion, and patient age (**Table 1**). Imaging is reserved for patients with physical examination findings suggesting extrauterine disease. Presence of metastatic adenopathy alters therapy and prognosis, and the risk of nodal metastases increases with the degree of myometrial invasion, tumor size, and the degree of histologic dedifferentiation. Surgery and adjuvant radiotherapy is effective for stage I and II cancers, with the alternative or additional administration of chemotherapy in high-risk patients. Despite adequate therapy, in approximately 15% of patients with stage I and II disease, there is recurrence, typically within 3 years of diagnosis.[1] Owing to lack of data indicating change in patient survival, the National Comprehensive Cancer Network (NCCN) guidelines for posttherapy surveillance do not recommend serial imaging but rather, periodic physical examinations and monitoring of onset of new symptoms. Patients who present with recurrent disease have a poor prognosis, as there are limited treatment options for this group of patients.

Table 1 FIGO staging: endometrial cancer	
Stage	**Description**
I	Tumor confined to corpus uteri
IA	Tumor <50% myometrial invasion
IB	Invasion $\geq$50% of myometrium
II	Invasion of cervical stroma, not beyond the uterus
III	Local or regional tumor spread
IIIA	Invasion of serosa or adnexae
IIIB	Vaginal or parametrial invasion
IIIC	Pelvic or para-aortic nodal metastases
IIIC1	(+) Pelvic nodes
IIIC2	(+) Para-aortic nodes $\pm$ pelvic nodes
IV	Bladder or bowel invasion or distant metastases
IVA	Invasion of bladder and/or bowel mucosa
IVB	Distant metastasis, including abdominal and/or inguinal nodes

From Pecorelli S. Revised FIGO staging for carcinoma of the vulva, cervix, and endometrium. Int J Gynaecol Obstet 2009;105:104; with permission.

Fludeoxyglucose PET–Computed Tomography: Role in Management of Endometrial Cancer

Factors influencing patient prognosis that can be evaluated by imaging techniques include depth of myometrial invasion, extent of involvement of the lower uterine segment and cervix, presence of pelvic and para-aortic nodal metastases, and presence of distant metastatic disease. Although FIGO staging is based on surgical findings, continuing improvements in imaging technology and development of molecular targets might potentially improve staging accuracy. Endometrial cancer displays increased ^{18}F FDG uptake, which when seen in a postmenopausal woman should trigger further investigation, as malignancy is likely. The limited resolution of ^{18}F FDG PET prohibits accurate detection of the presence or degree of endometrial and cervical stromal invasion, and this is best evaluated by MR imaging.[2–4] The likelihood of pelvic nodal metastases increased with degree of myometrial invasion. The incidence of lymph node metastases is as low as 1% in patients diagnosed with early-stage endometrial cancer but up to 36% in patients with poorly differentiated, locally invasive tumors. Microscopic disease is not detected by any current imaging modality. The sensitivity and specificity of ^{18}F FDG PET in detection of pelvic lymph node metastases range from 53% to 78% and

95% to 100%, respectively.[5,6] A large-scale retrospective analysis published by the National Cancer Institute, Surveillance, Epidemiology, and End Results (SEER) concluded that lymphadenectomy is associated with a statistically significant increase in survival in patients with both advanced stage (5-year survival increased from 63% to 74%) and poorly differentiated stage 1 disease (5-year survival increased from 85% to 90%).[7] These data emphasize the critical importance of accurate initial staging. Although ^{18}F FDG PET-CT sensitivity is insufficient to forego surgical lymphadenectomy in most patients, the high specificity and a negative predictive value of up to 100% may allow a tailored approach in patients who are poor surgical candidates.[8–10]

There are conflicting data suggesting a relationship between ^{18}F FDG PET-CT SUVmax of the primary endometrial neoplasm and patient prognosis. Several researchers have suggested that increasing SUVmax and MTV is associated with more aggressive histologic grade and worse prognosis.[11–14] Sadlecki and colleagues[15] report that the level of hypoxia-inducible factor-1 α (HF-1 α) increases according to clinical stage and is significantly associated with type 2 neoplasias and poorer prognosis. The presence of HF-1 α changes the tumor microenvironment and drives GLUT-1 expression. The level of HF-1 α is increased in the endometrium during the secretory phase of the menstrual cycle, possibly explaining the presence of ^{18}F FDG uptake that is seen in premenopausal women.[16] These studies may lead to development of targeted therapies that could improve outcomes in patients with late-stage disease.

Early detection of recurrent disease may provide an opportunity for initiation of therapies that could potentially affect survival or quality of life (**Fig. 1**).

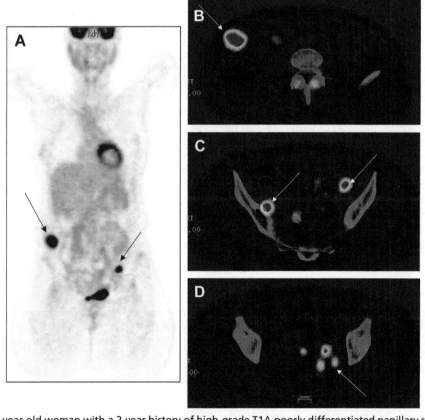

Fig. 1. A 61-year-old woman with a 2-year history of high-grade T1A poorly differentiated papillary serous endometrial carcinoma, status postlaparoscopic total abdominal hysterectomy with bilateral salpingo-oophorectomy and pelvic node dissection with initial pathology negative for parametrial, adnexal, and nodal metastases, treated, by choice, with only 3 courses of chemotherapy, presents with a mass in the abdominal wall and vaginal spotting. (*A*) Coronal ^{18}F FDG PET image reveals intense metabolic uptake in the right-side abdominal wall and left iliac nodal metastases (*arrows*). (*B*) Axial fused PET-CT image demonstrating the metastatic lesion in the right internal and external oblique muscles (*arrow*). (*C, D*) Axial fused PET-CT images reveal bilateral iliac nodal metastases and pelvic implants (*arrows*).

Based on only clinical assessment using physical examination, Pap smear, and serum tumor marker CA-125, metastatic disease is missed in up to approximately 70% of asymptomatic patients.[17] [18]F FDG PET-CT has been shown to provide better accuracy than CT and MR imaging, with reported high sensitivity (92%–100%) and specificity (88%–95%) in detection of recurrent disease in both symptomatic and asymptomatic patients with endometrial cancer (**Fig. 2**).[18–21] A potential scanning pitfall is detection of recurrent disease at the vaginal apex and vagina, and this region may be obscured by high activity within the bladder lumen. The combination of PET and CT images can facilitate identification of disease at this site by careful inspection of the anatomy in the surgical bed and comparison of findings with prior studies if available. Vaginal recurrences are the most frequent site of recurrent disease and can be successfully treated with a combination of brachytherapy and external beam radiation if diagnosed early (**Fig. 3**).[22]

Summary

Early diagnosis and therapy is the most critical factor in outcome for patients with endometrial cancer. [18]F FDG PET-CT can affect initial therapy in patients with advanced-stage malignancy by accurate detection of para-aortic lymph nodes or distant metastases. Initiation of treatment can be facilitated by early detection of recurrent disease in asymptomatic patients and may improve patient quality of life. Patients with recurrent, advanced disease, however, have limited treatment options and poor prognosis. Although higher ^{18}F FDG uptake in primary tumor is associated with poorer outcomes, the clinical value of SUVmax in determining prognosis is unclear.

OVARIAN CANCER

Epithelial ovarian cancer (EOC) is the second most common gynecologic malignancy and the most frequent cause of death in patients with gynecologic cancer. For the year 2014, the American Cancer Society estimates that 21,980 new cases of EOC will be diagnosed, with 14,270 deaths attributable to this disease. Ten percent of EOC is associated with an inherited genetic mutation, including breast-ovarian cancer syndrome (BRCA1, BRCA2) and Lynch syndrome type II (colorectal, ovarian, and endometrial). Ninety percent of EOC is sporadic. The poor survival of this malignancy is related to the lack of hallmark symptoms or accurate screening methods that result in up to 70% of patients being diagnosed with late-stage disease.[23] Patients present with nonspecific abdominal pain, bloating, increase in abdominal girth, increased urinary frequency, or other nonspecific complaint. Postmenopausal women who experience these symptoms for more than 3 weeks should be evaluated for possible ovarian pathology.

Ovarian cancer spreads along peritoneal and serosal surfaces and is not apparent on anatomic imaging until lesions are 5 mm or greater. Consequently, initial tumor staging is surgical and optimized primary cytoreductive surgery, that is, residual tumor less than 1 cm in diameter is associated with better survival (**Table 2**).[24] According to 2013 SEER statistics, for patients with disease limited to the ovary, the 5-year survival approaches 90%, whereas for patients presenting with advanced disease, survival rate at 5 years is 32% or less. NCCN guidelines version 3.2014 for primary treatment includes total abdominal hysterectomy with bilateral salpingo-oophorectomy with cytoreductive surgery for stages II to IV and neoadjuvant chemotherapy with platinum and taxanes

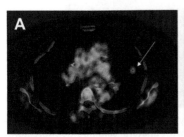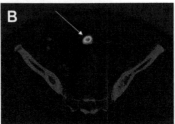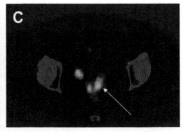

Fig. 2. A 64-year-old woman with a diagnosis of stage I grade 2, endometrioid adenocarcinoma, status post total abdominal hysterectomy with bilateral salpingo-oophorectomy. At diagnosis, the patient's tumor was 8 cm, extending to the lower uterine segment, and at the time of surgery, peritoneal washings were positive for tumor. The patient refused adjuvant therapy and missed follow-up oncology appointments. The following year, CA 125 was reported to be 645 U/mL and a PET-CT was ordered for restaging. (*A–C*) Fused axial PET-CT document pulmonary (*arrow*), mesenteric (*arrow*), and pelvic metastasis at the vaginal apex (*arrow*).

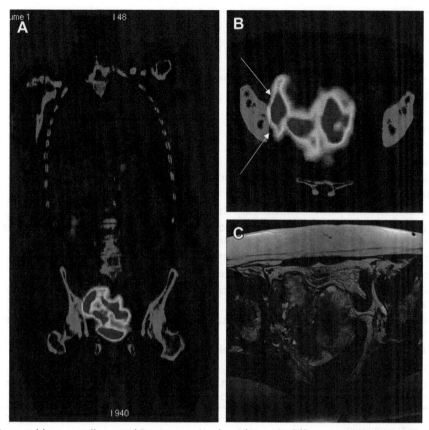

Fig. 3. A 71-year-old woman diagnosed 2 years previously with poorly differentiated endometrial cancer, status post total abdominal hysterectomy with bilateral salpingo-oophorectomy and 6 cycles of chemotherapy followed by pelvic external beam radiotherapy and brachytherapy. A CT scan, followed by pelvic MR imaging was performed for investigation of vague flank discomfort and nonspecific urinary symptoms. Discovery of a large pelvic mass prompted a restaging PET-CT. (*A*) Coronal fused PET-CT demonstrates intense metabolic uptake, with regions of photopenia in large pelvic mass. (*B*) Axial fused PET-CT images document extension of recurrent tumor to the right pelvic side wall (*arrows*). (*C*) T2 axial MR imaging for comparison reveals the complex nature of this mass and confirms invasion of the right pelvic side wall.

in patients with poor surgical risks. Prognosis is determined by tumor grade and cell type, tumor stage, volume of ascites, patient age, and amount of residual tumor after primary cytoreductive surgery.[25–27] Patients are monitored for 5 years, and surveillance includes serial physical examinations, serum tumor marker CA-125, and CT, MR imaging, or PET-CT when there is evidence of clinical relapse. Approximately 60% of patients have recurrence after primary therapy. In patients with platinum-sensitive disease, secondary cytoreductive surgery for recurrent tumor is associated with a significant improvement in overall survival (OS).[28,29]

Fludeoxyglucose PET–Computed Tomography: Role in Management of Ovarian Cancer

EOCs express GLUT-1 and therefore display varying degrees of ^{18}F FDG uptake based on tumor size and amount of solid components. Benign ovarian lesions such as endometriomas, thecomas, corpus luteum cysts, and serous cystadenomas also display increased ^{18}F FDG uptake.[30] The likelihood of malignant disease increases with increasing SUVmax. With a cut-off of 2.5 SUVmax, the sensitivity and specificity for detection of a malignant ovarian lesion is 80.6% to 82.4% and 76.9% to 94.6%.[31,32] The degree of GLUT-1 overexpression in EOC correlates with tumor proliferation and microvessel density and is associated with a poor prognosis and decreased likelihood of optimal cytoreduction.[33,34] Although primary ovarian neoplasm will display FDG uptake, overlap of patterns of metabolic uptake with benign lesions, variable sensitivity and specificity as well as costliness of the scan dictate that the procedure provides no additional value and has no role in diagnosis of ovarian cancer. Although ^{18}F FDG PET-CT is not a recommended imaging tool in

Table 2
FIGO staging: carcinoma of the ovary

Stage I: Tumor confined to ovaries	
IA	One ovary, capsule intact, no surface tumor. (−) washings
IB	Both ovaries and as IA
IC	One or both ovaries
IC1	Surgical spill
IC2	Capsule rupture or surface tumor
IC3	Malignant cells in ascites or washings
Stage II: Tumor in one or both ovaries with pelvic extension or primary peritoneal tumor	
IIA	Extension and/or implant on uterus and/or fallopian tubes
IIB	Extension to other pelvic intraperitoneal tissues
Stage III: One or both ovaries with cytologically or histologically confirmed spread to peritoneum outside pelvis and/or metastasis to retroperitoneal lymph nodes	
IIIA1	(+) Retroperitoneal nodes [IIIA1 (i) mets$\leq$10 mm/IIIA (ii) mets$\geq$10 mm]
IIIA2	Microscopic, extrapelvic peritoneal involvement $\pm$ retroperitoneal nodes
IIIB	Macroscopic, extrapelvic, peritoneal metastases $\leq$2 cm $\pm$ positive retroperitoneal nodes, includes capsule of liver and spleen
IIIC	Macroscopic, extrapelvic, peritoneal metastases >2 cm $\pm$ positive retroperitoneal nodes, includes capsule of liver and spleen
Stage IV: Distant metastases excluding peritoneal metastasis	
IVA	Pleural effusion with (+) cytology
IVB	Hepatic and/or splenic parenchymal metastasis, metastasis to extra-abdominal organs (includes inguinal nodes and extra-abdominal nodes)

From Prat J. Staging classification for cancer of the ovary, fallopian tube, and peritoneum. Int J Gynaecol Obstet 2014;124(1):2; with permission.

the initial staging of EOC, use of this modality in patients with advance-stage disease increases detection of extra-abdominal metastases and subsequent upstaging of disease.[35] Identification of the presence of pelvic and para-aortic nodal metastases improves staging accuracy of EOC, and the presence of para-aortic nodal metastases is associated with poorer 5-year survival.[36,37] The reported sensitivity, specificity, accuracy, positive predictive value, and negative predictive value of ^{18}F FDG PET-CT in the detection of nodal metastases is 83.3%, 98.2%, 95.6%, 90.9%, and 96.5%, respectively.[38] The high negative predictive value may allow avoidance of lymphadenectomy, which is associated with increased morbidity and cost.

The greatest value of ^{18}F FDG PET-CT lies in the high accuracy in the detection of residual disease after primary therapy and in the identification of recurrent disease in both symptomatic and asymptomatic patients (**Fig. 4**).[39] [18]F FDG PET-CT has higher accuracy than CA-125, CT, and MR imaging in the detection of metastatic disease.[40,41] Because of detection of disease not confirmed or identified on conventional imaging, including extra-abdominal and nodal sites, ^{18}F FDG PET-CT findings have been reported to lead to change in management in greater than 50% of

patients.[42–44] The high accuracy in detection of recurrent disease makes ^{18}F FDG PET-CT a useful tool for selection of patients who may benefit from secondary cytoreductive surgery.[45] Some centers use staging laparoscopy as part of treatment-selection protocols for patients with suspected recurrent EOC. [18]F FDG PET-CT and laparoscopy are complementary techniques, as ^{18}F FDG PET may detect disease in regions inaccessible to laparoscopy visualization resulting from abdominal adhesions (**Fig. 5**).[46,47] There are only limited data regarding the use of ^{18}F FDG PET-CT for monitoring response to neoadjuvant chemotherapy. A unified approach does not exist for determination of therapy response. With a post-treatment percentage change of SUV of 65%, Nishiyama and colleagues[48] achieved a sensitivity and specificity of 90% and 81.8%. Finally, a negative result on posttreatment ^{18}F FDG PET-CT scan has a high negative predictive value for the presence of disease and is associated with improved disease-specific survival (DSS) (**Fig. 6**).[49]

Summary

High ^{18}F FDG uptake in primary EOC is associated with more aggressive disease and poor survival.

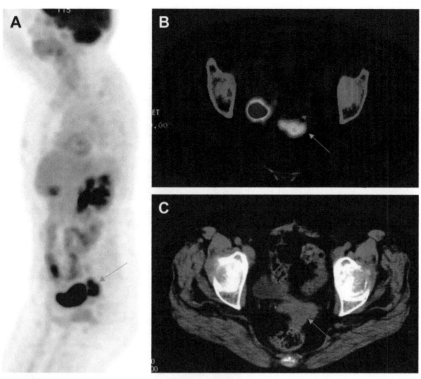

Fig. 4. A 72-year-old woman status post total abdominal hysterectomy with bilateral salpingo-oophorectomy for papillary serous carcinoma of the right ovary. At the time of surgery, metastatic implants were documented in the right fallopian tube, on the left ovary, and the uterine serosa. Patient was treated with 6 cycles of carboplatin/ Taxol (Paclitaxel). Approximately 1 year after completion of therapy, the patient presented with vaginal bleeding. PET-CT ordered for restaging reveals recurrent tumor at the vaginal apex. (*A*) Oblique PET maximum intensity projection demonstrates focal intense metabolic uptake in a mass posterior to the urinary bladder (*arrow*). (*B, C*) Axial fused PET-CT image and axial noncontrast CT of PET-CT examination shows a lobulated mass at the level of the vaginal apex (*arrows*).

The clinical application of this information at this time is undetermined. In initial staging of patients with advanced EOC, pretherapy imaging may detect disease that upstages the patient, which may lead to change in management or help direct surgical planning, thus aiding optimized cytoreduction. Because of the high accuracy in detection of recurrent disease and complementary role with laparoscopy, ^{18}F FDG PET-CT is an excellent tool for assessment of patients for secondary cytoreductive surgery. More data are needed to determine the utility of response patterns of ^{18}F FDG PET-CT in monitoring neoadjuvant therapy.

CERVICAL CANCER

Death rates from cervical cancer have decreased in industrialized nations as a result of adaptation of cancer screening programs using the Pap smear test. For the year 2014, the American Cancer Society predicts 12,360 cases of cervical cancer will be diagnosed in the United States and estimates 4020 deaths. The statistics are significantly worse in developing countries, with approximately 80,000 new cases of cervical cancer diagnosed each year and an estimated 60,000 deaths.[50] Eighty percent of cervical neoplasms are squamous cell carcinomas, and approximately 10% are of the adenocarcinoma type. Persistent infection with human papilloma virus (HPV), most frequently types 16 and 18, has been identified as the causative factor in the development of cervical cancer and is found in 70% of cervical cancers worldwide.[51] The strong association of HPV and cervical cancer led to the development of vaccines against HPV. The Centers for Disease Control and Prevention (CDC) recommends vaccination of preteen girls and girls up to age 26 years and boys from age 11 to 21 years. Other factors associated with increased risk of cervical cancer include young age at first intercourse, smoking, HIV infection, and socioeconomic status.[52–54]

Cervical cancer is a curable disease when discovered at an early stage and is limited to the cervix (**Table 3**). Although not a part of FIGO

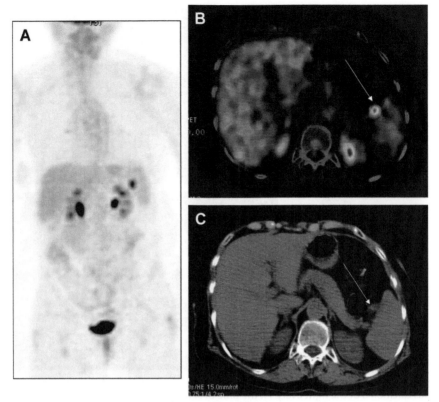

Fig. 5. A 65-year-old woman with diagnosis of stage IIIC papillary serous ovarian carcinoma treated with radical cytoreductive surgery followed by 6 cycles of chemotherapy, followed by a second cytoreductive surgery and peritoneal chemotherapy 6 years later for peritoneal recurrence. The patient remained stable without clinical or laboratory evidence of disease for 3 years. A surveillance PET-CT documents focal recurrent tumor in the left upper quadrant. CA 125 level at the time is 5.9 U/mL. (*A*) PET maximum intensity projection image reveals a single focus of hypermetabolic activity in the left upper quadrant. (*B*) Fused axial PET-CT image demonstrates a single focus of uptake anterior to the spleen (*arrow*), demonstrated to be a focal nodule (*arrow*) on the noncontract image (*C*) at the same level.

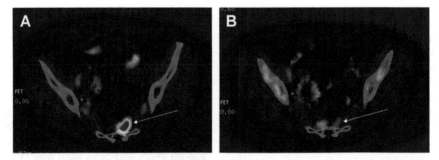

Fig. 6. A 61-year-old woman with a 10-year diagnosis of stage IIIC ovarian carcinoma treated with total abdominal hysterectomy with bilateral salpingo-oophorectomy and omentectomy followed by 6 cycles of Taxol and carboplatin. Patient underwent debulking surgery and additional chemotherapy for a left pelvic recurrence 2 years after diagnosis. Patient remained disease-free for 3 years. CA 125 levels remained normal. A routine restaging PET-CT revealed focal metastatic disease in the left ischiorectal fossa. (*A*) Fused axial PET-CT scan demonstrates focal intense metabolic uptake anterior to the sacrum and involving the medial aspect of the left piriformis muscle (*arrow*). (*B*) Fused axial PET-CT obtained 4 months after completion of external beam radiation, documenting almost complete resolution of disease (*arrow*).

Table 3
FIGO staging cervical cancer

Carcinoma of the cervix	
Stage I: Confined to uterus	
IA	Microscopic invasion, maximal stromal invasion of 5 mm and horizontal spread ≤7 mm
IA1	Microscopic invasion of ≤3 mm in depth and lateral spread ≤7 mm
IA2	Microscopic invasion of >3 mm and <5 mm with lateral spread ≤7 mm
IB	Clinically visible lesion confined to cervix
IB1	Clinically visible lesion ≤4 cm in greatest dimension
IB2	Clinically visible lesion >4 cm in greatest dimension
Stage II: Carcinoma invades beyond the uterus but not pelvic side wall or lower third vagina	
IIA	Without parametrial or vaginal involvement
IIA1	Tumor <4 cm in greatest dimension with involvement of <upper two-thirds of the vagina
IIA2	Tumor >4 cm in greatest dimension with involvement of <upper two-thirds of vagina
IIB	Parametrial involvement
Stage III: Extension to pelvic wall and/or involves lower third of vagina and/or hydronephrosis or nonfunctioning kidney	
IIIA	Lower third vagina, no pelvic side wall extension
IIIB	Extension to pelvic side wall and/or hydronephrosis or nonfunctioning kidney
Stage IV: Tumor invades pelvic organs and/or distant metastases	
IVA	Tumor invades mucosa of bladder or rectum and/or extends beyond the true pelvis
IVB	Distant metastasis (including peritoneal spread, supraclavicular, para-aortic nodes, liver, lung, bone

From Pecorelli S. Revised FIGO staging for carcinoma of the vulva, cervix, and endometrium. Int J Gynaecol Obstet 2009;105:104; with permission.

staging, the most significant prognostic factor for tumor recurrence is the presence of para-aortic nodal metastases, and primary surgery includes pelvic lymph node dissection with or without para-aortic node sampling or sentinel lymph node biopsy. The likelihood of pelvic and para-aortic nodal metastases increases with increasing tumor size, presence of lymphovascular invasion, and increasing tumor stage, and failure to detect para-aortic nodal metastases in the initial workup results in suboptimal treatment and decreased survival.[55–57] Micrometastatic nodal disease is documented to occur at a low rate even in FIGO stage IA2, and the incidence of pelvic node metastases in stage IB ranges from 11.5% to 21.7%.[58–61] Initial therapy is tailored to tumor stage and can be effectively treated with either surgery or radiotherapy, with more advanced disease treated with radiotherapy and adjuvant platinum-based chemotherapy, either curative or palliative. After treatment, patients are monitored serially over a 5-year period with physical examination, cervical and vaginal cytology, and imaging including CT, PET-CT, or MR imaging. Most recurrences occur within 2 years of diagnosis, and prognosis for these patients is poor as therapeutic options are limited. Trials with the antiangiogenic chemotherapy agent bevacizumab have shown limited improvement in median OS in patients with metastatic, recurrent, or persistent cancer.[62]

Fludeoxyglucose PET–Computed Tomography: Role in Management of Cervical Cancer

Systematic lymph node dissection is the most reliable diagnostic method in the detection of para-aortic lymph node metastasis, and the documentation of the presence of nodal metastases results in treatment change, including extension of radiation therapy fields to include the para-aortic node region. A complication rate of up to 30% has been reported with lymphadenectomy with a transperitoneal laparotomy approach and 4% to 18% using a retroperitoneal laparoscopic approach.[63] A noninvasive method for pretreatment evaluation of lymph node status is, therefore, desirable. Despite poor accuracy for diagnosis of micrometastases, ^{18}F FDG PET-CT is the single most accurate imaging modality for pretreatment detection of para-aortic lymph node metastases (**Fig. 7**).[64,65] Although sensitivity in stage 1 B disease is only 30% to 50%, sensitivity and specificity

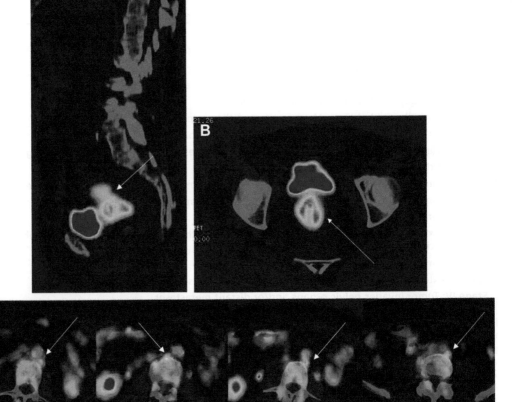

Fig. 7. A 70-year-old woman with new diagnosis of locally invasive squamous cell cancer of the cervix. PET-CT is performed for initial staging. (*A*) Sagittal fused and (*B*) axial fused PET-CT images demonstrate a large tumor involving the cervix with extension to the lower uterine segment (*arrows*). Poor resolution prohibits confident assessment of the tissue planes between the cervix and vagina. (*C*) Series of axial fused PET-CT images reveal foci of hypermetabolic uptake in multiple subcentimeter para-aortic nodes (*arrows*), consistent with para-aortic lymph node metastatic disease.

of 95% and 95% to 100% are documented in advanced-stage disease.[66–68]

Several studies have reported an association of cervical tumor SUVmax and MTV with patient prognosis, with a higher MTV associated with increased likelihood of lymph node metastases and reduced disease-free survival (**Fig. 8**).[69–71] The presence of ^{18}F FDG-PET positive cervical lymph node metastases is a better predictor of survival than FIGO stage.[72] The significance of these findings has led to suggestion of an ^{18}F FDG-PET-based nomogram to better predict patient-specific recurrence-free survival (RFS), DSS, and OS. Kidd and colleagues[73] included pretreatment PET-based factors of lymph node status, SUVmax, and MTV. The researchers found good predictive accuracy particularly for RFS and DSS. Approaches such as this may allow for

more effective patient-specific treatment pathways.

Owing to the high accuracy of ^{18}F FDG PET-CT in metastatic lymph node detection, the technique plays a significant role in radiation treatment planning, particularly when radiotherapy is the primary treatment modality. Accurate staging and determination of treatment field is critical for successful radiation therapy, and findings on ^{18}F FDG PET can result in change in tumor stage and radiation therapy planning volume changes or therapy change from curative to palliative.[74–76]

[18]F FDG PET-CT posttreatment imaging is an effective tool to determine treatment efficacy, and imaging results can predict patient outcome and should be obtained no sooner than 3 months after completion of therapy (**Fig. 9**).[77] Schwartz and colleagues[78,79] report that posttherapy [18]F

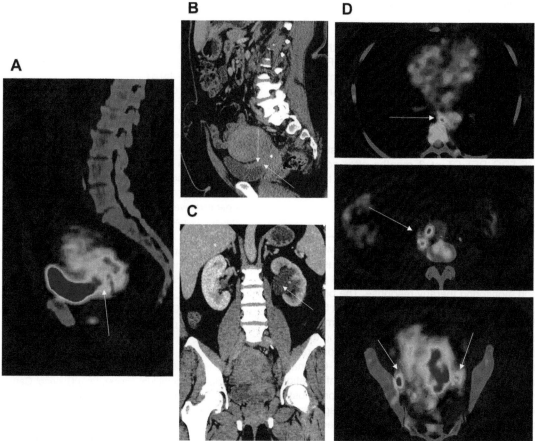

Fig. 8. A 52-year-old woman with diagnosis of stage IVA squamous cell carcinoma of the cervix with documented bladder invasion and left-side hydronephrosis by CT scan is imaged with PET-CT for initial staging and radiation treatment planning. (*A*) Sagittal fused PET-CT demonstrates a large cervical neoplasm extending to the lower uterine segment. Intense activity is contiguous with the posterior wall of the urinary bladder (*arrow*). (*B*) Sagittal and (*C*) coronal contrast-enhanced CT images document tumor invasion into the urinary bladder wall (*arrows*) and left-side hydronephrosis (*arrow*). (*D*) Series of axial fused PET-CT images reveal heterogeneous intense uptake in the cervical neoplasm, bilateral external iliac, left para-aortic, and posterior mediastinal metastatic adenopathy (*arrows*).

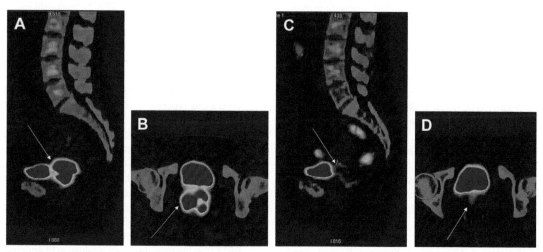

Fig. 9. A 46-year-old woman with diagnosis of stage IIIb squamous cell carcinoma of the cervix. Initial-staging PET-CT images in sagittal (*A*) and axial (*B*) planes reveal metabolic uptake within a large cervical mass. SUVmax is 18.9 (*arrows*). No extrauterine disease was found. The patient underwent external beam pelvic irradiation followed by high-dose brachytherapy. (*C, D*) Sagittal and axial images from a restaging PET-CT performed 7 months after completion of therapy documents a complete metabolic response (*arrows*).

FDG changes are predictive of both cause-specific and progression-free survival (PFS) after chemoradiation. A 78% PFS is documented in patients with complete metabolic response, 33% PFS in patients with partial metabolic response, and 0% PFS in patients with posttherapy scans documenting progressive disease. Complete metabolic response demonstrated on ^{18}F FDG PET-CT at 3 months after completion of therapy is associated with good long-term survival.

Summary

The treatment and follow-up of patients with cervical cancer is significantly affected by use of ^{18}F FDG PET-CT in initial staging, treatment planning, and monitoring therapy response. The prognostic information gleaned from primary lesion SUVmax, MTV, and extent of para-aortic nodal metastatic disease may play a critical role in tailoring therapy based on patient tumor-specific factors rather than on FIGO stage alone. [18]F FDG PET-CT imaging posttreatment provides accurate information regarding tumor response and valuable prognostic information that might direct more aggressive therapy or allow a more confident decision to choose palliation rather than cure.

REFERENCES

1. Sorbe B, Juresta C, Ahlin C. Natural history of recurrences in endometrial carcinoma. Oncol Lett 2014; 8(4):1800–6.
2. Antonsen SL, Jensen LN, Loft A, et al. MRI, PET/CT and ultrasound in the preoperative staging of andometrial cancer – a multicenter comparative study. Gynecol Oncol 2013;128(2):300–8.
3. Lin G, Ng KK, Chang JJ, et al. Myometrial invasion in endometrial cancer: diagnostic accuracy of diffusion-weighted 3.0-T MR imaging – initial experience. Radiology 2009;250(3):784–92.
4. Andreano A, Rechichi G, Rebora P, et al. MR diffusion imaging for preoperative staging of myometrial invasion in patients with endometrial cancer: a systematic review and meta-analysis. Eur Radiol 2014; 24(6):1327–38.
5. Chang MC, Chen JH, Liang JA, et al. 18-F FDG PET or PET/CT for detection of metastatic lymph nodes in patients with endometrial cancer: a systematic review and meta-analysis. Eur J Radiol 2012;81(11): 3511–7.
6. Kitajama K, Murakami K, Yamasaki E, et al. Accuracy of 18F-FDG PET/CT in detecting pelvic and para-aortic lymph node metastases in patients with endometrial cancer. AJR Am J Roentgenol 2008; 190(6):1652–8.
7. Denschlag D, Ulrich U, Emons G. The diagnosis and treatment of endometrial cancer. Dtsch Arztebl Int 2010;108(34–45):571–7.
8. Signorelli M, Guerra L, Buda A, et al. Role of the integrated FDG PET/CT in the surgical management of patients with high risk clinical early stage endometrial cancer: detection of pelvic nodal metastases. Gynecol Oncol 2009;115(2):231–5.
9. Park JY, Kim EN, Kim DY, et al. Comparison of the validity of magnetic resonance imaging and positron emission tomography/computed tomography in preoperative evaluation of patients with uterine corpus cancer. Gynecol Oncol 2008;58(1):24–38.
10. Crivellaro C, Signorelli M, Guerra L, et al. Tailoring systemic lymphadenectomy in high risk clinical early stage endometrial cancer: role of 18F-FDG PET/CT. Gynecol Oncol 2013;130(2):306–11.
11. Antonsen SL, Joft A, Fisker R, et al. SUV/max of 18FDG PET/CT as a predictor of high-risk endometrial cancer patients. Gynecol Oncol 2013;129(2): 298–303.
12. Nakamura K, Kodama J, Okumura Y, et al. The SUVmax of 18F-FDG PET correlates with histological grade in endometrial cancer. Int J Gynecol Cancer 2010;20(1):110–5.
13. Shim SH, Kim DY, Lee DY, et al. Metabolic tumor volume and total lesion glycolysis, measured using pre-operative 18F-FDG PET/CT, predict the recurrence of endometrial cancer. BJOG 2014;121(9): 1097–106.
14. Ghooshkhanei H, Treglia G, Sabouri G, et al. Risk stratification and prognosis determination using (18)F-FDG PET imaging in endometrial cancer patients: a systematic review and meta-analysis. Gynecol Oncol 2014;132(3):669–76.
15. Sadlecki P, Bodnar M, Grabiec M, et al. The role of hypoxia-inducible factor-1 α, glucose transporter-1 (GLUT-1) and carbon anhydrase IX in endometrial cancer patients. Biomed Res Int 2014;2014:616850.
16. Critchley HO, Osei J, Henderson TA, et al. Hypoxia-inducible factor-1 alpha expression in human endometrium and its regulation by protaglandin E-series prostanoid receptor 2 (EP2). Endocrinology 2006; 14(2):744–53.
17. Fung-Kee-Fung M, Dodge J, Elit L, et al. Follow-up after primary therapy for endometrial cancer: a systematic review. Gynecol Oncol 2006;101(3):520–9.
18. Ryu SY, Kim K, Kim K, et al. Detection of recurrence by 18F-FDG PET in patients with endometrial cancer showing no evidence of disease. J Korean Med Sci 2010;25(7):1029–33.
19. Ozcan KP, Kara T, Kaya B, et al. The value of FDG-PET/CT in the post-treatment evaluation of endometrial carcinoma: a comparison of PET/CT findings with conventional imaging and CA 125 as a tumour marker. Rev Esp Med Nucl Imagen Mol 2012; 31(5):257–60.

20. Sharma P, Kumar R, Singh H, et al. Carcinoma endometrium: role of 18-FDG PET/CT for detection of suspected recurrence. Clin Nucl Med 2012;37(7):649–55.

21. Kadkhodayan S, Shahriari S, Treglia G, et al. Accuracy of 18-F-FDG PET imaging in the follow up of endometrial cancer patients: systematic review and meta-analysis of the literature. Gynecol Oncol 2013;128(2):397–404.

22. Hasbini A, Haie Meder C, Morice P, et al. Outcome after salvage radiotherapy (brachytherapy +/- external) in patients with a vaginal recurrence from endometrial carcinomas. Radiother Oncol 2002;65(1):23–8.

23. Lu KH, Skates S, Hernandez MA, et al. A 2-stage ovarian cancer screening strategy using Risk of Ovarian Cancer Algorithm (ROCA) identifies early-stage incident cancers and demonstrates high predictive value. Cancer 2013;119(19):3454–61.

24. Elatter A, Bryant A, Winter-Roach BA, et al. Optimal primary surgical treatment for advanced epithelial ovarian cancer. Cochrane Database Syst Rev 2011;(8):CD007565.

25. Omura GA, Brady MF, Homesley HD, et al. Long-term follow-up and prognostic factor analysis in advanced ovarian carcinoma: the gynecologic oncology group experience. J Clin Oncol 1991;9(7):1138–50.

26. Thigpen T, Brady MF, Omura GA, et al. Age as a prognostic factor in ovarian carcinoma. The Gynecologic Oncology Group experience. Cancer 1993;71(2 Suppl):606–14.

27. Dembo AJ, Davy M, Stenwig AE, et al. Prognostic factors in patients with stage I epithelial ovarian cancer. Obstet Gynecol 1990;75(2):263–73.

28. Laas E, Luyckx M, De Cuypere M, et al. Secondary complete cytoreduction if recurrent ovarian cancer: benefit of optimal patient selection using scoring system. Int J Gynecol Cancer 2014;24(2):238–46.

29. Al Rawahi T, Lopes AD, Bristow RE, et al. Surgical cytoreduction for recurrent epithelial ovarian cancer. Cochrane Database Syst Rev 2013;(2):CD008765.

30. Fenchel S, Grab D, Nuessle K, et al. Asymptomatic adnexal masses: correlation of FDG PET and histopathologic findings. Radiology 2002;223:780–8.

31. Kitajama K, Suzki K, Senda M, et al. FDG-PET/CT for diagnosis of primary ovarian cancer. Nucl Med Commun 2011;32(7):549–53.

32. Tanzaki Y, Kobayashi A, Shiro M, et al. Diagnostic value of preoperative SUVmax on FDG-PET/CT for the detection of ovarian cancer. Int J Gynecol Cancer 2014;24(3):454–60.

33. Semaan A, Munkarah AR, Arabi H, et al. Expression of GLUT-1 in epithelial ovarian carcinoma: correlation with tumor proliferation, angiogenesis, survival and ability to predict optimal cytoreduction. Gynecol Oncol 2011;212(1):181–6.

34. Cho H, Lee YS, Kim J, et al. Overexpression of glucose transporter-1 (GLUT-1) predicts poor prognosis in epithelial ovarian cancer. Cancer Invest 2013;31(9):607–15.

35. Fruscio R, Sina F, Dolci C, et al. Preoperative 18F-FDG PET/CT in the management of advanced epithelial ovarian cancer. Gynecol Oncol 2013;131(3):689–93.

36. Li X, Xing H, Li L, et al. Clinical significance of para-aortic lymph node dissection and prognosis in ovarian cancer. Front Med 2014;8(1):96–100.

37. Bachmann C, Bachmann S, Fehm T, et al. Nodal status – its impact on prognosis in advanced ovarian cancer. J Cancer Res Clin Oncol 2012;138(2):261–7.

38. Signorelli M, Guerra L, Pirovano c, et al. Detection of nodal metastases by 18F-FDG PET/CT in apparent early stage ovarian cancer: a prospective study. Gynecol Oncol 2013;131(2):295–9.

39. Ghosh J, Thulkar S, Kumar R, et al. Role of FDG PET-CT in asymptomatic epithelial ovarian cancer with rising CA-125: a pilot study. Natl Med J India 2013;26(6):327–31.

40. Antunovic L, Cimitan M, Borsatti E, et al. Revisiting the clinical value of 18F-FDG PET/CT in detection of recurrent epithelial ovarian carcinomas: correlation with histology, serum CA-125 assay, and conventional radiological modalities. Clin Nucl Med 2012;37(8):e184–8.

41. Gu P, Pan LL, Wu SQ, et al. CA 125, PET alone, PET-CT, CT and MRI in diagnosing recurrent ovarian cancer: a systematic review and meta-analysis. Eur J Radiol 2009;71(1):164–74.

42. Bilici A, Ustaalioglu BB, Seker M, et al. Clinical value of FDG PET/CT in the diagnosis of suspected recurrent ovarian cancer: is there an impact of FDG PET/CT on patient management? Eur J Nucl Med Mol Imaging 2010;37(7):1259–69.

43. Fulham MJ, Carter J, Baldey A, et al. The impact of PET-CT in suspected recurrent ovarian cancer: a prospective multi-centre study as part of the Australian PET Data Collection Project. Gynecol Oncol 2009;112(3):462–8.

44. Simcock B, Neesham D, Quinn M, et al. The impact of PET/CT in the management of recurrent ovarian cancer. Gynecol Oncol 2006;103(1):271–6.

45. Ebina Y, Watari H, Kaneuchi M, et al. Impact of FDG PET in optimizing patient selection for cytoreductive surgery in recurrent ovarian cancer. Eur J Nucl Med Mol Imaging 2014;41(3):446–51.

46. Fagotti A, Fanafani F, Rossitto C, et al. A treatment selection protocol for recurrent ovarian cancer patients: the role of FDG-PET/CT and staging laparoscopy. Oncology 2008;75(3–4):152–8.

47. De Iaco P, Musto A, Orazi L, et al. FDG-PET/CT in advanced ovarian cancer staging: value and pitfalls in detecting lesions in different abdominal quadrants compared with laparoscopy. Eur J Radiol 2011;80(2):e98–103.

48. Nishiyama Y, Yamamoto Y, Kanenishi K, et al. Monitoring the neoadjuvant therapy response in gynecologic cancer patients using FDG PET. Eur J Nucl Med Mol Imaging 2008;35(2):287–95.

49. Hebel CB, Behrendt FF, Heinzel A, et al. Negative 18F-2-fluordeoxyglucose PET/CT predicts good cancer specific survival in patients with suspicion of recurrent ovarian cancer. Eur J Radiol 2014; 83(3):463–7.

50. Denny L. Cervical cancer: prevention and treatment. Discov Med 2012;14(75):125–31.

51. Ciesielska U, Nowinska K, Podhorska M, et al. The role of human papilloma virus in the malignant transformation of cervix epithelial cells and the importance of vaccination against this virus. Adv Clin Exp Med 2012;21(2):235–44.

52. Louie KS, de Sanjose S, Diaz M, et al. Early age at first sexual intercourse and early pregnancy are risk factors for cervical cancer in developing countries. Br J Cancer 2009;100(7):1191–7.

53. Natphopsuk S, Settheetham-Ishida W, Sinawat S, et al. Risk factors for cervical cancer in northeastern Thailand: detailed analysis of sexual and smoking behavior. Asian Pac J Cancer Prev 2012;13(11): 5489–95.

54. Holms RS, Hawes SE, Toure P, et al. HIV infection as a risk factor for cervical cancer and cervical intraepithelial neoplasia in Senegal. Cancer Epidemiol Biomarkers Prev 2009;18(9):2442–6.

55. Koleli IK, Ozdogan E, Sariibrahim B, et al. Prognostic factors affecting lymph node involvement in cervical cancer. Eur J Gynaecol Oncol 2014;35(4):4225–8.

56. Chism SE, Park RC, Keys HM. Prospects for para-aortic irradiation in treatment of cervical cancer. Cancer 1975;35:1505–9.

57. Delgado G, Bundy B, Zaino R, et al. Prospective surgical-pathological study of disease-free interval in patients with stage IB squamous cell carcinoma of the cervix: a Gynecologic Oncology Group study. Gynecol Oncol 1990;38:352–7.

58. Morice P, Castaigne D, Pautier P, et al. Interest of pelvic and para-aortic lymphadenectomy in patients with stage IB and II cervical carcinoma. Br J Cancer 1999;110(1):34–41.

59. Gein LT, Covens A. Lymph node assessment in cervical cancer: prognostic and therapeutic implications. J Surg Oncol 2009;99(4):242–7.

60. Buckley SL, Tritz DM, Van le L, et al. Lymph node metastases and prognosis in patients with stage A12 cervical cancer. Gynecol Oncol 1996;63(1):4–9.

61. Juretzka MM, Jensen KC, Longacre TA, et al. Detection of lymph node micrometastases in stage IA2-IB2 cervical cancer by immunohistochemical analysis. Gynecol Oncol 2004;93(1):107–11.

62. Tewari KS, Sill MW, Long HJ, et al. Improved survival with bevacizumab in advanced cervical cancer. N Engl J Med 2014;370(8):734–43.

63. Smits RM, Zusterzeel LM, Bekkers RL. Pretreatment retroperitoneal para-aortic lymph node staging in advanced cervical cancer. Int J Gynecol Cancer 2014;24(6):973–83.

64. Choi HJ, Ju W, Myung SK, et al. Diagnostic performance of computed tomography, magnetic resonance imaging, and positron emission tomography/computed tomography for detection of metastatic lymph nodes in patients with cervical cancer. Cancer Sci 2010;101(6):1471–9.

65. Lv K, Guo HM, Lu YJ, et al. Roles of 18F-FDG PET/CT in detecting pelvic lymph-node metastases in patients with early stage uterine cervical cancer: a comparison with MRI findings. Nucl Med Commun 2014;35(12):1204–11.

66. Signorelli M, Guerra L, Montanelli L, et al. Preoperative staging of cervical cancer: is 18F-FDG-PET/CT really effective in patients with early stage disease? Gynecol Oncol 2011;123(2):236–40.

67. Havrilesky LJ, Kulasingam SL, Matchar DB, et al. FDG-PET for management of cervical and ovarian cancer. Gynecol Oncol 2005;97(1):183–91.

68. Guo F, Yang R, Tian J, et al. The role of F-fluorodeoxyglucose (FDG) positron emission-computed tomography (PET/CT) in screening cervical cancer: a literature review. Cell Biochem Biophys 2014;69(2):197–201.

69. Kim BS, Kim IJ, Kim SJ, et al. The prognostic value of the metabolic tumor volume in FIGO stage IA to IIB cervical cancer for tumor recurrence: measured by F-18 FDG PET/CT. Nucl Med Mol Imaging 2011; 45(1):36–42.

70. Micco M, Vargas HA, Burger IA, et al. Combined pre-treatment MRI and 18F-FDG PET/CT parameters as prognostic biomarkers in patients with cervical cancer. Eur J Radiol 2014;83(7):1169–76.

71. Kidd EA, Siegal BA, Dehdashti F, et al. The standardized uptake value for F-18 fluorodeoxyglucose is a sensitive predictive biomarker for cervical cancer treatment response and survival. Cancer 2007; 110(8):1738–44.

72. Grigsby PW, Siegal BA, Dedashti F. Lymph node staging by positron emission tomography in patients with carcinoma of the cervix. J Clin Oncol 2001;19: 3745–9.

73. Kidd EA, El Naqa I, Siegal BA, et al. FDG-PET-based prognostic nomograms for locally invasive advanced cervical cancer. Gynecol Oncol 2012;127(1):136–40.

74. Lazzari R, Cecconi A, Jereczek-Fossa BA, et al. The role of [18F]FDG-PET/CT in staging and treatment planning for volumetric modulated Rapidarc radiotherapy in cervical cancer: experience of the European Institute of Oncology, Milan, Italy. Ecancermedicalscience 2014;8:409.

75. Cihoric N, Tapia C, Kruger K, et al. IMRT with FDG-PET/CT based simultaneous integrated boost for treatment of nodal positive cervical cancer. Radiat Oncol 2014;9:83–90.

76. Esthappan J, Mutic S, Malyapa RS, et al. Treatment planning guidelines regarding the use of CT/PET-guided IMRT for cervical carcinoma with positive para-aortic lymph nodes. Int J Radiat Oncol Biol Phys 2004;58(4):1289–97.

77. Bodurka-Bevers D, Morris M, Eifel P, et al. Posttherapy surveillance of women with cervical cancer and outcomes analysis. Gynecol Oncol 2000;78(2):187–93.

78. Schwartz JK, Grigsby PW, Dehdashti F, et al. The role of ^{18}F-FDG PET in assessing therapy response in cancer of the cervix and ovaries. J Nucl Med 2009;50:64S–73S.

79. Schwartz JK, Siegel BA, Dehdashti F, et al. Association of Posttherapy positron emission tomography with tumor response and survival in cervical carcinoma. JAMA 2007;298(19):2289–95.

PET/Computed Tomography in Neuroendocrine Tumor
Value to Patient Management and Survival Outcomes

Shamim Ahmed Shamim, MD[a], Abhishek Kumar, MD[b],
Rakesh Kumar, MD, PhD[b],*

KEYWORDS

- PET/CT • ^{18}F-DOPA • ^{68}Ga-DOTANOC • ^{18}F-FDG • Neuroendocrine tumors
- Medullary thyroid cancer • Pheochromocytoma • Paraganglioma

KEY POINTS

- Given the slow-growing nature of neuroendocrine tumors, they often do not show FDG uptake unless aggressive in behavior and hence the need for novel PET radiotracers, such as ^{18}F-DOPA and ^{68}Ga somatostatin peptide derivatives.
- Neuroendocrine tumors express somatostatin receptors and ^{68}Ga somatostatin peptide derivatives bind to these receptors and so are used in diagnosis and staging of these tumors.
- Expression of SSTR on PET provides and alternative option of treatment in the form of targeted radionuclide therapy.
- ^{68}Ga-DOTANOC is the agent of choice in GEP-NETs. ^{18}F-DOPA should be used as first radiotracer of choice in patients with medullary thyroid cancer and pheochromocytomas/paragangliomas.
- ^{18}F FDG-PET positivity is an indicator for poor prognosis in these patients and suggests a high proliferation index of the tumor.

INTRODUCTION

Neuroendocrine tumors (NETs) are neoplasms that arise from cells of the endocrine (hormonal) and nervous systems. Kulchitsky cells or similar enterochromaffin-like cells can give rise to NETs. These cells are abundantly found in the gastrointestinal system followed by the tracheobronchial tree and hence there is an abundance of these tumors in these areas. NETs are slow-growing tumors and have been reported in a wide range of organs. The most commonly encountered NETs in clinical practice are carcinoids of gut and lungs, pheochromocytomas/paragangliomas, and medullary thyroid cancer (MTC). Other rare tumors are neuroblastoma, schwannoma, and NET of the anterior pituitary. These tumors have secretory granules and may produce polypeptide hormones or biogenic amines depending on the parent organ, such as calcitonin in the case of MTC and serotonin in the case of carcinoids. The clinical presentation of these tumors depends on localization, hormone production, and extent of the disease. In the case of gut carcinoids, they may be diagnosed

The authors have nothing to disclose.
[a] Therapeutic Nuclear Medicine Division, Department of Nuclear Medicine, All India Institute of Medical Sciences, New Delhi 110029, India; [b] Diagnostic Nuclear Medicine Division, Department of Nuclear Medicine, All India Institute of Medical Sciences, New Delhi 110029, India
* Corresponding author.
E-mail address: rkphulia@yahoo.com

under evaluation for abdominal pain or discomfort, gastrointestinal bleeding, obstruction, or carcinoid syndrome caused by production of serotonin. MTC may initially manifest as neck swelling, whereas a lung carcinoid may present as cough and hemoptysis or may be diagnosed incidentally on chest radiography. It may also present as adrenocorticotropic hormone (ACTH)–dependent Cushing syndrome if it is secreting ACTH. These tumors are generally slow-growing tumors but do have potential for local and extensive distant metastasis. These NETs are rare tumors in clinical practice and early diagnosis of these tumors presents a challenge especially because in the case of metastatic NETs, treatment options are limited. Biochemical markers and routine radiology investigation by sonography, computed tomography (CT), and MR imaging have been used extensively in diagnosis and staging of these tumors. With the advent of PET/CT there has been a breakthrough in the early detection of these tumors. This article discusses PET/CT radiotracers for the diagnosis and staging of these tumors and possible use in response evaluation and predicting response to treatment.

^{18}F-DOPA/^{18}F-DOPAMINE PET/COMPUTED TOMOGRAPHY

PET using the catecholamine precursor 6-(fluoride-18)fluorolevodopa (^{18}F-DOPA) has emerged as a new imaging method for NETs.[1] These NETs take up amine precursors, such as ^{18}F-DOPA, and this forms the basis of uptake mechanism. Patients usually fast for about 6 hours before imaging. At our center a dose of 370 MBq is used for whole-body imaging followed by image acquisition after 60 minutes. Some centers advocate the use of carbidopa for reduction of tracer decarboxylation and subsequent renal clearance to increase tracer uptake in tumor cells.[2–4] A normal whole-body ^{18}F DOPA-PET/CT demonstrates high uptake in the urinary excretory system (kidney, ureter, and urinary bladder), gallbladder, sometimes common bile duct, and striatum. Low-level uptake may be seen in myocardium and liver. ^{18}F-DOPA has been used in diagnosis of gliomas, parkinsonism, gastroenteropancreatic NETs (GEP-NETs), lung carcinoids, pheochromocytoma, paragangliomas, and MTC. ^{18}F-dopamine is a catecholamine precursor that has been used in imaging of pheochromocytomas and paragangliomas.

GALLIUM 68 SOMATOSTATIN DERIVATIVES PET/COMPUTED TOMOGRAPHY

Gallium 68 (^{68}Ga)–labeled somatostatin analogues are generally short peptide analogues of somatostatin that are linked to the positron emitter ^{68}Ga by a bifunctional chelate, usually 1,4,7,10-tetraazacyclododecane-1,4,7,10-tetraacetic acid (DOTA). ^{68}Ga-labeled somatostatin derivatives (DOTA-NOC, DOTA-TOC, DOTA-TATE) are being used for imaging of tumors expressing somatostatin receptors (SSTR). SSTR expression has been seen in NETs, brain tumors, small cell lung cancer, lymphoma, and breast cancer.[5] These peptides are now being routinely used for imaging of NETs. These peptides can be labeled with ^{68}Ga, indium 111, and yttrium 86 for imaging of these tumors; when indicated, lutetium 177– or yttrium 90–labeled peptides can be used for therapy.[6–8] DOTA-NOC is one such peptide used for PET/CT imaging. At our center, a dose of 111 to 185 MBq is used for whole-body imaging followed by image acquisition 45 to 60 minutes postinjection. Physiologic uptake of ^{68}Ga-DOTA-NOC is seen in the pituitary gland, spleen, liver, and urinary tract (kidneys and urinary bladder). It is being used in PET/CT imaging of GEP-NET, lung carcinoids, pheochromocytomas, paragangliomas, meningiomas, and MTC.

Gastroenteropancreatic Neuroendocrine Tumors

GEP-NETs are rare tumors that are mostly clinically silent or may be detected because of mass effect. They synthesize, store, and secrete various peptides and neuroamines that might produce distinct clinical syndromes.[9–14] Clinical presentation also depends on site of tumor and presence of metastasis. These tumors are mostly sporadic but may present as part of familial syndromes, such as multiple endocrine neoplasia (MEN) IIa, von Hippel-Lindau disease, and neurofibromatosis type I.[15]

The GEP-NETs can be divided into carcinoids of the gut and pancreatic endocrine tumors, the former being more prevalent. The carcinoids are slow-growing tumors most commonly found in the small bowels, particularly the ileum (Fig. 1). In the gastrointestinal tract, up to 30% of NETs occur in the distal part of the ileum, followed by the rectum (21%–27%) and the appendix (17%–20%).[16] These tumors are mostly asymptomatic unless they are large enough to produce mass effect. Despite being slow growing they have the potential to metastasize, particularly to liver and regional lymph nodes. Some carcinoids, however, even if small in size may produce polypeptides or neuroamines and manifest as clinical syndromes, such as carcinoid syndromes. Carcinoid syndrome is most often seen in cases of midgut carcinoids, which produce serotonin (5-HT) or substance P and cause such symptoms as flushing, diarrhea,

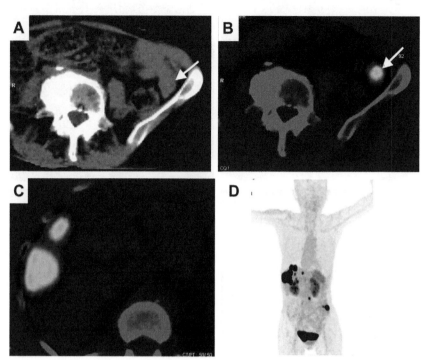

Fig. 1. Axial CT image shows soft tissue density lesion in left iliac fossa (*arrow*) in relation to iliac loops (*A*) with increased uptake in corresponding ^{68}Ga-DOTA-NOC-PET/CT fused image (*B*). In addition, fused ^{68}Ga-DOTA-NOC-PET/CT image shows increased radiotracer uptake in liver lesions (*C*). Whole-body MIP images of ^{68}Ga-DOTA-NOC-PET image shows increased uptake in primary and metastatic lesions (*D*). MIP, maximum intensity projection.

abdominal cramps, wheezing, palpitations, and occasionally congestive heart failure and peripheral edema. Gastric and duodenal carcinoids are associated with hypergastrinemia either caused by gastrin production from these tumors or secondary to chronic atrophic gastritis.[15] Duodenal carcinoids mostly secrete gastrin and cause Zollinger-Ellison syndrome, which might also be a part of spectrum of MEN I presentation.[17] However, it should be noted that most of these carcinoids are nonfunctioning and usually diagnosed late. Pancreatic endocrine tumors are also mostly nonfunctional, but may secrete insulin, glucagon, vasoactive intestinal polypeptide, or somatostatin and may produce symptoms according to the hormone secreted. The diagnosis of GEP-NET includes routine sonography; CT; MR imaging; biochemical tests, such as chromogranin A; and histopathology. The previously mentioned PET radiotracers (ie, ^{18}F-DOPA and ^{68}Ga-DOTA-NOC) have proved to be great tools to the clinician in diagnosis, staging, and follow-up of these patients. These tracers aid primary diagnosis and also provide metastatic work-up and follow-up for these patients (**Fig. 2**). Koopmans and colleagues[18] assessed 53 patients and reported a sensitivity of 100% for ^{18}F-DOPA in detection of carcinoids on

a patient-based analysis. On a region-wise analysis they reported sensitivity of 100% for pancreatic lesions and 96% for lesions of abdomen and pelvis. Sensitivity for liver lesions was 97% in this study. In another study, Becherer and colleagues[19] reported a sensitivity of 85% with a high specificity of nearly 100%. Sensitivity of 81.3% in detection of metastatic liver lesions, 90.9% for skeleton, and 100% for the mediastinum, pancreas, and lymph nodes was reported in this study. Hoegerle and colleagues[1] reported sensitivities of 88%, 87%, and 32% in detection of primary lesions, lymph node metastases, and organ metastases, respectively, in these patients with ^{18}F-DOPA. Detection of small subcentimetric metastatic lesions in lungs might be difficult because of respiratory movements and resolution of PET. [18]F DOPA-PET of pancreas has also been shown to distinguish between focal and diffuse forms of hyperinsulinism in infancy by Ribeiro and colleagues.[20] A high sensitivity has been reported in detection of insulinomas with ^{18}F-DOPA.[21]

[68]Ga-labeled somatostatin derivatives have been increasingly used in detection and staging of GEP-NETs. The most commonly used peptides are DOTA-NOC and DOTA-TATE. These tumors are well differentiated and frequently express SSTRs

414

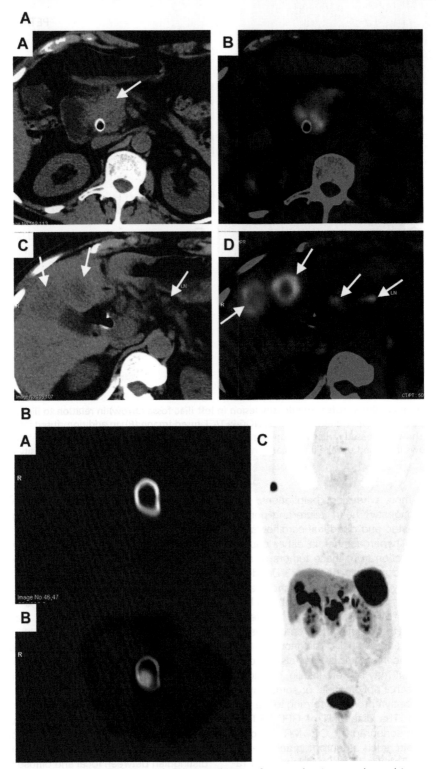

Fig. 2. (*A*) Pancreatic NET. Axial CT images of abdomen shows soft tissue density mass (*arrow*) in pancreatic head region (*a*). ⁶⁸Ga-DOTA-NOC fused PET/CT image (*b*) showing increased DOTA-NOC uptake in pancreatic head mass, suggestive of pancreatic NET. Axial CT images of abdomen show multiple peripancreatic lymph nodes (*small arrows*) and multiple hypodense lesions (*long arrows*) in the liver (*c*). ⁶⁸Ga-DOTA-NOC fused PET/CT image (*d*) showing increased DOTA-NOC uptake in peripancreatic lymph nodes (*small arrows*) and liver lesions (*arrows facing each other*) suggestive of multiple liver and regional lymph node metastases. (*B*) Axial CT image shows doubtful focal marrow lesion in right humerus (*a*). Fused ⁶⁸Ga-DOTA-NOC-PET/CT image increased radiotracer uptake suggestive of marrow metastasis (*b*). Whole-body MIP images of ⁶⁸Ga-DOTA-NOC-PET image shows increased uptake in primary and in metastatic lesions (*c*).

and hence these radiolabelled peptides are taken up by the tumor. ^{68}Ga-DOTA-NOC/DOTA-TATE PET studies have been used in detection of primary and metastatic lesions. Haug and colleagues[22] reported a sensitivity of 94% with a specificity of 89% with ^{68}Ga-DOTA-TATE in patients with GEP-NETs. Naswa and colleagues[23] reported sensitivity of 91% with sensitivity of 50% with ^{68}Ga-DOTA-NOC in patients with GEP-NETs on a patient-wise analysis. On region-wise analysis this study demonstrated sensitivities of 94%, 93%, 81%, and 75% in detecting primary lesion, lymph node, liver, and skeletal metastases, respectively. Haug and colleagues[24] demonstrated that in response evaluation of these patients ^{68}Ga-DOTA-TATE standardized uptake values may not indicate response. Patients positive on ^{68}Ga-DOTA-NOC have better prognosis than those positive on PET with fludeoxyglucose F 18 (^{18}F FDG-PET), probably indicating that FDG-PET–positive patients have high rate of proliferation. Also for a patient positive on ^{68}Ga-labeled somatostatin analogue, peptide receptor radionuclide therapy (PRRT) can be offered as a mode of treatment. Ambrosini and colleagues[25] compared ^{68}Ga-DOTA-NOC with ^{18}F-DOPA for evaluation of gastroenteropancreatic and lung NETs. Thirteen patients with biopsy-proved gastroenteropancreatic or pulmonary NET were prospectively enrolled and scheduled for ^{18}F-DOPA and ^{68}Ga-DOTA-NOC PET. The most common primary tumor site was pancreas (8 of 13) followed by ileum (2 of 13), lung (2 of 13), and duodenum (1 of 13). The carcinoma was well differentiated in 10 of 13 and poorly differentiated in 3 of 13 cases. ^{68}Ga-DOTA-NOC PET was positive, showing at least one lesion, in 13 of 13 cases, whereas ^{18}F DOPA-PET was positive in 9 of 13. On a lesions basis, ^{68}Ga-DOTA-NOC identified more lesions than ^{18}F-DOPA (71 vs 45), especially in liver, lung, and lymph node level. ^{68}Ga-DOTA-NOC correctly identified the primary site in six of eight nonoperated cases (in five cases, the primary was surgically removed before PET), whereas ^{18}F-DOPA identified the primary only in two of eight cases. They concluded that ^{68}Ga-DOTA-NOC is accurate for the detection of gastroenteropancreatic and lung NETs in either the primary or the metastatic site, and that it offers several advantages over ^{18}F-DOPA.

Thus, ^{18}F-DOPA and ^{68}Ga-labeled somatostatin analogues are good PET radiotracers in detection of primary and metastatic lesions in patients with GEP-NETs.

Pulmonary Neuroendocrine Tumors

Pulmonary NETs are the second most common site for NETs after GEP-NETs and account for 22% to 27% of such tumors. These pulmonary NETs express SSTRs and have amine precursor uptake mechanisms. Thus, ^{18}F-DOPA and ^{68}Ga-labeled somatostatin analogues are used in PET imaging of these tumors. There are limited published data on these radiotracers. Ambrosini and colleagues[26] evaluated ^{68}Ga-DOTA-NOC PET/CT in 11 patients with bronchial carcinoid. PET/CT detected at least one lesion in 9 of 11 patients and was negative in two. PET/CT and contrast enhanced computed tomography (CECT) were discordant in 8 of 11 patients. On a clinical basis, PET/CT provided additional information in 9 of 11 patients leading to the changes in the clinical management in three of nine patients. In a largest prospective study, involving 32 patients with clinical suspicion of bronchopulmonary carcinoid, we have demonstrated a sensitivity, specificity, and accuracy 96%, 100%, and 97%, respectively, of ^{68}Ga-DOTA-TOC PET/CT.[27]

Similarly, ^{18}F-DOPA has been used in detection of pulmonary NETs. Dubois and colleagues[28] reported a case of ACTH-dependent Cushing syndrome being detected as pulmonary carcinoid on ^{18}F DOPA-PET/CT. However, there are limited research data pertaining only to pulmonary NETs and most of the studies with ^{18}F-DOPA are mixed studies discussing NETs in general and further research is needed.

PET with Fludeoxyglucose F 18 in Neuroendocrine Tumors

FDG-PET/CT is not used for initial evaluation of NETs because they are slow-growing tumors and show less FDG avidity (**Fig. 3**). Binderup and coworkers[29] in a prospective study found a sensitivity of 58% with FDG-PET. However, uptake pattern of tumor changes in late stage of disease when tumor characteristic changes from well differentiated to poorly differentiated. At this stage they express less SSTRs and show high FDG uptake. Sensitivity of FDG-PET is higher in tumors having proliferation index greater than 15. Kayani and colleagues[30] in a retrospective study on 38 patients with primary and recurrent disease reported the sensitivity of 82%, 66%, and 92% for ^{68}Ga-DOTA-TATE PET/CT, FDG PET/CT, and combined, respectively. High-grade tumor has shown more FDG uptake, whereas low-grade tumors were more Ga-DOTA-TATE avid. They observed that high-grade NET are more FDG avid than 68Ga-DOTA-TATE.

Pheochromocytoma/Paraganglioma

Paragangliomas are tumors that develop from endocrine cells derived from pluripotent neural

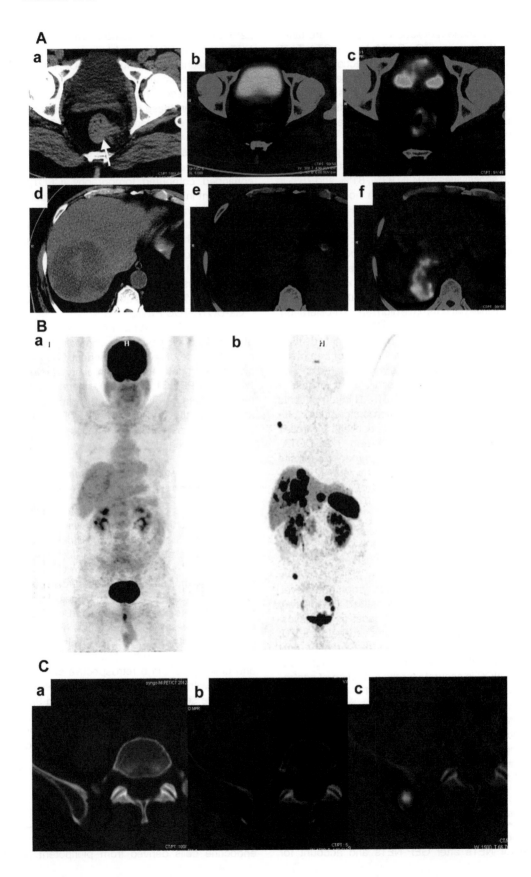

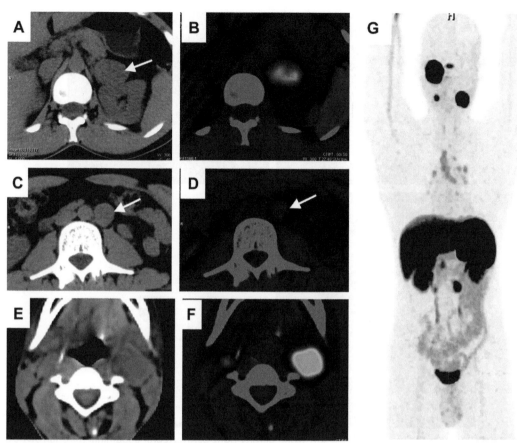

Fig. 4. Axial CT image shows a well-defined soft tissue density lesion (*arrow*) of left adrenal (*A*). Fused ⁶⁸Ga-DOTA-NOC-PET/CT image shows increased radiotracer uptake in left adrenal lesion suggestive of pheochromocytoma (*B*). CT image shows another well-defined soft tissue density lesion in left paravertebral region (*arrow*) (*C*). Fused ⁶⁸Ga-DOTA-NOC-PET/CT image shows increased radiotracer uptake in left paravertebral region suggestive of paraganglioma (*arrow*) (*D*). CT image shows well-defined soft tissue density mass bilateral carotid space (*E*). Fused ⁶⁸Ga-DOTA-NOC-PET/CT image shows increased radiotracer uptake in soft tissue density mass bilateral carotid space (*F*). Whole-body MIP images of ⁶⁸Ga-DOTA-NOC-PET image shows increased uptake in all lesions described previously (*G*).

crest stem cells and are associated with neurons of the autonomic nervous system (**Figs. 4** and **5**). Those developing from adrenal medulla are most common (~90%) and called pheochromocytoma.[31] These are mostly sporadic or may be genetic in origin; about 25% of paraganglioma are inherited or familial. It can be a part of rare syndromes, such as MEN2, neurofibromatosis type 1, von Hippel-Lindau disease, and familial paraganglioma syndrome. The classic symptoms of paraganglioma are high blood pressure, palpitations, headache, flushing, sweating, and anxiety or panic attacks. These symptoms are mainly caused by catecholamine overproduction. It

Fig. 3. (*A*) NET of rectum. Axial CT images of pelvis shows asymmetrical thickening (*arrow*) (*a*). Fused ¹⁸F FDG-PET/CT image does not show any significant FDG uptake (*b*). However, abnormal increased uptake of radiotracer is noted on ⁶⁸Ga-DOTA-NOC fused PET/CT image (*c*). Axial CT images of abdomen shows hypodense lesion in liver (*d*). Fused ¹⁸F FDG-PET/CT image does not show any significant uptake in liver lesion (*e*). However, abnormal increased uptake of radiotracer is noted on ⁶⁸Ga-DOTA-NOC fused PET/CT image (*f*). (*B*) Whole-body MIP images: ¹⁸F FDG-PET/CT study with no significant abnormal FDG uptake in whole-body image (*a*). ⁶⁸Ga-DOTA-NOC study shows increased uptake in primary and metastatic lesions (*b*). (*C*) Axial CT images of pelvis show no abnormality in right ileum (*a*). Fused ¹⁸F FDG-PET/CT image does not show any significant uptake (*b*). However, abnormal increased uptake of radiotracer is noted on ⁶⁸Ga-DOTA-NOC fused PET/CT image (*c*) suggestive of marrow metastasis.

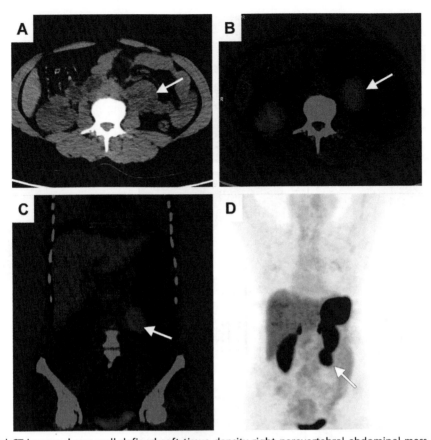

Fig. 5. Axial CT images shows well-defined soft tissue density right paravertebral abdominal mass (*arrow*) (*A*). Fused ^{68}Ga-DOTA-NOC-PET/CT image increased radiotracer uptake right paravertebral abdominal mass (*arrow*) (*B, C*). Whole-body MIP images of ^{68}Ga-DOTA-NOC-PET image shows increased uptake in right paravertebral abdominal mass (*D*). On each image lesion is depicted by *arrow*. Findings are suggestive of paraganglioma.

should be noted that catecholamine overproduction is mostly a feature of those paragangliomas arising from the sympathetic nervous system (abdominothoracic paraganglioma), whereas paragangliomas from the parasympathetic system (head and neck) rarely do so.[32] The diagnosis of pheochromocytoma is established biochemically by measuring the level of urinary and plasma catecholamines and their metabolites (24-h total metanephrine and/or catecholamine). Imaging is used for localization and evaluation for resectability. It also provides information if the disease is multicentric in origin. Routine radiologic procedures, such as sonography, CT, MR imaging, and iodine (I) 123/131 iobenguane (MIBG) have been used. Because of SSTR expression and ability for uptake of amine precursors, ^{68}Ga-labeled somatostatin analogues and ^{18}F DOPA-PET tracers have been used in localization, response to therapy, and detection of recurrence of these tumors. In comparison with MIBG scintigraphy these PET radiotracers provide advantage of higher spatial resolution. ^{18}F-DOPA does not show physiologic uptake in adrenals as compared with MIBG scintigraphy and ^{68}Ga-labeled somatostatin analogues and hence has a distinct advantage over these radiotracers. Hoegerle and colleagues[33] reported sensitivity of ^{18}F DOPA-PET to be 100% (17 of 17 tumors) and specificity of 100% (25 of 25 tumor-free adrenal and extra-adrenal regions). Their study compared this imaging modality with MIBG scintigraphy and MR imaging in 14 patients and showed that ^{18}F DOPA-PET is a reliable biochemical imaging approach that seemed superior to MIBG scintigraphy. It has sensitivity similar to MR imaging, whereas the specificity of ^{18}F DOPA-PET was similar to MIBG scintigraphy. Magnaldi and colleagues[34] attempted to describe appearance of pheochromocytomas on ^{18}F DOPA-PET and MR imaging and concluded that in the assessment of pheochromocytoma, the combination of ^{18}F DOPA-PET with MR imaging is superior to MR imaging alone. ^{18}F DOPA-PET/MR imaging may yield a higher diagnostic confidence for the detection of pheochromocytoma than ^{18}F DOPA-PET/CT. Rufini and colleagues[35] compared MIBG scintigraphy with ^{18}F-DOPA in known or suspected recurrent paraganglioma.[18]F-DOPA studies showed 100% sensitivity, whereas ^{123}I-MIBG studies had 75% sensitivity (P = not significant). ^{18}F-DOPA detected 98% of lesions, whereas 38% were detected with ^{123}I-MIBG (P = .04). ^{18}F-DOPA showed more lesions than ^{123}I-MIBG in eight patients, whereas in two patients ^{123}I-MIBG showed a greater number of lesions. A change in treatment planning was suggested by ^{18}F-DOPA in one patient.

It has been demonstrated through in vivo and in vitro studies that pheochromocytomas and paragangliomas express SSTRs 2, 3, and 4.[36] Even normal adrenals express these receptors and hence physiologic uptake is seen in somatostatin receptor scintigraphy (SRS) and ^{68}Ga-labeled somatostatin analogue study. Usually the expression of SSTR receptors is increased in malignant pheochromocytomas and paragangliomas.[37] Kroiss and colleagues[38] showed that ^{68}Ga-DOTA-TOC PET/CT provides accurate tumor extent in patients with extra-adrenal paraganglioma compared with ^{123}I-MIBG single-photon emission CT(SPECT)/CT. On a per-lesion basis, the overall sensitivity of ^{68}Ga-DOTA-TOC PET was 100% (McNemar, P<.5), that of planar ^{123}I-MIBG imaging was 3.4% (McNemar, P<.001), and that of SPECT/CT was 6.9% (McNemar, P<.001). They concluded that ^{68}Ga-DOTA-TOC PET/CT is superior to ^{123}I-MIBG SPECT/CT, particularly in head and neck and bone lesions, and that it provides valuable information for staging extra-adrenal paragangliomas.

Naswa and colleagues[39] from our center showed the superiority of ^{68}Ga-DOTA-NOC PET/CT over ^{131}I-MIBG in 35 patients with pheochromocytoma/paraganglioma. Naswa and colleagues[40] have also shown the use of ^{68}Ga-DOTA-NOC PET/CT for imaging of carotid body chemodectoma, by demonstrating additional lesions or metastasis. In another study, Kroiss and colleagues[41] compared ^{68}Ga-DOTA-TOC PET/CT with ^{18}F DOPA-PET/CT in patients with extra-adrenal paraganglioma. ^{68}Ga-DOTA-TOC PET and ^{18}F DOPA-PET each had a per-patient and per-lesion detection rate of 100% in nonmetastatic extra-adrenal paragangliomas. However, in metastatic or multifocal disease, the per-lesion detection rate of ^{68}Ga-DOTA-TOC was 100% and that of ^{18}F DOPA-PET was 56.0%. They mentioned that ^{68}Ga-DOTA-TOC PET may be superior to ^{18}F DOPA-PET and diagnostic CT in providing valuable information for pretherapeutic staging of extra-adrenal paragangliomas.

Other PET radiotracers that have been used in evaluation of pheochromocytomas and paragangliomas are ^{18}F-dopamine and carbon 11 hydroxyephedrine. The mechanism of uptake is catecholamine uptake and storage in the tumor cells. However, these tracers are not widely available and limited data are available regarding the accuracy of these PET radiotracers. Similarly ^{11}C-metomidate has been used in the detection of tumors of adrenal cortex; it is an analogue in corticosteroid synthesis pathway.

Medullary Thyroid Cancer

MTC arises from the parafollicular cells (C cells) of the thyroid gland, which are derived from cells of neural crest. These C cells produce calcitonin, levels of which are increased in this form of thyroid cancer and used in diagnostic evaluation and follow-up of these patients. MTC also produces polypeptide carcinoembryonic antigen, which is also used as tumor marker in these patients. MTC is mostly sporadic but about 20% to 25% of MTC are genetic in nature, caused by a mutation in the RET proto-oncogene and then classified as familial MTC. It can also be a part of MEN2 syndrome and is associated with tumors of the parathyroid gland pheochromocytoma. Lymph nodes are the most common site of metastases throughout the clinical course[42] followed by bones, liver, and lungs.[43] Surgery is the primary mode of treatment.[44]

Localization of recurrent tumor is difficult with radiologic morphology imaging. Radiotracers, such as technetium 99m (V)-dimercaptosuccinic acid, technetium 99m sestamibi, and [131/123]I-meta-iodobenzylguanidine, have been evaluated with variable success. PET radiotracers ^{18}F-DOPA, ^{68}Ga-DOTA-NOC, and ^{18}F-FDG have been used in evaluation of MTC. Being tumors of neuroendocrine origin they express SSTRs and have amine uptake mechanisms. Treglia and colleagues[45] compared ^{18}F-DOPA, ^{18}F-FDG, and ^{68}Ga-somatostatin analogue PET/CT in the evaluation of MTC and found a statistically significant difference in the number of lymph node, liver, and bone lesions detected with the three tracers (P<.01). They concluded that ^{18}F DOPA-PET/CT may be the most useful imaging method for detecting recurrent MTC lesions in patients with elevated serum calcitonin levels, and performed better than ^{18}F-FDG and ^{68}Ga-somatostatin analogue PET/CT. In case of aggressive tumors ^{18}F-FDG findings may complement ^{18}F-DOPA. In another study, Verbeek and colleagues[46] evaluated clinical relevance of ^{18}F FDG-PET and ^{18}F DOPA-PET in recurrent MTC. Calcitonin and carcinoembryonic antigen doubling times as markers for progression were compared with ^{18}F FDG-PET and ^{18}F DOPA-PET/CT, and assessment was done whether these imaging modalities could be of value in detecting progressive disease. There was a significant correlation with ^{18}F FDG-PET positivity. Doubling times were less than 24 months in 77% of ^{18}F FDG-PET–positive patients compared with 88% of ^{18}F FDG-PET–negative patients who had doubling times greater than 24 months (P<.001). Between doubling times and ^{18}F DOPA-PET positivity, no significant correlation existed. [18]F DOPA-PET detected significantly more lesions than ^{18}F-FDG. They concluded that ^{18}F FDG-PET positivity was an indicator for poor survival in these patients. They commented that ^{18}F-DOPA and ^{18}F FDG-PET/CT may be complimentary in tumor localization and behavior. Conry and colleagues[47] evaluated ^{68}Ga-DOTA-TATE and ^{18}F FDG-PET/CT in detection of recurrent MTC. ^{68}Ga-DOTA-TATE-PET/CT showed sensitivity of 72.2% (95% confidence interval, 46.4%–89.3%) versus 77.8% (95% confidence interval, 51.9%–92.6%) for ^{18}F-FDG (nonsignificant difference). They concluded that neither ^{18}F-FDG nor ^{68}Ga-DOTA-TATE-PET/CT can fully map the extent of disease in patients with recurrent MTC. They identified ^{68}Ga-DOTA-TATE-PET/CT as a useful complementary imaging tool and that it may serve as a guide for targeted radionuclide somatostatin analogue therapy. Thus, in case of MTC, all these tracers may have a role in staging and detection of recurrence. At our center, we routinely evaluate these patients with both ^{68}Ga-DOTA-NOC and ^{18}F-FDG as initial tests after clinical and biochemical work-up. However, more data are needed to identify the ideal PET radiotracer of choice in these patients.

REFERENCES

1. Hoegerle S, Altehoefer C, Ghanem N, et al. Whole-body 18F dopaPET for detection of gastrointestinal carcinoid tumors. Radiology 2001;220(2):373–80.
2. Brown WD, Oakes TR, DeJesus OT, et al. Fluorine-18-fluoro-L-DOPA dosimetry with carbidopa pretreatment. J Nucl Med 1998;39:1884–91.
3. Bergstrom M, Lu L, Eriksson B, et al. Modulation of organ up take of 11C-labelled 5-hydroxytryptophan. Biog Amines 1996;12:477–85.
4. Ishikawa T, Dhawan V, Chaly T, et al. Fluorodopa positron emission tomography with an inhibitor of catechol-O-methyltransferase: effect of the plasma 3-O-methyldopa fraction on data analysis. J Cereb Blood Flow Metab 1996;16:854–63.
5. Pettinato C, Sarnelli A, Di Donna M, et al. Bergamini. 68Ga-DOTANOC: biodistribution and dosimetry in patients affected by neuroendocrine tumors. Eur J Nucl Med Mol Imaging 2008;51:72–9.
6. Forster GJ, Engelbach M, Brockmann JJ, et al. Preliminary data on biodistribution and dosimetry for therapy planning of somatostatin receptor positive tumors: comparison of [86]Y-DOTATOC and ^{111}In-DTPA-octreotide. Eur J Nucl Med 2001;28:1743–50.
7. Cremonesi M, Ferrari M, Bodei L, et al. Dosimetry in peptide radionuclide receptors therapy: a review. J Nucl Med 2006;47:1467–75.
8. Cremonesi M, Ferrari M, Zoboli S, et al. Biokinetics and dosimetry in patients administered with[111]In-DOTA-Tyr[3]-octreotide: implications for internal radiotherapy with[90]Y-DOTATOC. Eur J Nucl Med 1999;26:877–86.
9. Modlin IM, Kidd M, Latich I, et al. Current status of gastrointestinalcarcinoids. Gastroenterology 2005;128:1717–51.
10. Tonnies H, Toliat MR, Ramel C, et al. Analysis of sporadicneuroendocrine tumours of the enteropancreatic system bycomparative genomic hybridisation. Gut 2001;48:536–41.
11. Thakker RV. Multiple endocrine neoplasia type 1. In: DeGroot LJ, Jamesson JL, editors. Endocrinology. 5th edition. Philadelphia: Elsevier Saunders; 2006. p. 3509–21.
12. Lollgen RM, Hessman O, Szabo E, et al. Chromosome 18 deletionsare common events in classical midgut carcinoid tumors. Int J Cancer 2001;92:812–5.
13. DeLellis RA, Lloyd RV, Heitz PU, et al, editors. World Health Organization classification of tumours, pathology and genetics of tumours of endocrine organs. Lyon (France): IARC Press; 2004.
14. Anlauf M, Perren A, Meyer CL, et al. Precursor lesions in patientswith multiple endocrine neoplasia type 1-associated duodenalgastrinomas. Gastroenterology 2005;128:1187–98.
15. Modlin IM, Oberg K, Chung DC, et al. Gastroenteropancreatic neuroendocrine tumours [review]. Lancet Oncol 2008;9(1):61–72.
16. Sahani DV, Bonaffini PA, Fernández-Del Castillo C, et al. Gastroenteropancreatic neuroendocrine tumors: role of imaging in diagnosis and management. Radiology 2012;266:38–61.
17. Kaltsas GA, Besser GM, Grossman AB. The diagnosis and medical management of advanced neuroendocrine tumors. Endocr Rev 2004;25(3):458–511.
18. Koopmans KP, de Vries EG, Kema IP, et al. Staging of carcinoid tumours with 18F-DOPA PET: a prospective, diagnostic accuracy study. Lancet Oncol 2006;7(9):728–34.
19. Becherer A, Szabó M, Karanikas G, et al. Imaging of advanced neuroendocrine tumors with ^{18}F-FDOPA PET. J Nucl Med 2004;45:1161–7.
20. Ribeiro MJ, De Lonlay P, Delzescaux T, et al. Characterization of hyperinsulinism in infancy assessed with PET and 18F-fluoro-L-DOPA. J Nucl Med 2005;46:560–6.
21. Otonkoski T, Näntö-Salonen K, Seppänen M, et al. Noninvasive diagnosis of focal hyperinsulinism of infancy with [18F]-DOPA positron emission tomography. Diabetes 2006;55(1):13–8.

22. Haug AR, Cindea-Drimus R, Auernhammer CJ, et al. Neuroendocrine tumor recurrence: diagnosis with 68Ga-DOTATATE PET/CT. Radiology 2014;270(2): 517–25.

23. Naswa N, Sharma P, Gupta SK, et al. Dual tracer functional imaging of gastroenteropancreatic neuroendocrine tumors using 68Ga-DOTA-NOC PET-CT and 18F-FDG PET-CT. Clin Nucl Med 2014;39(1):e27–34.

24. Haug AR, Rominger A, Mustafa M, et al. Treatment with octreotide does not reduce tumor uptake of 68Ga-DOTATATE as measured by PET/CT in patients with neuroendocrine tumors. J Nucl Med 2011;52: 1679–83.

25. Ambrosini V, Tomassetti P, Castellucci P, et al. Comparison between 68Ga-DOTA-NOC and 18F-DOPA PET for the detection of gastro-entero-pancreatic and lung neuro-endocrine tumours. Eur J Nucl Med Mol Imaging 2008;35:1431–8.

26. Ambrosini V, Castellucci P, Rubello D, et al. 68Ga-DOTA-NOC: a new PET tracer for evaluating patients with bronchial carcinoid. Nucl Med Commun 2009; 30:281–6.

27. Venkitaraman B, Karunanithi S, Kumar A, et al. Role of 68Ga-DOTATOC PET/CT in initial evaluation of patients with suspected bronchopulmonary carcinoid. Eur J Nucl Med Mol Imaging 2014;41(5):856–64.

28. Dubois S, Morel O, Rodien P, et al. Pulmonary adrenocorticotropin secreting carcinoid tumor localized by 6-Fluoro-[18F]L-dihydroxyphenylalanine positron emission/computed tomography imaging in a patient with Cushing's syndrome. J Clin Endocrinol Metab 2007;92(12):4512–3.

29. Binderup T, Knigge U, Loft A, et al. Functional imaging of neuroendocrine tumors: a head-to-head comparison of somatostatin receptor scintigraphy, 123I-MIBG scintigraphy, and 18F-FDG PET. J Nucl Med 2010;51(5):704–12.

30. Kayani I, Bomanji JB, Groves A, et al. Functional imaging of neuroendocrine tumors with combined PET/CT using 68Ga-DOTATATE (DOTA-DPhe1,Tyr3-octreotate) and 18F-FDG. Cancer 2008;112(11):2447–55.

31. Gifford RW Jr, Manger WM, Bravo EL. Pheochromocytoma. Endocrinol Metab Clin North Am 1994;23: 387–404.

32. Hinerman RW, Amdur RJ, Morris CG, et al. Definitive radiotherapy in the management of paragangliomas arising in the head and neck: a 35- year experience. Head Neck 2008;30:1431–8.

33. Hoegerle S, Nitzsche E, Altehoefer C, et al. Pheochromocytomas: detection with 18F DOPA whole body PET–initial results. Radiology 2002;222(2):507–12.

34. Magnaldi S, Mayerhoefer ME, Khameneh A, et al. (18)F-DOPA PET/CT and MRI: description of 12 histologically-verified pheochromocytomas. Anticancer Res 2014;34(2):791–5.

35. Rufini V, Treglia G, Castaldi P, et al. Comparison of 123I-MIBG SPECT-CT and 18F-DOPA PET-CT in the evaluation of patients with known or suspected recurrent paraganglioma. Nucl Med Commun 2011;32(7):575–82.

36. Ueberberg B, Tourne H, Redmann A, et al. Differential expression of the human somatostatin receptor subtypes sst1 to sst5 in various adrenal tumors and normal adrenal gland. Horm Metab Res 2005; 37:722–8.

37. Van der Harst E, de Herder WW, Bruining HA, et al. (123)I metaiodobenzylguanidine and (111) in octreotide uptake in begnign and malignant pheochromocytomas. J Clin Endocrinol Metab 2001;86:685–93.

38. Kroiss A, Shulkin BL, Uprimny C, et al. 68Ga-DOTATOC PET/CT provides accurate tumour extent in patients with extraadrenalparaganglioma compared to 123I-MIBG SPECT/CT. Eur J Nucl Med Mol Imaging 2015;42(1):33–41.

39. Naswa N, Sharma P, Nazar AH, et al. Prospective evaluation of 68Ga-DOTA-NOC PET-CT in phaeochromocytoma and paraganglioma: preliminary results from a single centre study. Eur Radiol 2012;22:710–9.

40. Naswa N, Kumar A, Sharma P, et al. Imaging carotid body chemodectomas with 68Ga-DOTA-NOC PET-CT. Br J Radiol 2012;85:1140–5.

41. Kroiss A, Putzer D, Frech A, et al. A retrospective comparison between 68Ga-DOTA-TOC PET/CT and 18F-DOPA PET/CT in patients with extra-adrenal paraganglioma. Eur J Nucl Med Mol Imaging 2013; 40(12):1800–8.

42. Dralle H, Damm I, Scheumann GF, et al. Frequency and significance of cervicomediastinal lymph node metastases in medullary thyroid carcinoma: results of a compartment-oriented microdissection method. Henry Ford Hosp Med J 1992;40:264–7.

43. Bergholm U, Adami HO, Bergstrom R, et al. Clinical characteristics in sporadic and familial medullary thyroid carcinoma: a nationwide study of 249 patients in Sweden from 1959 through 1981. Cancer 1989;63:1196–204.

44. Scollo C, Baudin E, Travagli JP, et al. Rationale for central and bilateral lymph node dissection in sporadic and hereditary medullary thyroid cancer. J Clin Endocrinol Metab 2003;88:2070–5.

45. Treglia G, Castaldi P, Villani MF, et al. Comparison of 18F-DOPA, 18F-FDG and 68Ga-somatostatin analogue PET/CT in patients with recurrent medullary thyroid carcinoma. Eur J Nucl Med Mol Imaging 2012;39(4):569–80.

46. Verbeek HH, Plukker JT, Koopmans KP, et al. Clinical relevance of 18F-FDG PET and 18F-DOPA PET in recurrent medullary thyroid carcinoma. J Nucl Med 2012;53(12):1863–71.

47. Conry BG, Papathanasiou ND, Prakash V, et al. Comparison of (68)Ga-DOTATATE and (18)F-fluorodeoxyglucose PET/CT in the detection of recurrent medullary thyroid carcinoma. Eur J Nucl Med Mol Imaging 2010;37(1):49–57.

18F-Flourodeoxy-Glucose PET/Computed Tomography in Brain Tumors
Value to Patient Management and Survival Outcomes

Rick Wray, MD[a], Lilja Solnes, MD[a], Esther Mena, MD[a],
Avner Meoded, MD[a],
Rathan M. Subramaniam, MD, PhD, MPH[a,b,c,*]

KEYWORDS

- Central nervous system neoplasm • PET • PET/computed tomography • Brain • Tumor • Cancer
- Survival outcomes • Patient management

KEY POINTS

- 18F-flourodeoxy-glucose (FDG) PET/computed tomography (CT) is useful in the diagnosis, pretherapy prognosis, and response to therapy evaluation in primary central nervous system lymphoma.
- FDG avidity correlates with tumor grade in gliomas.
- FDG PET/CT can be used to identify nonenhancing, low-grade gliomas undergoing malignant transformation.
- FDG PET/CT can differentiate radiation therapy effect from tumor recurrence.

INTRODUCTION

The annual incidence of intracranial central nervous system (CNS) tumors in the United States is 21.4 per 100,000 persons.[1] The 5-year survival rate of all primary brain tumors is 34%.[2] There are many types of primary brain tumors. Gliomas account for greater than 80% of adult primary brain tumors. Less frequent types, such as primary CNS lymphoma, represent 3% of adult primary brain tumors.[3] Metastatic disease to the CNS occurs much more frequently than primary CNS lesions, with an estimated incidence 10 times greater.

The initial presentations for all CNS lesions are similar, manifesting as seizures, headaches, and focal neurologic deficits related to the anatomic site of involvement. The course of disease, however, differs greatly and is influenced by the patterns of growth and anatomic location. Treatment is generally dictated by histopathologic classification. Biopsy is mandatory and key to diagnosis and treatment planning. Although tissue sampling is crucial, it represents a short stop along the pathway from diagnosis to outcome. The standard of care requires a multimodality approach of complementary imaging utilizing dedicated computed tomography (CT), MR imaging, and PET/CT examinations to provide the highest quality assessment.[4]

The authors have nothing to disclose.
[a] Russell H Morgan Department of Radiology and Radiological Sciences, Johns Hopkins School of Medicine, JHOC 3230, 601 North Caroline Street, Baltimore, MD 21287, USA; [b] Department of Oncology, Johns Hopkins School of Medicine, 401 North Broadway, Baltimore, MD 21231, USA; [c] Department of Health Policy and Management, Johns Hopkins Bloomberg School of Public Health, 624 North Broadway, Baltimore, MD 21205, USA
* Corresponding author. Russell H Morgan Department of Radiology and Radiological Sciences, Johns Hopkins Medical Institutions, 601 North Caroline Street/JHOC 3235, Baltimore, MD 21287.
E-mail address: rsubram4@jhmi.edu

MR IMAGING

As per National Comprehensive Cancer Center (NCCN) guidelines, MR imaging is the gold standard of brain imaging, providing high soft-tissue contrast and high-resolution anatomic images.[5]

In addition to anatomy, new developments in MR imaging technique allow functional and metabolic analysis through perfusion-weighted, diffusion-weighted sequences and MR spectroscopy. Although MR imaging does have some limitations - such as availability, cost, and artifacts, it is critical in the diagnostic evaluation and post-therapy assessment of all brain tumors. MR imaging is utilized for anatomic localization, delineation of tumor extent, determination of involvement of higher cortical structures, identifying optimal biopsy sites, tumor grading, assessment of response to therapy, and identifying recurrent/progressive disease.[6–10]

^{18}F-FLOURODEOXY-GLUCOSE PET/ COMPUTED TOMOGRAPHY

Traditionally, ^{18}F-flourodeoxy-glucose (FDG) PET/ CT has played a vital complementary role to MR imaging, supplementing interpretation in areas where MR imaging tended to be equivocal. FDG PET/CT has been shown to correlate with tumor grade, demonstrate malignant transformation, and differentiate tumor from radiation necrosis.[11,12] This article provides an up-to-date assessment of the value of FDG PET/CT to patient management and survival outcomes in primary brain tumors.

GLIOMAS

FDG uptake is typically increased in high-grade tumors.[13] Histologic grading is a means of predicting the biological behavior of a neoplasm, and in the case of gliomas, it is a key factor in diagnosis, prognosis, and treatment selection. Grading is based on the World Health Organization (WHO) criteria and divided into 4 grades. Grades I and II are considered low grade, and grades III and IV are considered high grade. The differentiation reflects not only proliferative activity but also a distinct change in survival outcomes and recurrence rates.

PATIENT MANAGEMENT AND SURVIVAL OUTCOME

Low-grade tumors, such as infiltrative astrocytomas and oligodendrogliomas, have a low proliferative potential, and depending on risk factor stratification, have a median overall survival outcome of 3.9 years for high risk and 10.8 years for low risk.[14] Diffuse astrocytomas were traditionally considered benign but are now considered malignant, because they may dedifferentiate and undergo malignant transformation over time.[15] Low-risk features include age less than 40 years, Karnofsky performance status of at least 70, minor or no neurologic deficits, oligodendroglioma or mixed oligoastrocytoma, tumor dimension less than 6 cm, 1p and 19q co-deletion, and IDH1/2 mutations.[5]

High-grade tumors, such as anaplastic astrocytomas and glioblastomas, demonstrate histologic evidence of malignancy with nuclear atypia and increased mitotic activity. Anaplastic astrocytomas have a 27% 5-year survival rate, and glioblastomas have less than a 5% 5-year survival rate.[16] These high-grade tumors infiltrate adjacent parenchyma, resulting in significant peri-lesional edema, frequently causing symptoms related to their size and subsequent increased intracranial pressure.

Temozolomide is now the standard of care with postoperative radiation therapy (RT) in younger patients with good performance status (PS), showing improved survival when compared with RT alone.[17] Current NCCN guidelines recommend gross tumor resection whenever possible. Aggressive surgery has been shown in multiple studies to be associated with a good prognosis.[18] Adjuvant chemoradiation therapies are based on grade, status of the 1p 19q loci, performance status, and age. Procarbazine, lomustine, and vincristine (PCV) with fractionated external beam radiation therapy (EBRT) are recommended for anaplastic oligodendroglioma or oligoastrocytoma with 1p 19q co-deletion.[19] For glioblastoma in patients younger than 70 with good PS, temozolomide with fractionated RT is given. For glioblastoma in older age patients with poor PS, the regimen vary.

IMAGING EVALUATION: TUMOR GRADE

In the evaluation of a primary CNS tumor, as per NCCN guidelines, MR imaging is performed first to aid diagnosis, then postoperatively within 72 hours, and every 3 to 6 months for 5 years.[5] As grading is a critical factor in patient management and survival outcome, noninvasive radiologic determination of grade has potential to add great value to patient care. The principle that MR imaging exploits to determine enhancement is directly related to the integrity of the blood–brain barrier (BBB). Breakdown of the BBB allows contrast to enter, and this manifests as enhancement. Typically high-grade gliomas are associated with breakdown of the BBB and show enhancement, while low-grade gliomas do not show enhancement. However, this does not always hold true. Some glioblastomas do not show enhancement early in their course, and some anaplastic tumors may not disrupt the BBB. In these cases, the metabolic function of the tumor can become more representative of the grade rather than enhancement on MR imaging.

FDG PET/CT can supplement MR imaging to better determine the grade of a lesion. Evidence for the correlation between FDG avidity and tumor grade in primary brain neoplasms was originally described by Di Chiro in the early 1980s, before generalized use of MR imaging, and it was subsequently shown to predict survival outcome.[13] Since then, the idea has evolved and the concept of a metabolic biopsy generating prognostic information from a lesion's metabolic profile has become an important aspect of the noninvasive oncologic workup.[20] Padma and colleagues[11] were able to predict pathology demonstrating that 86% of patients with tumor uptake less than contralateral white matter on FDG PET had low-grade gliomas (grade I, II) and 94% of patients with tumor uptake greater than contralateral white matter had high-grade gliomas (grade III, IV). Furthermore, the level of uptake had increasing significance on survival with 94% of patients, with low uptake surviving greater than 1 year, and only 29% with high uptake surviving greater than 1 year.

After recurrence of a low-grade glioma, FDG PET/CT can add prognostic value over time. Greater than 60% of astrocytomas and 40% to 50% of oligodendrogliomas will eventually undergo malignant transformation to a higher grade.[15,21,22] Therefore, the histologic features of a low-grade glioma may not reflect the long-term clinical course; however, higher glucose utilization of the tumors with more malignant potential is similar to high-grade gliomas.[23] De Witte and colleagues[24] showed that 19 of 19 (100%) patients with hypometabolic low-grade gliomas survived after 5 years of follow-up compared with only 3 of 9 (33%) patients with hypermetabolic low-grade gliomas. Increased FDG uptake in a previously diagnosed low-grade lesion is highly suggestive of malignant transformation, and this noninvasive finding signifies a decrease in survival outcome.

IMAGING EVALUATION: RECURRENCE VERSUS PSEUDOPROGRESSION AND TUMOR NECROSIS

The treatment for high-grade glioma consists of surgical excision and subsequent radiation therapy with or without chemotherapy for grade IV and grade III disease, respectively.[25] The sequelae of these interventions result in a complex series of events including cell death and vascular injury,

hypoxia, upregulation of vascular endothelial growth factor, and increased vascular permeability.[26] This dynamic process can result in worsening inflammation and edema over time, giving the appearance of worsening disease, a process that has been labeled pseudoprogression.[27] Once the BBB has been significantly violated, surveillance imaging performed with serial MR imaging scans can no longer rely on contrast enhancement to distinguish pseudoprogression from recurrence (**Fig. 1**).[28]

Based on the idea that increased glucose uptake is expected in cancer and not in necrotic or edematous tissue, FDG PET/CT can help differentiate between post-therapy necrosis and tumor recurrence (**Figs. 2** and **3**). Doyle and colleagues[29] demonstrated 100% sensitivity and specificity in 9 patients using lesion to adjacent brain ratios of greater than 1 as positive and less than 1 as negative for tumor with histopathological correlation in 7 of 9 cases. However, additional studies with larger sample sizes have not reproduced these exemplary results, and have been criticized for lack of histopathological

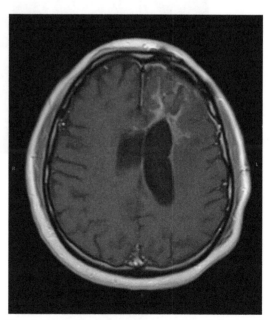

Fig. 1. 36-year-old male patient with a left frontal lobe high-grade glioma status postsurgical resection and chemoradiation. This is an axial slice of a gadolinium postcontrast sequence T1W MR imaging of the brain. There is residual postcontrast enhancement within the left frontal periventricular white matter around the resection cavity, along the ependymal surface of the left lateral ventricle and minimally across the genu of the corpus callosum. These findings raise the possibility of residual disease, but postradiation changes cannot be excluded.

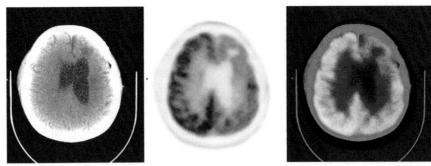

Fig. 2. Follow-up axial PET/CT images after the MR imaging examination of the patient noted in **Fig. 1**. CT attenuation correction images on the left, PET images in the center, PET/CT fused images on the right. Decreased FDG activity in the region of the left, middle, and superior frontal gyri compatible with postsurgical changes status after resection. There is no abnormal hypermetabolism localizing to the enhancement within the left frontal periventricular white matter or ependymal surface noted on the previous MR imaging. These findings are not consistent with residual high-grade glioma and strongly support postradiation changes as the cause for the enhancement on MR imaging.

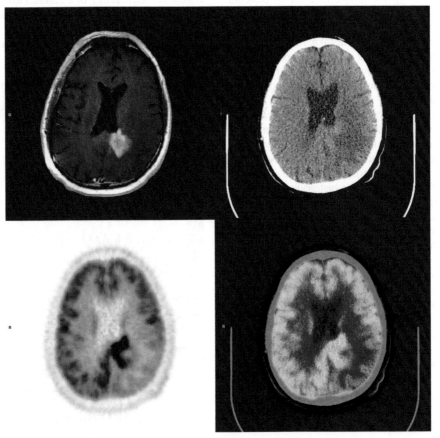

Fig. 3. 53-year-old male patient with a left parietal grade IV glioblastoma status after radiation therapy. Axial slice of a gadolinium postcontrast sequence T1W MR imaging of the brain (*top left*) demonstrates a heterogeneously enhancing mass along the atrium of the left lateral ventricle. This suggests recurrent malignancy, but post-radiation changes cannot be excluded. On CT images (*top right*), there is relative left posterior periventricular hyperdensity. On PET images (*bottom left and right*), this area is associated with focal intense FDG activity relative to the cortex. This intense activity is strongly suggestive of recurrent malignancy and can be used in follow-up evaluation after subsequent treatment.

correlation. Chao and colleagues[30] found sensitivity and specificity of 75% and 81%, respectively, in 47 patients, only 18 with pathologic correlation. Van Laere and colleagues[31] reported sensitivity of 95% and specificity of 50% in a study with 30 patients, only 5 of whom had pathologic correlation. Unfortunately, these more recent reports of heterogenous lower specificities are not useful in the clinical setting and seem to align with anecdotal reports from clinical practice. This has created a desire for new tracers that operate on different principles specifically tailored to brain imaging and primary CNS malignancies.

NOVEL RADIOTRACERS

The current state-of-the art human brain tumor imaging radiotracers are shifting from energy metabolism toward amino acid and nucleic acid metabolism. L-[methyl-11C] methionine (MET) and 8F-fluoroethyl-tyrosine (FET) are amino acid derivatives taken up in larger quantities by tumor cells via system L amino acid transporters (LATs).[32] This pathway has an advantage over FDG, specifically in primary CNS neoplasms, due to its low uptake in normal brain cells.[33]

Despite this advantage, MET PET has shown great differences in diagnostic accuracy but has

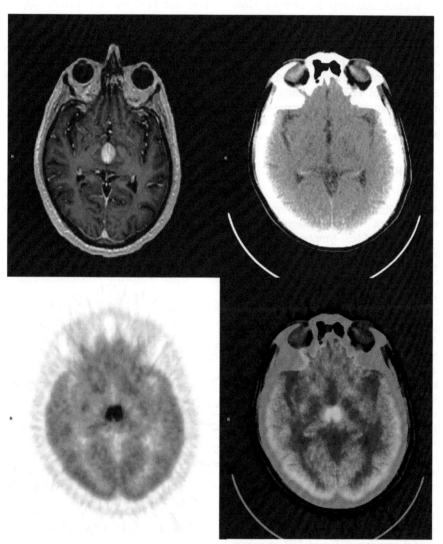

Fig. 4. 76-year-old male patient with progressive memory decline, confusion, and lethargy. Axial slice of a gadolinium postcontrast sequence T1W MR imaging of the brain (*top left*) demonstrates homogeneously an enhancing mass within the midbrain involving the bilateral medial cerebral peduncles at the floor of the third ventricle. These findings are concerning for malignancy, inflammation, or a paraneoplastic syndrome. On PET images (*bottom left and right*), there is intense FDG activity localizing to the bilateral medial cerebral peduncles. On biopsy, this was proven to be primary CNS lymphoma, diffuse large B-cell type.

shown improvements in prediction of outcome when compared with FDG PET. Terakawa and colleagues[34] showed a sensitivity and specificity of 75% in 77 patients when comparing MET with FDG to differentiate tumor recurrence from radiation necrosis. Singhal and colleagues[35] was able to show that MET predicted survival in patients non enhancing lesions and that patients with low grade gliomas who had high uptake (tumor/normal cortex >1.51) had a poorer prognosis than those with low uptake.

FET PET on the other hand has been able to better differentiate between tumor and therapy-associated changes when compared to FDG PET as well as predict outcome in primary CNS neoplasms. Rachinger and colleagues[36] demonstrated a sensitivity and specificity of 100% and 92.9%, respectively in 44 patients with high-grade gliomas, 32 of whom had pathologic correlation. Jansen and colleagues[37] showed that on dynamic evaluation of FET PET, early minimal time to peak was associated with a worse survival outcome comparable to the prognostic significance of WHO grade.

PRIMARY CENTRAL NERVOUS SYSTEM LYMPHOMA

FDG PET/CT has its most distinctive impact on patient management in the diagnosis and follow-up of primary CNS lymphoma. Primary CNS lymphoma is intensely FDG avid, demonstrating standard uptake values (SUVs) significantly greater than gray matter and other CNS neoplasms (**Fig. 4**). Either qualitatively or more precisely by utilizing an SUV cutoff value, primary CNS lymphoma can be reliably distinguished from glioblastoma and brain metastases. Kosaka and colleagues[38] studied 34 patients with CNS tumors and found that utilizing a SUVmax quantitation was a valuable method to distinguish primary CNS lymphoma from primary glioma and metastases. They reported 100% sensitivity when utilizing the lowest SUV (max and average) measurements for CNS lymphomas. When using an SUVmax of 15, there was only one false positive, which proved on biopsy to represent a high-grade glioma. Analogous to the prognostic value of therapy evaluation in systemic lymphoma, which demonstrates a metabolic response to therapy before anatomic response may be detected by conventional imaging (CT and MR imaging), application of this follow-up routine demonstrates similar prognostic advantages in primary CNS lymphoma.[39,40] The standard of care for primary CNS lymphoma is methotrexate therapy. FDG PET/CT allows earlier imaging and response

assessment directing continued therapy or modification with second-line approaches. Kawai and colleagues[41] demonstrated that in immunocompromised patients with primary CNS lymphoma, those who had low-to-moderate FDG uptake were found to have significantly lower overall survival and progression-free survival.

SUMMARY

FDG PET/CT is most useful in the evaluation of primary CNS lymphoma, important in diagnosis, pretherapy prognosis, and therapy response evaluation. Utility in working up gliomas is less effective, and FDG PET/CT is most helpful when MR imaging is unclear. FDG avidity correlates with the grade of gliomas. FDG PET/CT can be used to noninvasively identify malignant transformation. Establishing this change in the disease process has significant effects on patient management and survival outcome.

REFERENCES

1. Ostrom QT, Gittleman H, Liao P, et al. CBTRUS statistical report: primary brain and central nervous system tumors diagnosed in the United States in 2007-2011. Neuro Oncol 2014;16(Suppl 4):iv1–63.
2. Surveillance, Epidemiology, and End Results Program SEER*Stat Databases. Accessed March 13, 2015.
3. Kumar V, Abbas AK, Aster JC. The central nervous system. In: Frosch MP, Anthony DC, De Girolami U, editors. Robbins and cotran pathologic basis of disease. Philadelphia: Elsevier Saunders; 2013. p. 1252–317.
4. Fulham MJ, Mohamed A. Central nervous system. In: Wahl R, editor. Principles and practices of PET and PET/CT. Philadelphia: Lippincott Williams & Wilkins; 2009. p. 199–220.
5. National Comprehensive Cancer Network. Available at: http://www.nccn.org/professionals/physician_gls/pdf/cns.pdf. Accessed March 13, 2015.
6. Wen PY, Macdonald DR, Reardon DA, et al. Updated response assessment criteria for high-grade gliomas: response assessment in neuro-oncology working group. J Clin Oncol 2010;28:1963–72.
7. Rees J. Advances in magnetic resonance imaging of brain tumours. Curr Opin Neurol 2003;16:643–50.
8. Keogh BP, Henson JW. Clinical manifestations and diagnostic imaging of brain tumors. Hematol Oncol Clin North Am 2012;26:733–55.
9. Upadhyay N, Waldman AD. Conventional MRI evaluation of gliomas. Br J Radiol 2011;84(Spec No 2): S107–11.
10. Horska A, Barker PB. Imaging of brain tumors: MR spectroscopy and metabolic imaging. Neuroimaging Clin N Am 2010;20:293–310.

11. Padma MV, Said S, Jacobs M, et al. Prediction of pathology and survival by FDG PET in gliomas. J Neurooncol 2003;64:227–37.

12. Kim EE, Chung SK, Haynie TP, et al. Differentiation of residual or recurrent tumors from post-treatment changes with F-18 FDG PET. Radiographics 1992; 12:269–79.

13. Di Chiro G. Positron emission tomography using [18F] fluorodeoxyglucose in brain tumors. A powerful diagnostic and prognostic tool. Invest Radiol 1987;22:360–71.

14. Daniels TB, Brown PD, Felten SJ, et al. Validation of EORTC prognostic factors for adults with low-grade glioma: a report using intergroup 86-72-51. Int J Radiat Oncol Biol Phys 2011;81:218–24.

15. Piepmeier J, Christopher S, Spencer D, et al. Variations in the natural history and survival of patients with supratentorial low-grade astrocytomas. Neurosurgery 1996;38:872–8 [discussion: 878–9].

16. Ostrom QT, Gittleman H, Farah P, et al. CBTRUS statistical report: primary brain and central nervous system tumors diagnosed in the United States in 2006–2010. Neuro Oncol 2013;15(Suppl 2):ii1–56.

17. Stupp R, Mason WP, van den Bent MJ, et al. Radiotherapy plus concomitant and adjuvant temozolomide for glioblastoma. N Engl J Med 2005;352: 987–96.

18. Laws ER, Parney IF, Huang W, et al. Survival following surgery and prognostic factors for recently diagnosed malignant glioma: data from the Glioma Outcomes Project. J Neurosurg 2003;99:467–73.

19. Medical Research Council Brain Tumor Working Party. Randomized trial of procarbazine, lomustine, and vincristine in the adjuvant treatment of high-grade astrocytoma Medical Research Council trial. J Clin Oncol 2001;19:509–18.

20. Hain SF, Curran KM, Beggs AD, et al. FDG-PET as a "metabolic biopsy" tool in thoracic lesions with indeterminate biopsy. Eur J Nucl Med 2001;28: 1336–40.

21. McCormack BM, Miller DC, Budzilovich GN, et al. Treatment and survival of low-grade astrocytoma in adults—1977-1988. Neurosurgery 1992;31:636–42 [discussion: 642].

22. Scott JN, Rewcastle NB, Brasher PM, et al. Which glioblastoma multiforme patient will become a long-term survivor? A population-based study. Ann Neurol 1999;46:183–8.

23. Francavilla TL, Miletich RS, Di Chiro G, et al. Positron emission tomography in the detection of malignant degeneration of low-grade gliomas. Neurosurgery 1989;24:1–5.

24. De Witte O, Levivier M, Violon P, et al. Prognostic value positron emission tomography with [18F] fluoro-2-deoxy-D-glucose in the low-grade glioma. Neurosurgery 1996;39:470–6 [discussion: 476–7].

25. Stupp R, Roila F. Malignant glioma: ESMO clinical recommendations for diagnosis, treatment and follow-up. Ann Oncol 2009;20(Suppl 4):126–8.

26. Caroline I, Rosenthal MA. Imaging modalities in high-grade gliomas: pseudoprogression, recurrence, or necrosis? J Clin Neurosci 2012;19:633–7.

27. Brandsma D, Stalpers L, Taal W, et al. Clinical features, mechanisms, and management of pseudoprogression in malignant gliomas. Lancet Oncol 2008;9:453–61.

28. Chaskis C, Neyns B, Michotte A, et al. Pseudoprogression after radiotherapy with concurrent temozolomide for high-grade glioma: clinical observations and working recommendations. Surg Neurol 2009; 72:423–8.

29. Doyle WK, Budinger TF, Valk PE, et al. Differentiation of cerebral radiation necrosis from tumor recurrence by [18F]FDG and 82Rb positron emission tomography. J Comput Assist Tomogr 1987;11: 563–70.

30. Chao ST, Suh JH, Raja S, et al. The sensitivity and specificity of FDG PET in distinguishing recurrent brain tumor from radionecrosis in patients treated with stereotactic radiosurgery. Int J Cancer 2001;96: 191–7.

31. Van Laere K, Ceyssens S, Van Calenbergh F, et al. Direct comparison of 18F-FDG and 11C-methionine PET in suspected recurrence of glioma: sensitivity, inter-observer variability and prognostic value. Eur J Nucl Med Mol Imaging 2005;32:39–51.

32. Huang C, McConathy J. Radiolabeled amino acids for oncologic imaging. J Nucl Med 2013;54:1007–10.

33. Kinoshita M, Arita H, Goto T, et al. A novel PET index, 18F-FDG-11C-methionine uptake decoupling score, reflects glioma cell infiltration. J Nucl Med 2012;53: 1701–8.

34. Terakawa Y, Tsuyuguchi N, Iwai Y, et al. Diagnostic accuracy of 11C-methionine PET for differentiation of recurrent brain tumors from radiation necrosis after radiotherapy. J Nucl Med 2008;49:694–9.

35. Singhal T, Narayanan TK, Jacobs MP, et al. 11C-methionine PET for grading and prognostication in gliomas: a comparison study with 18F-FDG PET and contrast enhancement on MRI. J Nucl Med 2012;53:1709–15.

36. Rachinger W, Goetz C, Popperl G, et al. Positron emission tomography with O-(2-[18F]fluoroethyl)-l-tyrosine versus magnetic resonance imaging in the diagnosis of recurrent gliomas. Neurosurgery 2005;57:505–11 [discussion: 505–11].

37. Jansen NL, Suchorska B, Wenter V, et al. Prognostic significance of dynamic 18F-FET PET in newly diagnosed astrocytic high-grade glioma. J Nucl Med 2015;56:9–15.

38. Kosaka N, Tsuchida T, Uematsu H, et al. 18F-FDG PET of common enhancing malignant brain tumors. AJR Am J Roentgenol 2008;190:W365–9.

39. Mikhaeel NG, Hutchings M, Fields PA, et al. FDG-PET after two to three cycles of chemotherapy predicts progression-free and overall survival in high-grade non-Hodgkin lymphoma. Ann Oncol 2005;16:1514–23.

40. Palmedo H, Urbach H, Bender H, et al. FDG-PET in immunocompetent patients with primary central nervous system lymphoma: correlation with MRI and clinical follow-up. Eur J Nucl Med Mol Imaging 2006;33:164–8.

41. Kawai N, Zhen HN, Miyake K, et al. Prognostic value of pretreatment 18F-FDG PET in patients with primary central nervous system lymphoma: SUV-based assessment. J Neurooncol 2010;100:225–32.

18-Fluoro-deoxyglucose–PET/Computed Tomography in Infection and Aseptic Inflammatory Disorders

Value to Patient Management

Sandip Basu, DRM, DNB, MNAMS*, Rohit Ranade, MBBS, DRM

KEYWORDS

- 18-fluoro-deoxyglucose–PET/computed tomography • Inflammation • Infection
- Pyrexia of unknown origin

KEY POINTS

- The role of 18-fluoro-deoxyglucose (FDG)-PET/computed tomography (CT) in infection and aseptic inflammatory disorders continues to evolve.
- In addition to multiple reviews, the joint guidance by The European Association of Nuclear Medicine/Society of Nuclear Medicine and Molecular Imaging (EANM/SNMMI) published in 2012 is a recent combined endeavor to look at the promising areas could translate into the routine management of these treatable conditions and it is imperative that further versions would evolve based upon growing evidence of its utility in the literature.
- In addition to its diagnostic role, FDG-PET can be potentially used for assessing early treatment response that could be useful in tailoring the treatment.

INTRODUCTION

Despite a number of published reports, the routine clinical application of 18-fluoro-deoxyglucose (FDG)-PET/computed tomography (CT) in infection and aseptic inflammatory disorders has been a subject of contention; the utility has been examined and highlighted by various investigators and in reviews and guidelines,[1–11] while others have expressed reservations on preferring FDG-PET-CT over radiolabeled leukocyte imaging (the traditional gold standard). Also, concerns have been raised over using an expensive investigation like PET-CT for a benign condition. However, over the years, the potential utility of this FDG-PET/CT application has grown steadily in the literature, in the form of original papers, case reports, and case series, with several reports underscoring its importance in solving difficult situation.

With several reviews already in literature,[1–11] the authors have provided a brief overview and enumerated the most important areas and practical utilities that can be foreseen from a patient management viewpoint in this group of disorders. Relevant important discussions and references are drawn from literature in fever of unknown origin (FUO) and pyrexia of unknown origin (PUO).

The authors have nothing to disclose.
Radiation Medicine Centre, Bhabha Atomic Research Centre, Tata Memorial Centre Annexe, Jerbai Wadia Road, Parel, Mumbai, Maharashtra 400012, India
* Corresponding author. Radiation Medicine Centre, Bhabha Atomic Research Centre, Tata Memorial Hospital Annexe, Jerbai Wadia Road, Parel, Mumbai, Maharashtra 400012, India.
E-mail address: drsanb@yahoo.com

FEVER OF UNKNOWN ORIGIN/PYREXIA OF UNKNOWN ORIGIN

Whole-body FDG-PET/CT has been increasingly utilized by the clinicians with encouraging results; sensitivity and nonspecificity (as it concentrates in infectious, noninfectious inflammation, as well as malignancy, the three major causes of FUO) of FDG-PET/CT are the major strengths of this modality, which have resulted in its superiority compared with other diagnostic modalities in this domain. The most recent meta-analysis,[12] published in 2013, analyzed 15 studies comprising a total of 595 patients and reported a pooled sensitivity of 85%. The European Association of Nuclear Medicine (EANM)/Society of Nuclear Medicine and Molecular Imaging (SNMMI) joint guidelines[1] state this indication to be having Cochrane grade B level of evidence. Interestingly, in addition to the classical FUO, the guidance mentions the forme-fruste entities, such as postoperative fever and recurrent sepsis, immunodeficiency (both induced and acquired)-related FUO, neutropenic fever, and isolated acute-phase inflammation markers. Furthermore, the role has been also suggested in surveying to detect metastatic infection in high-risk patients with bacteremia,[1,13–15] with a few studies demonstrating its positive impact on both

lowering relapse rates and mortality and also in terms of cost-effectiveness.

Future Clinical Role

It can be envisaged that with encouraging results in FUO and its forme-fruste, FDG-PET/CT would emerge as the imaging examination of first choice, when it is available, followed by FDG-PET/CT finding guided more specific investigations to clinch the diagnosis. Being a whole-body examination, the findings on PET-CT could also serve as an adjunct for therapeutic decision making and monitoring therapeutic efficacy in a given setting.

SPINAL INFECTION

In a limited number of reported studies and experience, FDG-PET/CT has shown promising results in this clinical setting and has been proposed to be the radionuclide examination of choice. The EANM/SNMMI guidelines[1] have proposed this indication to be having Cochrane grade B level of evidence. The high-resolution tomographic images further enhanced with PET/CT fusion enable precise localization of sites of infection (**Fig. 1**). This is in addition to its obvious advantage over the white blood cell (WBC) scanning

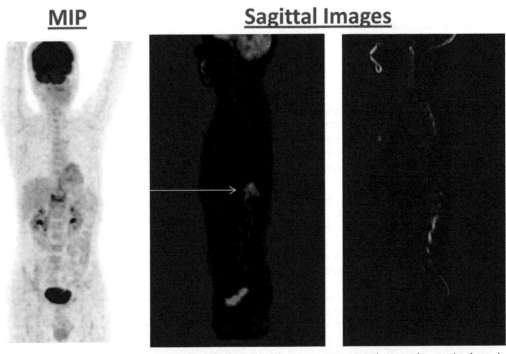

Fig. 1. In this 46-year-old man, a proven case of multiple tuberculomas on MRI recently started on anti-tubercular treatment (ATT) (initially presenting with fever, chills, and severe headache) FDG PET/CT demonstrating metabolically active lesion in dorsal and lumbar vertebrae D10-L1 vertebrae (*arrow*), subsequently proven to be Koch spine.

because of normal uptake of the tracer in the axial skeleton, and hence clearly proves FDG-PET/CT to be superior compared with WBC count.

Future Clinical Role

The meta-analysis by Prodromou and colleagues[16] reported encouraging results (from 12 comprising of 224 patients) with pooled sensitivity, specificity, positive predictive value, and negative predictive value of 97%, 88%, 96%, and 85%, respectively. However, a few points need to be clarified: increased FDG uptake related to degenerative disease, fracture, and presence of a foreign body such

as synthetic vertebral fixation devices. All of these might result in a noninfectious inflammatory response. CT features could be utilized as a powerful tool in these situations, and further studies are needed to clarify these concerns.

GRANULOMATOUS DISORDERS

Monitoring disease activity with FDG-PET/CT, assessing response to administered treatment, and tailoring therapy (rather than making a diagnosis) have been the primary purposes for employing FDG-PET/CT (**Figs. 2** and **3**) in this group of disorders.[8,9] However, akin to malignancy, the

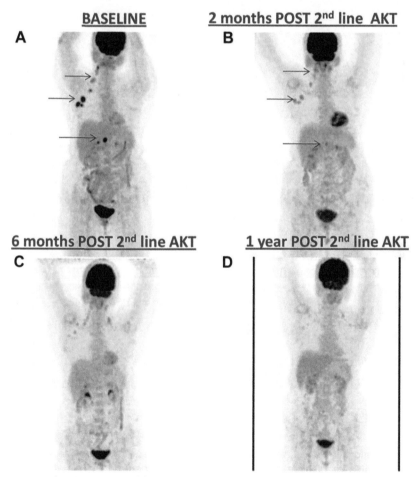

Fig. 2. The response evaluation to second-line anti-tubercular treatment (ATT) is demonstrated in a 47-year-old woman, who initially presented with right-sided neck swelling. Cervical nodal biopsy revealed it as granulomatous reaction with culture positive for mycobacterial species. The patient failed to respond to first-line treatment with HRZE (H, isoniazid; R, rifampin; Z, pyrazinamide; E, ethambutol) regimen and was designated to harbor multi-drug resistant (MDR) TB. FDG-PET/CT was considered for evaluating response to second-line ATT. Repeat PET-CT at 2 months showed complete resolution of right cervical, retropectoral and paracaval lymphadenopathy. There was decrease in metabolic activity of supraclavicular, axillary, and para-aortic lymphadenopathy. The figures show serial PET-CT done at baseline (A), PET-CT at 2 months (B), 6 months (C) and at 1 year (D), following second-line ATT, which showed gradual decrease in the indicated metabolically active lymph node groups (arrows) with complete resolution at end of 1 year after treatment. (E–H) Demonstrates response of individual lymph node regions in fused PET-CT Bransaxial format.

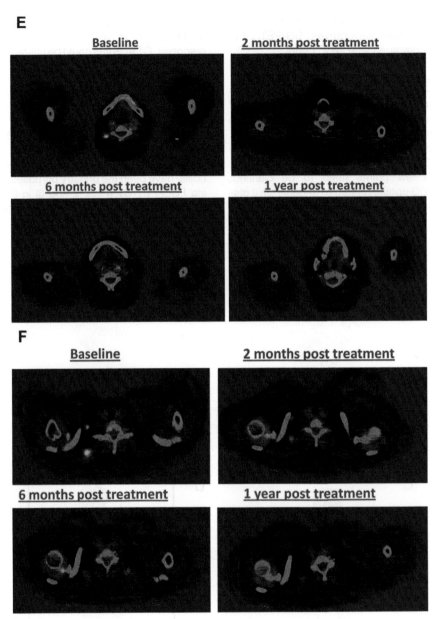

Fig. 2. (*continued*)

whole-body examination could not uncommonly reveal unexpected sites of disease involvement in these systemic disorders.[17]

In the joint guidance,[1] the cumulative sensitivity from 7 studies and 173 patients of sarcoidosis was 93.5%, and accuracy was 95.5%. In the setting of drug-resistant tuberculosis, assessment of metabolic activity of the lesions could be of substantial advantage. The exact time of response assessment is not clear, but 2 months following initiation of therapy is 1 point when the treating physician considers shifting from the 4-drug to 2-drug regimen, and

would find an imaging evidence of response to serve as useful parameter. This would be particularly true for nonpulmonary lesions, where sputum examination will not be helpful; invasive biopsy is not feasible, and hence, metabolic disease activity on FDG-PET/CT can be particularly valuable.[17] An area of particular interest is monitoring response in patients with high incidence of drug resistance such as those with human immunodeficiency virus (HIV)-associated tuberculosis, where FDG-PET/CT examination has demonstrated particular promise.[18,19]

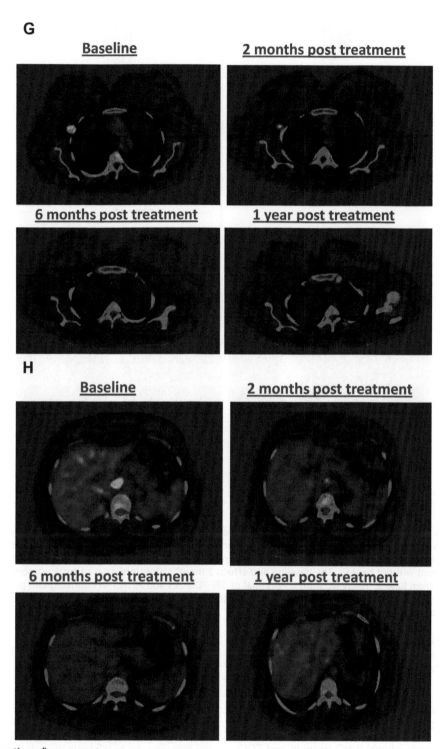

Fig. 2. (*continued*)

Future Clinical Role

FDG-PET/CT imaging could be utilized for assessing treatment response early in the disease course (both in sarcoidosis and tuberculosis)[17,19–21] and thus help in modifying/tailoring therapy. It could be particularly useful in tuberculosis in those patients who are at higher risk of drug resistance and also those with nonpulmonary involvement in whom the traditional sputum examination and

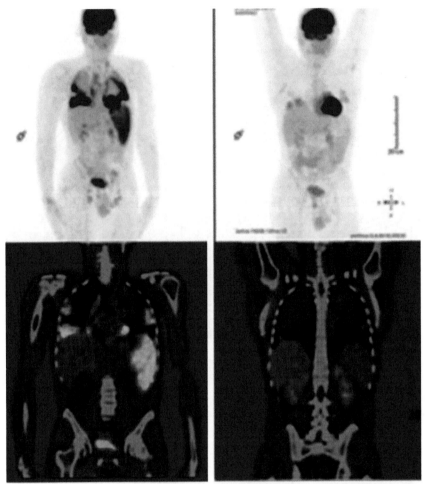

Baseline : Pre Rx   Post Rx: 2 Months

Fig. 3. Early treatment response monitoring of a 44-year-old man, diagnosed case of sarcoidosis who initially presented with cough; serum angiotensin converting enzyme (ACE) was 115 IU/L. He presented with expectoration, low-grade fever, and breathlessness on exertion and had earlier undergone with antibiotics and antitubercular treatment without benefit. The baseline and effects 2 months after initiation of corticosteroid therapy are illustrated. (*From* Basu S, Yadav M, Joshi J. Potential of 18F-FDG-PET and PET/CT in nonmalignant pulmonary disorders: much more than currently perceived? Making the case from experience gained in the Indian scenario. Nucl Med Commun 2014;35(7):4; with permission.)

culture is not be useful. The whole-body survey is an additional advantage and can help in assessing whole-body disease burden.

PERIPHERAL BONE OSTEOMYELITIS INCLUDING DIABETIC FOOT

While both conventional WBC imaging and FDG-PET/CT have demonstrated equivalent results, the latter is emerging as the preferred modality because of several advantages:

Completion of the examination within a short period of time (1.5–2 hours)
High target-to-background contrast ratios

Better interobserver agreement
Technically less demanding

The analysis by the joint guidelines[1] documents high efficacy for peripheral bone osteomyelitis examined in 8 original articles describing 287 patients with sensitivity of 94.6%, specificity of 91.5%, and accuracy of 94.5%, with relatively modest results in diabetic foot (5 papers, 220 patients, sensitivity 70.6%, specificity 84.4%, and accuracy 80.0%).

Future Clinical Role

In the authors' view, the superior resolution tomographic images of FDG-PET/CT can be of potential use in differentiating soft tissue infection and osteomyelitis (particularly it would have a high negative predictive value), while in the diabetic foot, in addition to the aforementioned benefits (**Fig. 4**), it can be potentially utilized in differentiating Charcot neuroarthropathy from osteomyelitis,[22] especially in difficult cases in which diagnosis is not clear.

INFECTION RELATED TO PROSTHESIS: JOINT PROSTHESIS (HIP AND KNEE), VASCULAR PROSTHESIS AND GRAFT INFECTION

The literature is divided in the following scenario. In the analysis of the joint guidance,[1] for skeletal joint prosthesis infection, in a total of 17 studies comprising of 770 patients, the cumulative sensitivity documented was 95.0%, while the specificity was 98.0%, with an overall accuracy of 78.0%. For vascular prosthesis, the calculated figures were 88.9%, 64.6%, and 74.5%, respectively calculated from 5 studies with 189 patients. Based upon the aforementioned results, the joint guidance concluded that it is unclear whether FDG-PET/CT could be preferred compared with the conventional WBC-based infection imaging.

Future Clinical Role

Although there has been some debate in these areas, the authors believe that with appropriate adjunctive correlation and defining criterion (especially joint prosthesis infection such as hip prosthesis), the results will be improved in the future.

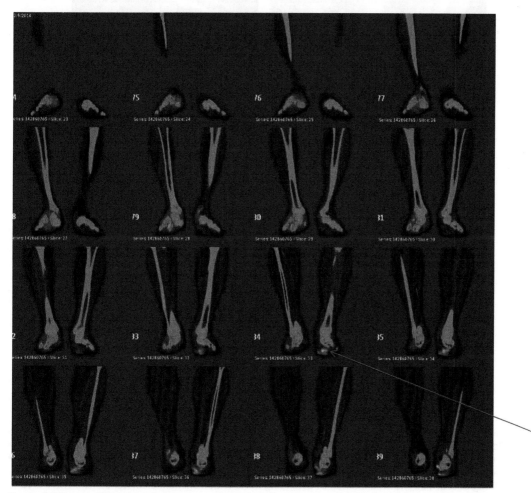

Fig. 4. A 54 –year-old man is a known case of type 2 diabetes on antidiabetic medication since the age of 12 years. He had a nonhealing ulcer in the left foot about 1 month previous. Radiograph of the left foot showed a soft tissue swelling in the left foot and predominantly around the ankle posteriorly. He was referred for FDG-PET/CT to look for any bony involvement. Coronal PET-CT images shows intense FDG uptake, primarily in the ulcer and soft tissue of the left foot (*arrows*) with the bone uninvolved ruling out osteomyelitis.

OTHER SOFT TISSUE INFECTIONS AND INFLAMMATION INCLUDING VASCULITIS

Assessing disease activity in vasculitis (such as giant cell arteritis, aortoarteritis) has been underscored by a number of reports in the literature.[1,23–26] FDG-PET can be potentially used for assessing early treatment response to steroid therapy (**Fig. 5**) and thus could be useful in tailoring the dose of treatment. This application of FDG-PET/CT has been graded to have Cochrane grade B level of evidence by the joint guidelines.[1]

The other promising areas, in which the precise role is not yet clear, but could be potentially useful include infected liver and kidney cysts in polycystic disease, and AIDS-associated opportunistic infections.[1] Evidence of a relatively lesser degree has been reported in endocarditis and inflammatory bowel disease (IBD), though in the authors' experience, it can be useful in difficult settings in the former,[27] while in the latter, using quantitative approach, the authors recently reported[28] a possibility of calculating indices of regional and global Chron's disease (CD) activity, which correlated

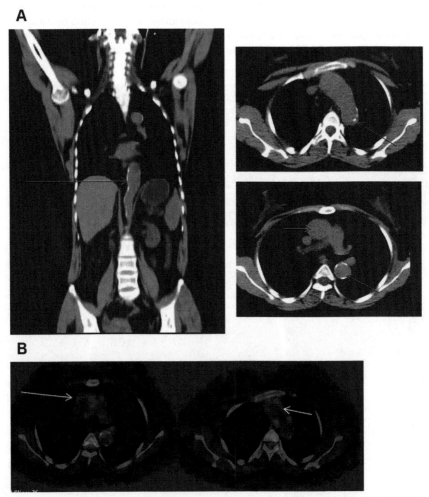

Fig. 5. Assessing disease activity in proven patient of aortoarteritis already on steroid therapy. The patient, a 26-year-old woman, initially presented with abdominal pain. She was subsequently confirmed to have renovascular hypertension and diagnosed to have aortoarteritis with right renal artery total occlusion and a history of left renal angioplasty. At the time of FDG-PET/CT she was asymptomatic and was on maintenance dose of prednisolone 10 mg/d. ceCT had shown dilatation of ascending aorta with maximum diameter 3.9 cm. There is calcification in the arch of aorta, especially in the posterior arch with associated intimal thickening (*arrow*). Also there is calcification and dilatation of thoracic part of abdominal aorta (*arrow*) with maximum diameter of 3.1 cm. Additionally, there is sudden change of caliber of the descending aorta just below the diaphragm (*A*). FDG-PET CT (*B*) on steroid showed persistence of low-grade metabolism in the lesions in ascending aorta and arch of aorta (*arrows*), consistent with her clinically asymptomatic status.

well with both clinical and pathologic disease activity in patients of IBD. This could be useful for tailoring therapy to the appropriate level.

REFERENCES

1. Jamar F, Buscombe J, Chiti A, et al. EANM/SNMMI guideline for 18F-FDG use in inflammation and infection. J Nucl Med 2013;54(4):647–58.

2. Alavi A, Zhuang H. Finding infection–help from PET. Lancet 2001;358(9291):1386.

3. Basu S, Zhuang H, Torigian DA, et al. Functional imaging of inflammatory diseases using nuclear medicine techniques. Semin Nucl Med 2009;39(2):124–45.

4. Basu S, Chryssikos T, Moghadam-Kia S, et al. Positron emission tomography as a diagnostic tool in infection: present role and future possibilities. Semin Nucl Med 2009;39(1):36–51.

5. Kumar R, Basu S, Torigian D, et al. Role of modern imaging techniques for diagnosis of infection in the era of 18F-fluorodeoxyglucose positron emission tomography. Clin Microbiol Rev 2008;21(1):209–24.

6. Love C, Tomas MB, Tronco GG, et al. FDG PET of infection and inflammation. Radiographics 2005; 25(5):1357–68.

7. Basu S, Saboury B, Werner T, et al. Clinical utility of FDG-PET and PET/CT in non-malignant thoracic disorders. Mol Imaging Biol 2011;13(6):1051–60.

8. Basu S, Alavi A. Emerging role of FDG-PET for optimal response assessment in infectious diseases and disorders. Expert Rev Anti Infect Ther 2011; 9(2):143–5.

9. Basu S. 18F-FDG PET/CT as a sensitive and early treatment monitoring tool: will this become the major thrust for its clinical application in infectious and inflammatory disorders? J Nucl Med 2012;53(1):165.

10. Alavi A, Saboury B, Basu S. Imaging the infected heart. Sci Transl Med 2011;3(99):99fs3.

11. Hess S, Hansson SH, Pederson KT, et al. FDG-PET/CT in infectious and inflammatory diseases. PET Clin 2014;9(4):497–519.

12. Hao R, Yuan L, Kan Y, et al. Diagnostic performance of 18F-FDG PET/CT in patients with fever of unknown origin: a meta-analysis. Nucl Med Commun 2013;34(7):682–8.

13. Bleeker-Rovers CP, Vos FJ, Wanten GJ, et al. 18F-FDG PET in detecting metastatic infectious disease. J Nucl Med 2005;46(12):2014–9.

14. Vos FJ, Bleeker-Rovers CP, Kullberg BJ, et al. Cost-effectiveness of routine (18)F-FDG PET/CT in high-risk patients with gram-positive bacteremia. J Nucl Med 2011;52(11):1673–8.

15. Vos FJ, Bleeker-Rovers CP, Sturm PD, et al. 18F-FDG PET/CT for detection of metastatic infection in gram-positive bacteremia. J Nucl Med 2010; 51(8):1234–40.

16. Prodromou ML, Ziakas PD, Poulou LS, et al. FDG PET is a robust tool for the diagnosis of spondylodiscitis: a meta-analysis of diagnostic data. Clin Nucl Med 2014;39(4):330–5.

17. Basu S, Yadav M, Joshi J. Potential of 18F-FDG-PET and PET/CT in nonmalignant pulmonary disorders: much more than currently perceived? Making the case from experience gained in the Indian scenario. Nucl Med Commun 2014;35(7):689–96.

18. Sathekge M, Maes A, Kgomo M, et al. Use of 18F-FDG PET to predict response to first-line tuberculostatics in HIV-associated tuberculosis. J Nucl Med 2011;52:880–5.

19. Sathekge M, Maes A, Kgomo M, et al. FDG uptake in lymph-nodes of HIV1 and tuberculosis patients: implications for cancer staging. Q J Nucl Med Mol Imaging 2010;54:698–703.

20. Tirpude S, Basu S, Joshi JM. FDG-PET scan in management of pulmonary sarcoidosis. J Assoc Physicians India 2013;61(4):276.

21. Basu S, Asopa RV, Baghel NS. Early documentation of therapeutic response at 6 weeks following corticosteroid therapy in extensive sarcoidosis: promise of FDG-PET. Clin Nucl Med 2009;34(10):689–90.

22. Basu S, Chryssikos T, Houseni M, et al. Potential role of FDG PET in the setting of diabetic neuro-osteoarthropathy: can it differentiate uncomplicated Charcot's neuroarthropathy from osteomyelitis and soft-tissue infection? Nucl Med Commun 2007;28: 465–72.

23. Webb M, Chambers A, AL-Nahhas A, et al. The role of 18F-FDG PET in characterising disease activity in Takayasu arteritis. Eur J Nucl Med Mol Imaging 2004;31:627–34.

24. Förster S, Tato F, Weiss M, et al. Patterns of extracranial involvement in newly diagnosed giant cell arteritis assessed by physical examination, colour coded duplex sonography and FDG-PET. Vasa 2011;40: 219–27.

25. Hautzel H, Sander O, Heinzel A, et al. Assessment of large-vessel involvement in giant cell arteritis with 18F-FDG PET: introducing an ROC-analysis-based cutoff ratio. J Nucl Med 2008;49:1107–13.

26. Meller J, Strutz F, Siefker U, et al. Early diagnosis and follow-up of aortitis with [18F]FDG PET and MRI. Eur J Nucl Med Mol Imaging 2003;30:730–6.

27. Moghadam-Kia S, Nawaz A, Millar BC, et al. Imaging with 18F-FDG-PET in infective endocarditis: promising role in difficult diagnosis and treatment monitoring. Hell J Nucl Med 2009;12:165–7.

28. Saboury B, Salavati A, Brothers A, et al. FDG PET/CT in Crohn's disease: correlation of quantitative FDG PET/CT parameters with clinical and endoscopic surrogate markers of disease activity. Eur J Nucl Med Mol Imaging 2014;41(4):605–14.

Cardiac PET/Computed Tomography Applications and Cardiovascular Outcome

CrossMark

Thomas Hellmut Schindler, MD*

KEYWORDS

- Coronary circulation • CAD • Hibernating myocardium • Myocardial blood flow
- Myocardial flow reserve • PET/CT • Prognosis • Sarcoid disease

KEY POINTS

- Cardiac PET/computed tomography (CT) in conjunction with different blood flow tracers is increasingly applied for the assessment of myocardial perfusion and myocardial flow reserve (MFR) in the detection of the coronary artery disease (CAD) process and its characterization in patients with suspected or known CAD.
- The concurrent ability of PET/CT to noninvasively determine regional myocardial blood flow in milliliters per gram per minute at rest and during vasomotor stress allows the calculation of the MFR, which carries important prognostic information in patients with subclinical forms of cardiomyopathy.
- The measured MFR optimizes the identification and characterization of the extent and severity of CAD burden, and contributes to the flow-limiting effect of single lesions in multivessel CAD.

INTRODUCTION

Although cardiac single-photon emission computed tomography (SPECT) and SPECT/computed tomography (CT) are still the mainstays for the detection of hemodynamically obstructive coronary artery disease (CAD) in clinical routine, cardiac PET/CT with positron-emitting perfusion tracers is increasingly applied for CAD detection and cardiovascular risk prediction in patients with suspected or known CAD.[1–3] While regional reductions in radiotracer uptake during hyperemic flow stimulation compared with rest commonly identifies downstream flow-limiting effects of the most severe epicardial narrowing, the hemodynamic obstructive effects of less

severe obstructive CAD lesions in multivessel disease and/or the presence of subclinical and non-obstructive CAD may remain unidentified.[2–5] In this respect, the concurrent ability of PET/CT in concert with various positron-emitting radiotracers, such as ^{13}N-ammonia, [82]rubidium, ^{15}O-water, and 18F-flurpiridaz, to determine regional myocardial blood flow (MBF) in milliliters per gram per minute during different forms of vasomotor stress and at rest allows the noninvasive assessment of the myocardial flow reserve (MFR).[1,3,6] The MFR reflects the vasodilator capacity of the coronary circulation and integrating flow dynamics of both the epicardial and coronary microcirculations. The added value of hyperemic MBF and MFR to the conventional visual

Disclosures: Dr Schindler acknowledges all sources of funding as follows: Departmental fund (no. 175470) from Johns Hopkins University, Baltimore, Maryland, USA, and Research grant no. 3200B0-122237 from the Swiss National Science Foundation (SNF; Dr Schindler), with contributions of the Clinical Research Center, University Hospital, and Faculty of Medicine, Geneva and the Louis-Jeantet Foundation; Swiss Heart Foundation; and Gustave and Simone Prévot fund.
Division of Nuclear Medicine, Department of Radiology SOM, Johns Hopkins University School of Medicine, Baltimore, MD, USA
* Division of Cardiovascular Nuclear Medicine, Department of Radiology and Radiological Science SOM, Johns Hopkins University School of Medicine, JHOC 3225, 601 North Caroline Street, Baltimore, MD 21287.
E-mail address: tschind3@jhmi.edu

analysis of myocardial perfusion has been realized (1) in the identification of an impairment of coronary circulatory function, as a functional precursor of the CAD process,[7–9] and its potential to noninvasively monitor its response to lifestyle intervention and/or preventive medical intervention[1,10,11]; (2) in prognostication in patients with subclinical and clinically manifest CAD as well as in cardiomyopathy[1,2,12] (3); in optimization of the identification and characterization of the extent and severity of CAD burden[13]; and (4) in the detection of the flow-limiting effect of single lesions in multivessel CAD (**Box 1**).[1,4,14] Apart from the increased use of cardiac PET/CT for CAD detection and cardiovascular risk stratification in clinical routine,[1,2] its role also extends to the identification of hibernating-stunning myocardium in ischemic cardiomyopathy[15]; cardiac sarcoid involvement; and, potentially in the near future, to the detection of inflammatory, and thus vulnerable, coronary plaque burden.[16–18]

This article discusses the contributions of cardiac PET/CT in the identification and characterization of subclinical or clinically manifest CAD, including its diagnostic and prognostic implications, its potential influence on the clinical decision-making process in patients with CAD with ischemic cardiomyopathy and cardiac sarcoid involvement, and its clinical outcome.

PERFUSION AND FLOW IN CORONARY ARTERY DISEASE DETECTION

Contrast CT coronary angiography with 128-slice, or more recently dual-source, CT has evolved clinically as a mainstay in the noninvasive exclusion or identification of the CAD process.[19] In contrast, invasive coronary angiography with quantitative evaluation of luminal stenosis still remains the gold standard for the evaluation of the severity of flow-obstructive CAD lesions.[20] Pioneering work in the 70th by Gould and colleagues[21–23] outlined that resting MBF remains normal and is related to cardiac workload[24] unless an epicardial stenosis attains a severity of 90%. Despite increasing severity of CAD-induced epicardial narrowing up to 90%, resting coronary or myocardial flow may still be maintained because of a compensatory vasodilation of the coronary microcirculation, compensating for the increase in epicardial vascular resistance. However, during hyperemic flow increase owing to pharmacologic vasodilation, an increasing severity of epicardial lesions with greater than or equal to 50% luminal obstruction is inversely associated with decreases of hyperemic flow and MFR, respectively.[25–28] However, the observed inverse relationship between epicardial stenosis severity and hyperemic flows does not necessarily apply in the presence of collateral flow supply and/or preserved MFR related to physical exercise and/or beneficial effects of preventive medical care with statins and/or angiotensin-converting enzyme (ACE) inhibitors.[1,25,27,29] This situation again contributes to a distinct variability of hyperemic flow increases and, thus, MFR, confounding the classic inverse association between the severity of obstructive CAD lesions and hyperemic flow increases.[25–27,30–33] In the clinical scenario, the decision-making process regarding interventional or surgical procedures to restore coronary flow is generally based on the identification of stress-induced myocardial ischemia, or invasively measured fractional MFR.[1,34,35] In this respect, PET/CT in concert with tracer kinetic modeling enables clinicians to concurrently determine regional MBF in milliliters per gram per minute at rest and during pharmacologically stimulated hyperemic flow increases, and thus the MFR (the ratio of hyperemic to resting MBF). This ability increases the scope of conventional myocardial perfusion imaging from the detection of advanced and flow-limiting epicardial CAD lesions to the identification and description of CAD burden in multivessel disease, as well as to early functional stages of the atherosclerotic process or microvascular dysfunction (see **Box 1**).[1,3,14]

ENHANCED IDENTIFICATION OF CORONARY ARTERY DISEASE BURDEN

Analyzing the regional radiotracer uptake on stress-rest scintigraphic perfusion images of the left ventricle in relative terms may underestimate the severity and extent of CAD burden in multivessel disease. Because a decrease in regional radiotracer uptake during stress compared with

---

Box 1
Clinical use of PET-determined MFR

1. Identification and characterization of subclinical CAD and its response to preventive medical intervention

2. Prognostic information in subclinical and clinically manifest CAD, as well as in cardiomyopathy

3. Characterization of the extent and severity of CAD burden in multivessel disease

4. Unraveling of balanced reduction in MBF owing to 3-vessel or main-stem CAD[a]

[a] Effects of diffuse myocardial ischemia need to be confirmed by a peak stress transient cavity dilation of the left ventricle during maximal vasomotor stress on gated PET images.

rest identifies advanced hemodynamically obstructive CAD lesions, the flow-limiting effects of other lesions but with less severe epicardial narrowing may be missed because the radiotracer uptake may still be homogeneous or normal, as in the reference region. Adding the concurrently determined regional hyperemic MBF and MFR to the conventional analysis of scintigraphic myocardial perfusion images may unmask not only the most advanced or culprit lesion, as signified by the stress-induced regional perfusion defect but also the flow-limiting effects of the other CAD stenoses of lesser severity in regions without stress-induced perfusion defects on visual perfusion analysis, as shown by markedly reduced MFRs (**Fig. 1**).[1,14] Yet, reductions in hyperemic MBFs are not only related to downstream effects of epicardial narrowing but also, at least in part, to cardiovascular risk factor–induced microvascular dysfunction.[3–5] In addition, because of differences in methodology and the positron-emitting tracers applied, the optimal cutoff values of PET-determined MFR are still a matter of debate.[1,4] For the positron-emitting tracers ^{13}N-ammonia or $H_2^{15}O$, the thresholds for abnormal reductions in MFR are commonly defined as 2.0 and 2.5, respectively.[36,37] However, the nonspecificity of reductions in regional hyperemic MBFs and MFRs[4,29] necessitates that the evaluation of flow values is performed in conjunction with known coronary anatomy and/or microvascular dysfunction in individuals with cardiovascular risk and/or CAD.[1,29] More recently, it has been suggested that, in the presence of an epicardial stenosis greater than or equal to 70%, reductions in MFR of less than 1.7 can be widely related to stenosis-induced increases in epicardial resistance using PET with ^{13}N-ammonia or ^{82}rubidium as myocardial flow tracer.[38] In contrast, a normal MFR carries a high negative predictive value (97%) for the exclusion of high-risk CAD, defined as 2-vessel disease (≥70% stenosis), including the proximal left anterior descending artery; 3-vessel disease; or left main CAD (≥50% stenosis).[29] There is a novel emerging suggestion that a PET-measured longitudinal decrease in hyperemic MBFs from the base to the apex of the heart may be a reflection of increases in epicardial resistance caused by diffuse or focal CAD-related epicardial narrowing.[39] This novel diagnostic approach to the assessment of longitudinal decrease in hyperemic MBFs from the base to the apex may yield more specific information on epicardial resistance than is gained from the conventional MFR,[4,6,40–42] and therefore may evolve as noninvasive fractional flow reserve but needing further clinical validation.

IDENTIFICATION OF DIFFUSE ISCHEMIA

Diffuse myocardial ischemia caused by flow-limiting effects of significant left main-stem lesion or 3-vessel diseases may remain undetected with the conventional approach of myocardial scintigraphic perfusion imaging to assess the relative distribution of the radiotracer uptake in the left ventricle. Under such conditions, the relative radiotracer uptake of the left ventricle during pharmacologically induced hyperemic flows remains widely homogeneous because reductions in hyperemic flows are balanced in all 3 major coronary territories of the left anterior descending (LAD), left circumflex artery (LCx), and right coronary artery (RCA). Consequently, the relative distribution of myocardial perfusion remains widely reduced homogeneously in the entire left ventricular myocardium during vasomotor stress.[43] This distribution again hampers the identification of 3-vessel CAD and/or left main-stem lesion because the radiotracer uptake of the left ventricle during hyperemic flows may stay homogeneous. It has been reported that, in patients with angiographically proven 3-vessel CAD, conventional myocardial perfusion scintigraphy (MPS) with SPECT could identify only 10% of patients (14 of 143) having stress-induced regional perfusion defects.[44] In contrast, when regional wall motion abnormalities on post–stress-gated SPECT were added to myocardial perfusion imaging in the evaluation, the detection for 3-vessel CAD increased but only to 25%. In another investigation, Berman and colleagues[45] investigated 101 patients with left main CAD (≥50% stenosis) without prior myocardial infarction or coronary revascularization who underwent gated exercise or adenosine stress technetium 99m sestamibi SPECT myocardial perfusion. When analyzing myocardial perfusion visually and semiquantitatively, a high-risk feature with moderate to severe perfusion defects (>10% myocardium at stress) was noted in 56% and 59% of patients, respectively. In contrast, no significant stress-induced perfusion defect (≥5% myocardium) was appreciated in 13% to 15% of patients. Conversely, combining abnormal perfusion and wall motion on post–stress-gated SPECT, 83% of patients were detected as high-risk individuals.[45] In this way, adding the PET/CT-determined reductions in hyperemic MBF and MFR may be of further help to directly interpret balanced ischemia of the left ventricular myocardium caused by severe 3-vessel CAD or significant stenosis of the left main coronary artery.[1,3,14] Because diffuse decreases in hyperemic MBF or MFR may also be related to microvascular dysfunction in individuals with cardiovascular risk, stress-induced and balanced

A

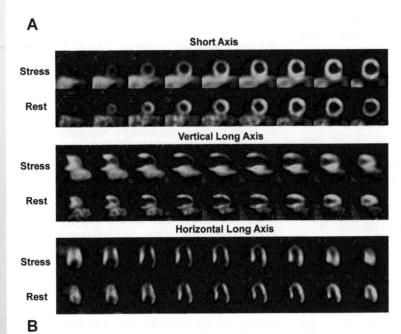

Fig. 1. ^{13}N-ammonia PET in the evaluation of multivessel CAD. (A) Myocardial perfusion study with ^{13}N-ammonia PET/CT during dipyridamole stimulation and at rest in a 61-year-old patient with arterial hypertension and type 2 diabetes mellitus. On stress images, there is a moderately decreased perfusion defect involving the mid to distal anterior, anteroseptal, and apical regions of the left ventricle, which becomes reversible on the rest images. Uptake is preserved in the lateral and inferior regions. (B) Regional MBF quantification and MFR calculation with ^{13}N-ammonia PET/CT and tracer kinetic modeling. The summarized quantitative data suggest a marked impairment of the MFR not only in the left anterior descending artery (LAD) territory but also in the right coronary artery (RCA) and left circumflex artery (LCx) vascular territories (regional MFR [rMFR] <2.0). (C) Invasive coronary angiography in this patient showed a proximal occlusion of the LAD, 80% stenosis in the proximal segments of the LCx (left panel), and sequential 50% to 60% lesions in the RCA (right panel). Corresponding regional MFRs are indicated for each vascular territory. (From Schindler TH, Schelbert HR, Quercioli A, et al. Cardiac PET imaging for the detection and monitoring of coronary artery disease and microvascular health. JACC Cardiovasc Imaging 2010;3(6):629; with permission.)

B

PET/CT and MBF quantification with radiotracer N-13 Ammonia

Coronary Territory	Rest MBF (mL/g/min)	Stress MBF (mL/g/min)	MFR (Stress / Rest)
LAD	1.09	1.31	1.20
LCx	1.10	1.55	1.41
RCA	1.22	1.65	1.35

C

Coronary Angiography Unmasking Multivessel Disease

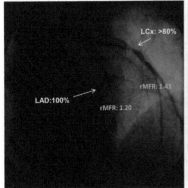

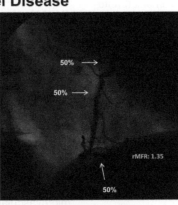

Left Coronary Tree   Right Coronary Tree

ischemia should always be confirmed by a peak stress transient ischemic cavity dilation of the left ventricle associated with a global hypokinesis on gated PET images.[46,47]

IDENTIFICATION OF SUBCLINICAL CORONARY ARTERY DISEASE AND PROGNOSTIC IMPLICATIONS

As mentioned earlier, conventional MPS is most valuable to detect hemodynamically obstructive CAD in patients with known or suspected CAD,[1,2] whereas an abnormal function of the coronary circulation, commonly regarded as functional precursor of the CAD process,[7,8] remains undetected in individuals with cardiovascular risk.[48] Subclinical stages of CAD commonly reveal a homogeneous or mild heterogeneity in relative myocardial uptake of the radiotracer during vasomotor stress[6,40,41] and homogeneously impaired hyperemic MBF increases that remain unnoted.[39] However, PET perfusion and flow imaging can signify early functional disturbances of the coronary circulation by interpreting homogeneously reduced hyperemic MBF and MFR, which is likely to promote the development of structural CAD.[8,42,49,50] An abnormal function of the coronary circulation commonly starts at the site of the endothelium, so that an endothelium-dependent or flow-mediated coronary vasodilation is impaired, whereas vascular smooth muscle cell function may still be operational in individuals with various cardiovascular risk factors.[1,51] In asymptomatic insulin-resistant individuals with normal stress-rest myocardial perfusion on PET images, concurrent MBF quantification has identified disturbances in endothelium-related MBF responses to cold pressor testing (CPT), whereas pharmacologically induced hyperemic flow increase was still maintained.[52] These observations confirm the possibility that early stages of the arterial wall may affect only the endothelium,[53–55] whereas, in more advanced stages of cardiovascular risk factors states, commonly associated with increases in oxidative stress burden, an impairment in smooth muscle cell vasodilator function of the coronary arteriolar vessels may ensue.[50,56,57] Such an abnormal function of the coronary circulation carries important diagnostic and prognostic information, as numerous PET flow studies outline.[7–9] As was initially noted, a dysfunction of the coronary endothelium in individuals with cardiovascular risk but with normal coronary angiograms, as determined with PET-measured flow responses to sympathetic stimulation with CPT and its MFR, was associated with a higher risk for cardiovascular events compared with those individuals with normal flow increases.[7] Note that the incidence of cardiovascular events increased with progressive worsening of endothelium-related MBF responses to CPT (**Fig. 2**). Subsequently, the prognostic value of reduced hyperemic MBF responses in

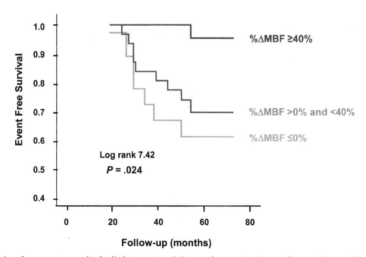

Fig. 2. PET-determined coronary endothelial vasoreactivity and prognosis. Kaplan-Meier analyses in patients with cardiovascular risk factors and normal coronary angiograms undergoing assessment of MBF response to CPT with PET. Attenuation of PET-measured and endothelium-related MBF responses to sympathetic stimulation with CPT are associated with a higher risk for cardiac events (during long-term follow-up) compared with those with normal flow increases; normal (%ΔMBF ≥40%), impaired (%ΔMBF >0% and <40%), and decreased (%ΔMBF ≤0%). (*From* Schindler TH, Nitzsche EU, Schelbert HR, et al. PET-measured abnormal responses of myocardial blood flow to sympathetic stimulation are associated with the risk of developing cardiovascular events. J Am Coll Cardiol 2005;45(9):1505–12; with permission.)

individuals with cardiovascular risk with and without CAD was also investigated.[8,9,58-60] For example, Herzog and colleagues[8] reported that reduced hyperemic MBFs in individuals with cardiovascular risk without clinically manifest CAD was also associated with a higher risk for cardiovascular events. In contrast, a normal hyperemic MBF response or MFR conferred a so-called warranty period of event-free survival of about 3 years. In addition, even when patients had stress-induced regional myocardial perfusion defects and abnormally reduced MFR, impaired MFR provided incremental information to the stress ^{13}N-ammonia perfusion imaging for the prediction of adverse cardiovascular outcome (**Fig. 3**). In a more extended clinical investigation, whereby 704 patients were prospectively enrolled for prognostic evaluation using [82]rubidium-PET for assessment of myocardial perfusion and MBF, the observations shown in **Fig. 3** were also confirmed by Ziadi and colleagues[9] For individuals with cardiovascular risk with normal perfusion imaging and decreased MFR compared with those with normal MFR, there was a higher incidence of cardiovascular events (**Fig. 4**). In contrast, among patients with stress-induced perfusion defects, individuals with an MFR less than 2.0 compared with those with a normal MFR also had a significantly higher cardiovascular event rate. These observations of an incremental predictive value of MFR for cardiac death were also reported for specific risk populations like patients with diabetes mellitus,[58] chronic kidney disease,[60] and ischemic or idiopathic cardiomyopathy.[12,61] These outcome data in individuals

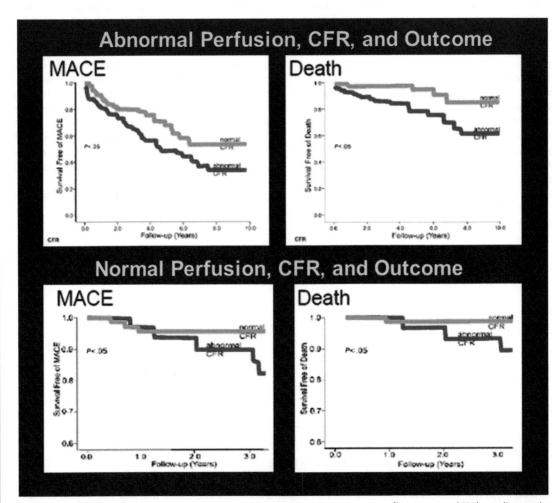

Fig. 3. Myocardial perfusion, coronary flow reserve, and prognosis. Coronary flow reserve (CFR) predicts major cardiovascular events (MACE) such as cardiac death, nonfatal myocardial infarction, and hospitalization for any cardiac reasons, including late percutaneous coronary intervention or late coronary artery bypass grafting in the study population. (*From* Herzog BA, Husmann L, Valenta I, et al. Long-term prognostic value of 13N-ammonia myocardial perfusion PET added value of coronary flow reserve. J Am Coll Cardiol 2009;54(2):150–6; with permission.)

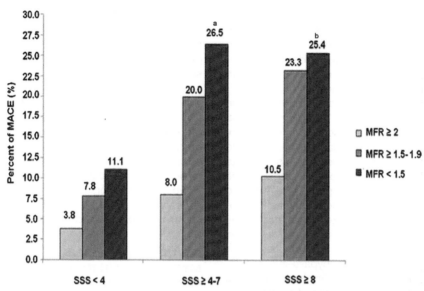

Fig. 4. Prognostic value of PET-determined MFR within subgroups of summed stress score (SSS) for different levels of MFR. At any level of SSS, the prevalence of MACE is higher in patients with the lowest MFR (<1.5) and statistically significantly different compared with MFR greater than or equal to 2 among patients with ischemia. [a]$P = $.028 for SSS greater than or equal to 4 to 7 and MFR less than 1.5 versus MFR greater than or equal to 2. [b]$P = $.002 for SSS greater than or equal to 8 and MFR less than 1.5 versus MFR greater than or equal to 2. (*From* Ziadi MC, Dekemp RA, Williams KA, et al. Impaired myocardial flow reserve on rubidium-82 PET imaging predicts adverse outcomes in patients assessed for myocardial ischemia. J Am Coll Cardiol 2011;58(7):740–8; with permission.)

with cardiovascular risk with subclinical or clinically manifest CAD emphasize a reduced MFR or coronary circulatory dysfunction as an integrating index of the overall stress burden imposed by various coronary risk factors on the arterial wall.[3,62] Beyond the described incremental prognostic value of reduced MFR, an impairment of hyperemic MBF increase and MFR has also been shown to predict future cardiovascular outcome in patients with idiopathic or hypertrophic cardiomyopathy.[12,61,63]

MONITORING REDUCTIONS IN CARDIOVASCULAR RISK WITH PET

PET assessment of MBF at rest and during different forms of vasomotor stress have been used to verify and follow up the effects of alterations in lifestyle, loss of body weight, and/or preventive medical care on coronary circulatory function in individuals with subclinical or with clinically manifest CAD.[3,14,64] Flow responses to vasomotor stress or the coronary vasodilator capacity could be improved with antioxidant challenges, regular exercise, preventive medical care, and euglycemic control with antidiabetic medication in individuals with cardiovascular risk.[65–69] More specifically, angiotensin II receptor blocker (ARB) with olmesartan was shown to restore endothelium-related MBF responses to CPT stimulation in patients with essential hypertension.[70] This improvement in coronary

endothelial function could be related to ARB-induced increases in superoxide dismutase levels. Thus, specific antioxidative effects of ARB inhibition, potentially conferred by inhibition of endothelial nicotinamide adenine dinucleotide phosphate (NADPH) oxidase activation accompanied by a decrease in reactive oxygen species or increases in antioxidative superoxide dismutase levels, are likely to have conferred beneficial effects on the function of the coronary endothelium in hypertensive patients. Epidemiologic investigations have shown that obesity is associated with increased cardiovascular morbidity and mortality.[71] A progressive worsening of coronary circulatory function with increasing body weight could reflect a mechanistic link between obesity and reduced cardiovascular outcome.[10,50,57,72,73] More recently, increases in endocannabinoid plasma levels have been identified as a cause for abnormal coronary endothelial function in obesity, which may trigger the initiation and/or progression of the CAD process.[10,57,72] In order to provide causal proof of increases in endocannabinoid plasma levels and coronary endothelial dysfunction, the effects of surgical bypass–induced weight loss in morbidly obese individuals (body mass index [BMI] $\geq$40 kg/m^2) on coronary circulatory dysfunction were also investigated.[10] After a median follow-up period of 22 months, gastric bypass induced a decrease in BMI from a median of 44.8 kg/m^2 to 30.8 kg/m^2. The gastric bypass–

related weight loss in initially morbidly obese individuals was accompanied by beneficial alterations in lipid profile, increase in insulin sensitivity, and decrease in chronic inflammation and endocannabinoid plasma levels, whereas a normalization of both endothelium-related MBF responses to CPT and hyperemic MBFs during pharmacologic vasodilation was noted, respectively (**Fig. 5**). In particular, the weight loss–induced decrease in plasma levels of endocannabinoids, such as anandamide, correlated with the observed restoration of MBF responses to CPT (**Fig. 6**). This close association between the decrease in anandamide plasma levels and improvement in coronary endothelial function provides direct in vivo proof of potential adverse effects of increased endocannabinoid plasma levels on coronary function in obese individuals.[57,72] Of further interest, the gastric bypass–induced increase in adiponectin plasma levels was followed by a restoration of hyperemic flow increases (**Fig. 7**), which emphasizes the favorable and most likely nitric oxide–mediated effect of increases in adiponectin plasma levels in concert with metabolic alterations and decreases in systemic inflammation on coronary circulatory function.[10] In another PET flow study, the effects of glucose-lowering intervention with glyburide and/or metformin on coronary artery calcifications (CAC) and coronary circulatory function over a mean follow-up period of 14 months in 22 individuals with type 2 diabetes mellitus were also investigated.[11] After the follow-up, plasma glucose levels had markedly decreased to 160 ± 44 mg/dL from an initial 205 ± 72 mg/dL because of glucose-lowering treatment. The noted decrease in plasma glucose levels after a 1-year follow-up was associated with a lower progression of CAC and increases in endothelium-related MBF responses to CPT and hyperemic MBFs, respectively ($r = 0.46$; $P = .038$ and $r = 0.36$; $P = .056$). These observations are unique in that they show favorable effects of euglycemic control not only on the function but also on the structure of the arterial wall. Of particular interest, the magnitude of increases in endothelium-related flow responses to CPT and slowed progression of CAC closely correlated (**Fig. 8**). When adjusting for metabolic parameters by multivariate analysis, the improvement of coronary endothelial dysfunction after glucose-lowering medical intervention remained an independent predictor of a slowed progression of CAC in these individuals with type 2 diabetes mellitus.[11] Such observations are first to signify that an improvement in coronary endothelial dysfunction in type 2 diabetes mellitus may confer, at least in part, direct preventive effects on the progression of diabetic vasculopathy. In another direction, PET flow measurements also provided unique insight into the effects of hormone replacement therapy (HRT) on coronary circulatory dysfunction in postmenopausal women.[49,54,74] HRT applying estrogen alone or in concert with progesterone in postmenopausal women, in addition to standard preventive medical treatment of traditional cardiovascular risk factors, helped to preserve a proper function of the coronary endothelium (**Fig. 9**).[49] Because disturbances in coronary circulatory function have been widely realized as functional precursors of the CAD process, its improvement or even normalization after lifestyle intervention and/or preventive medical care, for example by statin and/or ACE inhibitors, is assumed to manifest as an improved cardiovascular outcome; however, this assumption awaits clinical confirmation.

IDENTIFICATION OF HIBERNATING-STUNNING MYOCARDIUM IN ISCHEMIC CARDIOMYOPATHY

Ischemic heart disease is a prevalent cause of heart failure symptoms, followed by idiopathic cardiomyopathy (CMP) and valvular and hypertensive heart disease.[75] The increasing prevalence of ischemic CMP caused by an increasingly elderly population and improved survival of patients with acute coronary syndrome constitutes a major public health concern. Despite advancements in medical treatment of heart failure with β-blockers, ACE inhibition, angiotensin II type 1 receptor blockers, and aldosterone favorably altering morbidity and mortality, the 5-year mortality for CMP still remains as high as 50%.[75] It has been widely appreciated that ischemic left ventricular dysfunction may be maintained by repeated episodes of ischemia during times of increased metabolic demand or exercise. This so-called myocardial stunning may proceed to myocardial ischemia at rest and is referred to as myocardial hibernation.[15,76–78] In the clinical setting, stunned and hibernating myocardium commonly cannot be differentiated. However, timely revascularization of such ischemic compromised myocardium may completely or partially regain function in most patients with CAD with CMP.[76,77,79,80] Clinically, the term hibernating-stunning myocardium has been widely replaced by myocardial viability, which refers to an impairment of regional myocardial contractile dysfunction that is reversible if coronary flow is restored.[81–83] Fluorine-18–labeled fluorodeoxyglucose (FDG) PET has been widely accepted as the reference standard for the identification of viable myocardium in patients with ischemic CMP.[78,80,83] Applying FDG-PET for the detection of viable myocardium in these patients, a mean sensitivity and specificity of 92% and 63%, respectively, has been reported.[83,84] However, viable and

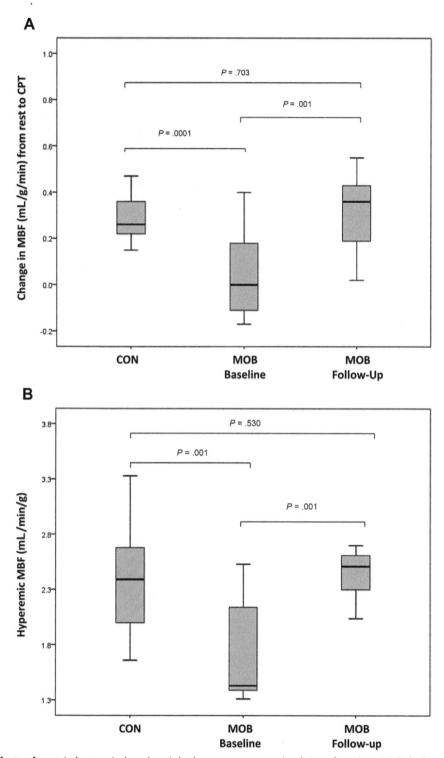

Fig. 5. Effects of gastric bypass–induced weight loss on coronary circulatory function. MBF during vasomotor stress in controls (CON) and morbidly obese (MOB) individuals. (*A*) Change in MBF to CPT from rest, and (*B*) in hyperemic MBF in CON and in MOB individuals at baseline and at the follow-up. (*From* Quercioli A, Montecucco F, Pataky Z, et al. Improvement in coronary circulatory function in morbidly obese individuals after gastric bypass-induced weight loss: relation to alterations in endocannabinoids and adipocytokines. Eur Heart J 2013;34(27):2063–73; with permission.)

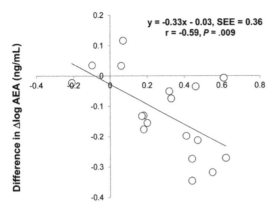

Fig. 6. Relationship between the decrease in ananda-mide (AEA) plasma levels and coronary circulatory function after gastric bypass–induced weight loss. Association between the differences in Δlog AEA and endothelium-related ΔMBF to CPT between base-line and follow-up. SEE, standard error of the esti-mate. (*From* Quercioli A, Montecucco F, Pataky Z, et al. Improvement in coronary circulatory function in morbidly obese individuals after gastric bypass-induced weight loss: relation to alterations in endo-cannabinoids and adipocytokines. Eur Heart J 2013;34(27):2063–73; with permission.)

ischemic jeopardized myocardium is detected and characterized with PET alone or in concert with SPECT perfusion imaging.[80,83] The term match is assigned to nonviable myocardium when blood

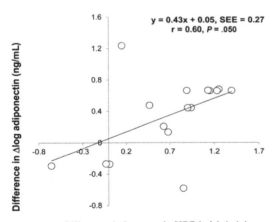

Fig. 7. Relationship between the increase in adipo-nectin plasma levels and coronary circulatory function after gastric bypass–induced weight loss. Association between the differences in Δlog adiponectin and hyperemic MBF between baseline and follow-up. (*From* Quercioli A, Montecucco F, Pataky Z, et al. Improvement in coronary circulatory function in morbidly obese individuals after gastric bypass-induced weight loss: relation to alterations in endo-cannabinoids and adipocytokines. Eur Heart J 2013;34(27):2063–73; with permission.)

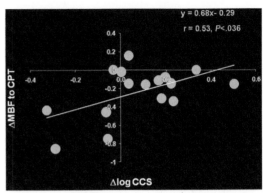

Fig. 8. Relationship between improvement in coro-nary endothelial dysfunction and slowed CAD pro-gression in response to glucose-lowering therapy in type 2 diabetes mellitus after a 1-year follow-up. Asso-ciation between the differences in ΔMBF to CPT and in Δlog-CCS (coronary calcium score) between baseline and follow-up (negative values on the x-ordinate indicate a progression of CAC). (*From* Schindler TH, Cadenas J, Facta AD, et al. Improvement in coronary endothelial function is independently associated with a slowed progression of coronary artery calcifica-tion in type 2 diabetes mellitus. Eur Heart J 2009;30(24):3064–73; with permission.)

flow is concurrently reduced with glucose utilization or FDG uptake. In contrast, mismatch findings describe viable myocardium with reduced blood flow in concert with an enhanced glucose utilization pattern (**Fig. 10**). A pooled analysis of 17 studies (including SPECT perfusion imaging and FDG-PET) showed increased diagnostic perfor-mance with a positive predictive value of 76% (range, 52%–100%) and a negative predictive value of 82% (range, 67%–100%).[80,83–85] Numerous investigations have shown a close asso-ciation between the assessment of viability with FDG-PET and different clinical outcome parame-ters.[78,80] There is overwhelming evidence to show an improvement of regional and global left ventric-ular ejection fraction after successful restoration of coronary flow to viable myocardial segments iden-tified with FDG-PET.[77,80,84–86] Notably, seminal in-vestigations of Di Carli and colleagues[85] have shown that the preoperative extent of a flow-metabolism mismatch was closely related to the magnitude of improvement in postrevascularization heart failure symptoms ($r = 0.65$; $P<.001$). The proof of a viability extent of greater than or equal to 18% had a sensitivity of 76% and a specificity of 78% for the greatest clinical benefit to improve the functional status.[85]

The amount of viable myocardium needed for a functional recovery after restoration of coronary flow remains controversial.[15,78,80] Nevertheless, it

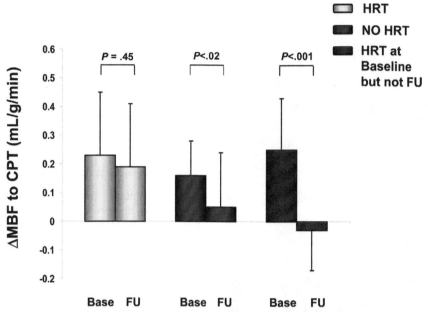

HRT
NO HRT
HRT at Baseline but not FU

Fig. 9. Hormone replacement and PET-determined coronary endothelial vasoreactivity in postmenopausal women. Effect of HRT on coronary endothelial dysfunction in postmenopausal women with medically treated cardiovascular risk factors. The endothelium-related change in ΔMBF from rest to CPT at baseline (Base) and follow-up (FU) among different groups are shown. In postmenopausal women with HRT at baseline and follow-up, the ΔMBF response to CPT was generally maintained, whereas in the women without HRT there was a significant decrease in ΔMBF to CPT. The ΔMBF to CPT in postmenopausal women who had discontinued HRT during follow-up was even worse than in those women who had never been on HRT, perhaps suggesting a rebound phenomenon on coronary endothelial (dys)function. (*From* Schindler TH, Campisi R, Dorsey D, et al. Effect of hormone replacement therapy on vasomotor function of the coronary microcirculation in postmenopausal women with medically treated cardiovascular risk factors. Eur Heart J 2009;30(8):978–86; with permission.)

has been widely accepted that, when more than 20% of viable, but ischemic jeopardized, myocardium of the left ventricle is identified, then it can be regarded as functionally significant, and has the potential to regain contractile function after restoration of blood flow.[87] When applying such criteria, functionally significant viability can be expected in 25% of patients with ischemic CMP and these patients are highly likely to benefit from timely coronary revascularization.[88] In contrast, ischemic jeopardized myocardium can be deemed as only prognostically significant when less than 20% of the left ventricle is affected.[87] This threshold has been challenged by a more recent investigation[89] that reported a threshold of 7% to 8% of dysfunctional but viable myocardium as prognostically significant. Apart from the potential prognostic and functional benefits of restoration of coronary flow to viable but ischemic compromised myocardium, it may also favorably influence the left ventricular remodeling process.[78,83,90]

Because most of these clinical investigations assessing the association between coronary revascularization of dysfunctional but viable myocardium and improvement in left ventricular function, symptoms, and prognosis were retrospective, a certain evaluation bias cannot be excluded. Consequently, the STICH (Surgical Treatment for Ischemic Heart Failure) trial[91] was set up and performed in 1212 patients with ischemic heart failure. These patients were randomly assigned to receive medical therapy alone or medical therapy plus coronary artery bypass grafting. In 601 of these patients, myocardial viability was determined with SPECT, dobutamine echocardiography, or both.[91] As expected, the presence of viable myocardium was observed to be associated with a greater likelihood of survival in patients with CAD and left ventricular dysfunction. However, after adjustment for other baseline clinical variables, this relationship no longer held.[91] At first sight, these observations may be surprising and contradictory to previous investigations in the assessment of myocardial viability in patients with ischemic heart failure.[76–78,80] However, several factors may reconcile this controversy in viability assessment, treatment, and clinical outcome of patients with ischemic

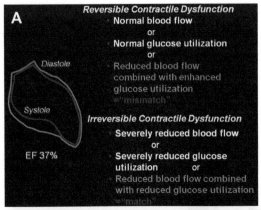

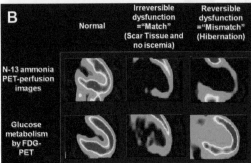

Fig. 10. Reversible and irreversible contractile dysfunction and PET imaging. (*A*) Reversible and irreversible contractile dysfunction in akinetic myocardial segments as defined by SPECT and/or PET assessment of myocardial perfusion and metabolism. (*B*) Examples of normal perfusion and FDG uptake (*left panel*), match finding with concordant reduction in perfusion and metabolism in the anteroapical and inferior wall, indicating nontransmural and transmural scar without ischemia (*middle panel*), and mismatch finding with reduced resting perfusion anteroapical, apical and inferoapical, and preserved metabolism, suggesting classical hibernating myocardium (*right panel*). EF, ejection fraction. (*From* Valenta I, Quercioli A, Ruddy TD, et al. Assessment of myocardial viability after the STICH trial: still viable? Cardiovasc Med 2013;16(11):289–98; with permission.)

CMP, such as (1) the timing of coronary revascularization; (2) absence or presence of ischemic, compromised, but viable myocardium; (3) stage of the myocardial remodeling process; and (4) intravenous use of suboptimal imaging protocols and techniques to determine the presence or absence of ischemic, jeopardized, but viable myocardium.[15,79,90,92–94]

From the clinical point of view, cardiac FDG-PET/CT or PET is most efficiently used in patients with ischemic CMP with a left ventricular ejection fraction less than or equal to 35% who present a stress-rest fixed perfusion defect of greater than or equal to 4 and akinetic or dyskinetic segments

of the left ventricle as determined with SPECT or PET/CT perfusion imaging. By adding FDG-PET/CT, 4 more conditions can be identified and assigned to 2 groups (see **Fig. 10**).

When there is a match finding between perfusion and viability, the assessment is noted and it signifies following[15]:

1. Transmural necrosis
2. Nontransmural necrosis and no ischemic component

Mismatch findings denote:

3. Nontransmural necrosis with viable but ischemic, compromised myocardium
4. Completely viable and ischemic, compromised myocardium

In about 20% to 40% of these patients with ischemic CMP,[84,88] FDG-PET/CT is likely to identify a reasonable extent of viable but ischemic jeopardized myocardium (list items 3 and 4) or hibernating-stunning myocardium. If large enough (≥4 segments), this dysfunctional area of hibernating-stunning myocardium may benefit from coronary revascularization both prognostically and functionally.[15,80,84] In contrast, if no sufficient amount of hibernating-stunning myocardium is identified, the patient may instead be referred to optimal medical heart failure treatment. If a patient with CMP presents a further worsening of left ventricular function over time despite all optimal medical heart failure care, heart transplantation as the final treatment option may be taken into account.

PET/COMPUTED TOMOGRAPHY IN CARDIAC SARCOID INVOLVEMENT

Sarcoidosis is a multisystem granulomatous disease of unknown cause that leads to the formation of noncaseating granuloma in affected organs.[95,96] Although the exact cause of cardiac sarcoidosis remains to be further elucidated, environmental, occupational, and infectious causes are assumed to trigger an immunologic response in genetically predisposed individuals.[96] The prevalence of sarcoid disease is estimated to be around 10 to 40 per 100,000 persons in the United States and Europe. This prevalence contrasts with a marked increased prevalence of sarcoidosis in African American compared with white people, with a ratio ranging from 10:1 to 17:1.[95] There also seems to be a higher prevalence of sarcoid disease in white people elsewhere, with 50 to 60 per 100,000 individuals in the Scandinavian population. In 1 out of 4 patients with sarcoid disease, cardiac involvement may manifest clinically through conduction abnormalities, arrhythmias, congestive heart failure, and sudden cardiac death.[97] The diagnosis of cardiac sarcoid involvement may be challenging and frequently still depends on the integration of both clinical and imaging findings. Based on the Japanese Ministry of Health and Welfare Diagnostic Guidelines,[98] the diagnosis of cardiac sarcoid involvement is stated either through a direct biopsy-proven confirmation of cardiac sarcoidosis or direct histologically proven extracardiac sarcoidosis combined with indirect evidence of an inflammatory myocardial lesion. FDG-PET/CT is commonly used to identify and describe systemic sarcoid disease[98–100] because in sarcoid disease an upregulation of

glucose metabolism at the sites of macrophage-mediated inflammation is noted, which can be used for the detection of an active and inflammatory cardiac sarcoid involvement. In a meta-analysis, the sensitivity and specificity of FDG-PET in the identification of cardiac sarcoid involvement was as high as 89% and 78%, respectively.[101] Imaging of inflammation with cardiac FDG-PET/CT is geared to identify the presence of ^{18}F-FDG uptake as an abnormal finding. A normal cardiac FDG-PET/CT study is therefore defined by a complete absence of myocardial FDG uptake under fasting conditions in order to avoid some physiologic uptake of about 20% to 30% caused by glucose metabolism of the heart.

Rest Perfusion	FDG	Frequency	Example		Interpretation / Comment
			Perfusion	FDG	
Normal perfusion and metabolism					
Normal	Normal (negative)	32 (27%)	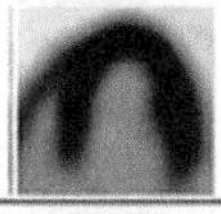	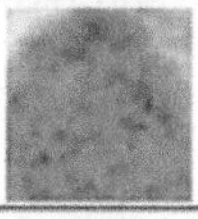	Normal
Normal	Diffuse (non-specific)	15 (12%)	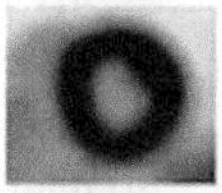	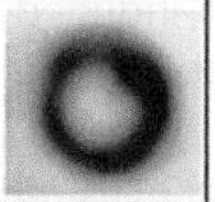	Diffuse FDG most likely due to failure to suppress FDG from normal myocardium
Abnormal perfusion or metabolism					
Normal	Focal	20 (17%)	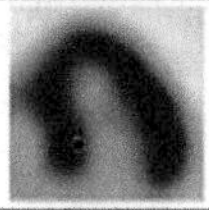	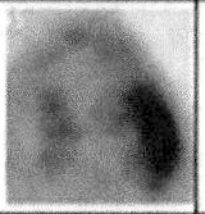	Nonspecific pattern; focal increase in FDG may represent early disease vs. normal variant
Positive	Negative	17 (14%)	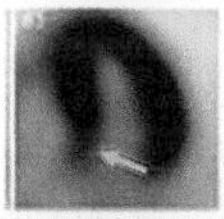	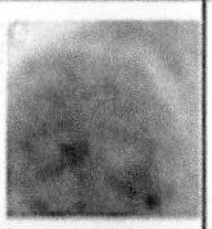	Rest perfusion defect may represent scar from cardiac sarcoidosis or other etiologies
Abnormal perfusion and metabolism					
Positive	Focal increase ("mismatch pattern")	23 (19%)	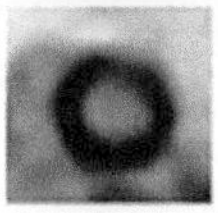	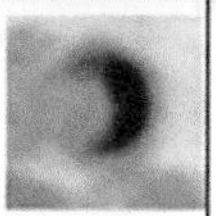	Presence of active inflammation ± scar in the same location
Positive	Focal on diffuse	6 (5%)	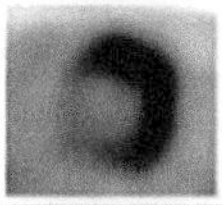	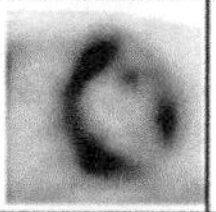	Similar to above but also areas of inability to suppress FDG from normal myocardium vs. diffuse inflammation
Positive	Focal increase (different area)	5 (4%)	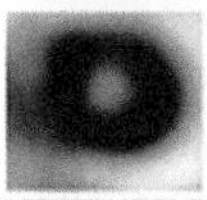	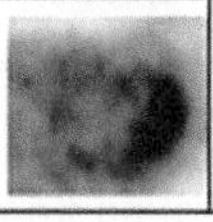	Presence of both scar and inflammation but in different segments

Fig. 11. Classification of cardiac PET/CT perfusion and metabolism imaging for the detection of cardiac sarcoid involvement. Normal perfusion and metabolism (category 1), abnormal perfusion or metabolism (category 2), abnormal perfusion and metabolism (category 3). (*From* Blankstein R, Osborne M, Naya M, et al. Cardiac PET enhances prognostic assessments of patients with suspected cardiac sarcoidosis. J Am Coll Cardiol 2014;63(4):329–36; with permission.)

Dietary modifications and intravenous heparin administration have been included in the protocols to reinforce a sufficient suppression of physiologic FDG uptake in the heart by stimulating the free fatty acid (FFA) uptake. In general, a low-carbohydrate meal the evening before scanning with at least an overnight fast is recommended.[98] In addition, unfractionated heparin can be administered intravenously leading to an increase in FFA plasma levels and its utilization in the myocardium instead of glucose. The effect of unfractionated heparin to markedly increase FFA plasma levels is related to the activation of the lipoprotein lipase with lipolytic effects. The protocol for the use of intravenous heparin to stimulate an FFA loading before the PET scanning can vary, whereas the administration of 700 to 1000 IU intravenously in divided doses 30 and 15 minutes before scanning in patients is a widely used option. In contrast with the fasting ^{18}F-FDG-PET/CT, which provides information about an inflammatory active state of cardiac sarcoid involvement, the assessment of myocardial perfusion is intended to detect regional perfusion defects at rest, indicating myocardial areas with fibrosis or caused by inflammation-induced edema associated with a compression of the coronary arteriolar vessels.[99]

Abnormalities in myocardial perfusion and myocardial inflammation are not only most helpful in signifying cardiac sarcoid involvement (**Fig. 11**) but they also carry important prognostic information (**Fig. 12**). For example, Blankstein and colleagues[99] investigated 118 consecutive patients without known CAD who were referred for FDG-PET and [82]rubidium-PET for assessment of cardiac sarcoid involvement, following a high-fat/low-carbohydrate diet to suppress normal myocardial glucose uptake. Forty percent had normal and 60% had abnormal cardiac PET findings, respectively. Patients were followed up over a median of 1.5 years and 31 (26%) adverse events (27 ventricular tachycardia and 8 deaths) ensued.

Cardiac PET findings were predictive of adverse events, and the presence of both a regional myocardial perfusion defect and abnormal ^{18}F-FDG uptake (29% of patients) was associated with a hazard ratio of 3.9 (P<.01). Even after adjustment for left ventricular ejection fraction and clinical criteria, perfusion abnormalities and/or abnormal FDG uptake on cardiac PET images remained independent predictors for the occurrence of ventricular tachycardia and cardiac death.[99] In contrast, extracardiac FDG uptake observed in 26% of patients was not accompanied by an adverse outcome. Overall, these initial observations strongly suggest that abnormal cardiac PET findings in patients with sarcoid disease allow a prognostication that goes beyond the Japanese Ministry of Health and Welfare clinical criteria, the presence of extracardiac sarcoidosis, and left ventricular ejection fraction.

Initial results of monitoring the success of immunosuppressive treatment in concert with standard heart failure therapy signifies that the reduction in the intensity and extent of myocardial inflammation on FDG-PET is associated with an

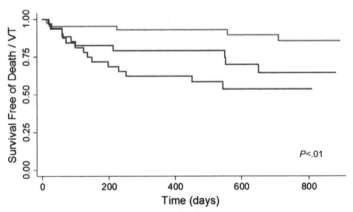

Fig. 12. Survival free of death or ventricular tachycardia (VT) stratified by cardiac PET examination results. Myocardial perfusion defects at rest, as indicating structural alterations such as interstitial fibrosis and/or edema. In addition, an inflammatory active myocardial state on FDG-PET was associated with a pronounced lower survival free of death or ventricular tachycardia compared with normal cardiac PET findings. Normal perfusion and FDG (*green line*), abnormal perfusion or FDG (*blue line*), and abnormal perfusion and FDG (*red line*). (*From* Blankstein R, Osborne M, Naya M, et al. Cardiac PET enhances prognostic assessments of patients with suspected cardiac sarcoidosis. J Am Coll Cardiol 2014;63(4):329–36; with permission.)

improvement in left ventricular ejection fraction.[100] A longitudinal regression analysis showed a significant inverse linear relationship between maximum standardized uptake value (SUV) and ejection fraction (EF) with an expected increase in EF of 7.9% per SUV reduction of 10 g mL^{-1} ($P = .008$). These observations emphasize that serial PET scanning may help to identify the success of immunosuppressive treatment in the prevention and treatment of heart failure caused by cardiac sarcoid involvement. Although this PET-guided approach to identifying and guiding treatment success in cardiac sarcoidosis is likely to improve the clinical outcome in these patients, further clinical evaluation is needed.

SUMMARY

The assessment of viable (or hibernating-stunning) myocardium in ischemic cardiomyopathy with PET/CT has emerged as an indispensable tool to justify and guide interventional and/or surgical coronary revascularization procedures. More recently, the possibility of measuring the MFR in conjunction with myocardial perfusion with PET/CT imaging has improved the detection and characterization of CAD burden in subclinical and clinically manifest CAD, respectively, and it also allows cardiovascular risk stratification in these patients. Although an improvement or even normalization of the MFR or coronary circulatory dysfunction after lifestyle intervention and/or preventive medical care is assumed to manifest as an improved cardiovascular outcome, it still awaits clinical validation. In addition, initial observations emphasize a unique role of PET/CT imaging for the detection of cardiac sarcoid involvement and the monitoring of its response to appropriate immunosuppressive treatment. Thus, cardiac PET/CT expands its clinical role beyond the identification of hibernating-stunning myocardium in ischemic cardiomyopathy to an optimized identification and characterization of CAD burden and cardiovascular prognostication as well as cardiac sarcoid involvement and, thereby, continues to emerge as unique tool to guide and individualize cardiovascular therapy for an improved clinical outcome in these patients.

REFERENCES

1. Schindler TH, Schelbert HR, Quercioli A, et al. Cardiac PET imaging for the detection and monitoring of coronary artery disease and microvascular health. JACC Cardiovasc Imaging 2010; 3(6):623–40.

2. Bengel FM. Leaving relativity behind: quantitative clinical perfusion imaging. J Am Coll Cardiol 2011;58(7):749–51.

3. Schindler TH, Quercioli A, Valenta I, et al. Quantitative assessment of myocardial blood flow-clinical and research applications. Semin Nucl Med 2014;44(4):274–93.

4. Valenta I, Quercioli A, Schindler TH. Diagnostic value of PET-measured longitudinal flow gradient for the identification of coronary artery disease. JACC Cardiovasc Imaging 2014;7(4):387–96.

5. Rahmim A, Tahari AK, Schindler TH. Towards quantitative myocardial perfusion PET in the clinic. J Am Coll Radiol 2014;11(4):429–32.

6. Valenta I, Quercioli A, Vincenti G, et al. Structural epicardial disease and microvascular function are determinants of an abnormal longitudinal myocardial blood flow difference in cardiovascular risk individuals as determined with PET/CT. J Nucl Cardiol 2010;17(6):1023–33.

7. Schindler TH, Nitzsche EU, Schelbert HR, et al. Positron emission tomography-measured abnormal responses of myocardial blood flow to sympathetic stimulation are associated with the risk of developing cardiovascular events. J Am Coll Cardiol 2005;45(9):1505–12.

8. Herzog BA, Husmann L, Valenta I, et al. Long-term prognostic value of 13N-ammonia myocardial perfusion positron emission tomography added value of coronary flow reserve. J Am Coll Cardiol 2009;54(2):150–6.

9. Ziadi MC, Dekemp RA, Williams KA, et al. Impaired myocardial flow reserve on rubidium-82 positron emission tomography imaging predicts adverse outcomes in patients assessed for myocardial ischemia. J Am Coll Cardiol 2011; 58(7):740–8.

10. Quercioli A, Montecucco F, Pataky Z, et al. Improvement in coronary circulatory function in morbidly obese individuals after gastric bypass-induced weight loss: relation to alterations in endocannabinoids and adipocytokines. Eur Heart J 2013;34(27):2063–73.

11. Schindler TH, Cadenas J, Facta AD, et al. Improvement in coronary endothelial function is independently associated with a slowed progression of coronary artery calcification in type 2 diabetes mellitus. Eur Heart J 2009;30(24):3064–73.

12. Neglia D, Michelassi C, Trivieri MG, et al. Prognostic role of myocardial blood flow impairment in idiopathic left ventricular dysfunction. Circulation 2002;105(2):186–93.

13. Ziadi MC, Dekemp RA, Williams K, et al. Does quantification of myocardial flow reserve using rubidium-82 positron emission tomography facilitate detection of multivessel coronary artery disease? J Nucl Cardiol 2012;19(4):670–80.

14. Valenta I, Dilsizian V, Quercioli A, et al. Quantitative PET/CT measures of myocardial flow reserve and atherosclerosis for cardiac risk assessment and predicting adverse patient outcomes. Curr Cardiol Rep 2013;15(3):344.

15. Valenta I, Quercioli A, Ruddy TD, et al. Assessment of myocardial viability after the STICH trial: still viable? Cardiovasc Med 2013;16(11):289–98.

16. Tahara N, Mukherjee J, de Haas HJ, et al. 2-deoxy-2-[18F]fluoro-D-mannose positron emission tomography imaging in atherosclerosis. Nat Med 2014; 20(2):215–9.

17. Dweck MR, Chow MW, Joshi NV, et al. Coronary arterial 18F-sodium fluoride uptake: a novel marker of plaque biology. J Am Coll Cardiol 2012;59(17): 1539–48.

18. Joshi NV, Vesey AT, Williams MC, et al. 18F-fluoride positron emission tomography for identification of ruptured and high-risk coronary atherosclerotic plaques: a prospective clinical trial. Lancet 2014; 383(9918):705–13.

19. Fuchs TA, Stehli J, Bull S, et al. Coronary computed tomography angiography with model-based iterative reconstruction using a radiation exposure similar to chest X-ray examination. Eur Heart J 2014;35(17):1131–6.

20. Leber AW, Knez A, von Ziegler F, et al. Quantification of obstructive and nonobstructive coronary lesions by 64-slice computed tomography: a comparative study with quantitative coronary angiography and intravascular ultrasound. J Am Coll Cardiol 2005;46(1):147–54.

21. Gould KL. Quantification of coronary artery stenosis in vivo. Circ Res 1985;57(3):341–53.

22. Gould KL. Noninvasive assessment of coronary stenoses by myocardial perfusion imaging during pharmacologic coronary vasodilatation. I. Physiologic basis and experimental validation. Am J Cardiol 1978;41(2):267–78.

23. Gould KL, Lipscomb K, Calvert C. Compensatory changes of the distal coronary vascular bed during progressive coronary constriction. Circulation 1975;51(6):1085–94.

24. Czernin J, Muller P, Chan S, et al. Influence of age and hemodynamics on myocardial blood flow and flow reserve. Circulation 1993;88(1):62–9.

25. Uren NG, Melin JA, De Bruyne B, et al. Relation between myocardial blood flow and the severity of coronary-artery stenosis. N Engl J Med 1994; 330(25):1782–8.

26. Krivokapich J, Czernin J, Schelbert HR. Dobutamine positron emission tomography: absolute quantitation of rest and dobutamine myocardial blood flow and correlation with cardiac work and percent diameter stenosis in patients with and without coronary artery disease. J Am Coll Cardiol 1996;28(3):565–72.

27. Di Carli M, Czernin J, Hoh CK, et al. Relation among stenosis severity, myocardial blood flow, and flow reserve in patients with coronary artery disease. Circulation 1995;91(7):1944–51.

28. Demer LL, Gould KL, Goldstein RA, et al. Assessment of coronary artery disease severity by positron emission tomography. Comparison with quantitative arteriography in 193 patients. Circulation 1989;79(4):825–35.

29. Naya M, Murthy VL, Taqueti VR, et al. Preserved coronary flow reserve effectively excludes high-risk coronary artery disease on angiography. J Nucl Med 2014;55(2):248–55.

30. Goldstein RA, Kirkeeide RL, Demer LL, et al. Relation between geometric dimensions of coronary artery stenoses and myocardial perfusion reserve in man. J Clin Invest 1987;79(5):1473–8.

31. Marcus ML, Harrison DG, White CW, et al. Assessing the physiologic significance of coronary obstructions in patients: importance of diffuse undetected atherosclerosis. Prog Cardiovasc Dis 1988;31(1):39–56.

32. Marcus ML, Skorton DJ, Johnson MR, et al. Visual estimates of percent diameter coronary stenosis: a battered gold standard. J Am Coll Cardiol 1988;11(4):882–5.

33. Vogel RA. Assessing stenosis significance by coronary arteriography: are the best variables good enough? J Am Coll Cardiol 1988;12(3):692–3.

34. Kern MJ. Coronary physiology revisited: practical insights from the cardiac catheterization laboratory. Circulation 2000;101(11):1344–51.

35. Kern MJ, Donohue TJ, Aguirre FV, et al. Assessment of angiographically intermediate coronary artery stenosis using the Doppler flowire. Am J Cardiol 1993;71(14):26D–33D.

36. Fiechter M, Ghadri JR, Gebhard C, et al. Diagnostic value of 13N-ammonia myocardial perfusion PET: added value of myocardial flow reserve. J Nucl Med 2012;53(8):1230–4.

37. Danad I, Raijmakers PG, Harms HJ, et al. Impact of anatomical and functional severity of coronary atherosclerotic plaques on the transmural perfusion gradient: a [15O]H2O PET study. Eur Heart J 2014;35(31):2094–105.

38. Gould KL, Johnson NP, Bateman TM, et al. Anatomic versus physiologic assessment of coronary artery disease. Role of coronary flow reserve, fractional flow reserve, and positron emission tomography imaging in revascularization decision-making. J Am Coll Cardiol 2013;62(18): 1639–53.

39. Gould KL, Nakagawa Y, Nakagawa K, et al. Frequency and clinical implications of fluid dynamically significant diffuse coronary artery disease manifest as graded, longitudinal, base-to-apex myocardial perfusion abnormalities by noninvasive

positron emission tomography. Circulation 2000; 101(16):1931–9.

40. Sdringola S, Loghin C, Boccalandro F, et al. Mechanisms of progression and regression of coronary artery disease by PET related to treatment intensity and clinical events at long-term follow-up. J Nucl Med 2006;47(1):59–67.

41. Sdringola S, Patel D, Gould KL. High prevalence of myocardial perfusion abnormalities on positron emission tomography in asymptomatic persons with a parent or sibling with coronary artery disease. Circulation 2001;103(4):496–501.

42. Schindler TH, Facta AD, Prior JO, et al. Structural alterations of the coronary arterial wall are associated with myocardial flow heterogeneity in type 2 diabetes mellitus. Eur J Nucl Med Mol Imaging 2009;36(2):219–29.

43. Beller GA. Underestimation of coronary artery disease with SPECT perfusion imaging. J Nucl Cardiol 2008;15(2):151–3.

44. Lima RS, Watson DD, Goode AR, et al. Incremental value of combined perfusion and function over perfusion alone by gated SPECT myocardial perfusion imaging for detection of severe three-vessel coronary artery disease. J Am Coll Cardiol 2003; 42(1):64–70.

45. Berman DS, Kang X, Slomka PJ, et al. Underestimation of extent of ischemia by gated SPECT myocardial perfusion imaging in patients with left main coronary artery disease. J Nucl Cardiol 2007;14(4):521–8.

46. Dorbala S, Hachamovitch R, Curillova Z, et al. Incremental prognostic value of gated Rb-82 positron emission tomography myocardial perfusion imaging over clinical variables and rest LVEF. JACC Cardiovasc Imaging 2009;2(7): 846–54.

47. Dorbala S, Vangala D, Sampson U, et al. Value of vasodilator left ventricular ejection fraction reserve in evaluating the magnitude of myocardium at risk and the extent of angiographic coronary artery disease: a 82Rb PET/CT study. J Nucl Med 2007; 48(3):349–58.

48. Schwaiger M, Muzik O. Assessment of myocardial perfusion by positron emission tomography. Am J Cardiol 1991;67(14):35D–43D.

49. Schindler TH, Campisi R, Dorsey D, et al. Effect of hormone replacement therapy on vasomotor function of the coronary microcirculation in postmenopausal women with medically treated cardiovascular risk factors. Eur Heart J 2009;30(8): 978–86.

50. Schindler TH, Cardenas J, Prior JO, et al. Relationship between increasing body weight, insulin resistance, inflammation, adipocytokine leptin, and coronary circulatory function. J Am Coll Cardiol 2006;47(6):1188–95.

51. Schindler TH, Zhang XL, Vincenti G, et al. Role of PET in the evaluation and understanding of coronary physiology. J Nucl Cardiol 2007;14(4):589–603.

52. Quinones MJ, Hernandez-Pampaloni M, Schelbert HR, et al. Coronary vasomotor abnormalities in insulin-resistant individuals. Ann Intern Med 2004;140(9):700–8.

53. Campisi R, Czernin J, Schoder H, et al. L-Arginine normalizes coronary vasomotion in long-term smokers. Circulation 1999;99(4):491–7.

54. Campisi R, Nathan L, Pampaloni MH, et al. Noninvasive assessment of coronary microcirculatory function in postmenopausal women and effects of short-term and long-term estrogen administration. Circulation 2002;105(4):425–30.

55. Schindler TH, Nitzsche EU, Olschewski M, et al. Chronic inflammation and impaired coronary vasoreactivity in patients with coronary risk factors. Circulation 2004;110(9):1069–75.

56. Munzel T, Daiber A, Ullrich V, et al. Vascular consequences of endothelial nitric oxide synthase uncoupling for the activity and expression of the soluble guanylyl cyclase and the cGMP-dependent protein kinase. Arterioscler Thromb Vasc Biol 2005;25(8):1551–7.

57. Quercioli A, Pataky Z, Vincenti G, et al. Elevated endocannabinoid plasma levels are associated with coronary circulatory dysfunction in obesity. Eur Heart J 2011;32(11):1369–78.

58. Murthy VL, Naya M, Foster CR, et al. Association between coronary vascular dysfunction and cardiac mortality in patients with and without diabetes mellitus. Circulation 2012;126(15):1858–68.

59. Murthy VL, Naya M, Foster CR, et al. Improved cardiac risk assessment with noninvasive measures of coronary flow reserve. Circulation 2011;124(20): 2215–24.

60. Murthy VL, Naya M, Foster CR, et al. Coronary vascular dysfunction and prognosis in patients with chronic kidney disease. JACC Cardiovasc Imaging 2012;5(10):1025–34.

61. Tio RA, Dabeshlim A, Siebelink HM, et al. Comparison between the prognostic value of left ventricular function and myocardial perfusion reserve in patients with ischemic heart disease. J Nucl Med 2009;50(2):214–9.

62. Bonetti PO, Lerman LO, Lerman A. Endothelial dysfunction: a marker of atherosclerotic risk. Arterioscler Thromb Vasc Biol 2003;23(2):168–75.

63. Cecchi F, Olivotto I, Gistri R, et al. Coronary microvascular dysfunction and prognosis in hypertrophic cardiomyopathy. N Engl J Med 2003; 349(11):1027–35.

64. Valenta I, Dilsizian V, Quercioli A, et al. The influence of insulin resistance, obesity, and diabetes mellitus on vascular tone and myocardial blood flow. Curr Cardiol Rep 2012;14(2):217–25.

65. Czernin J, Barnard RJ, Sun KT, et al. Effect of short-term cardiovascular conditioning and low-fat diet on myocardial blood flow and flow reserve. Circulation 1995;92(2):197–204.

66. Baller D, Notohamiprodjo G, Gleichmann U, et al. Improvement in coronary flow reserve determined by positron emission tomography after 6 months of cholesterol-lowering therapy in patients with early stages of coronary atherosclerosis. Circulation 1999;99(22):2871–5.

67. Gould KL, Martucci JP, Goldberg DI, et al. Short-term cholesterol lowering decreases size and severity of perfusion abnormalities by positron emission tomography after dipyridamole in patients with coronary artery disease. A potential noninvasive marker of healing coronary endothelium. Circulation 1994;89(4):1530–8.

68. Bennett SK, Smith MF, Gottlieb SS, et al. Effect of metoprolol on absolute myocardial blood flow in patients with heart failure secondary to ischemic or nonischemic cardiomyopathy. Am J Cardiol 2002;89(12):1431–4.

69. Schindler TH, Facta AD, Prior JO, et al. Improvement in coronary vascular dysfunction produced with euglycaemic control in patients with type 2 diabetes. Heart 2007;93(3):345–9.

70. Naya M, Tsukamoto T, Morita K, et al. Olmesartan, but not amlodipine, improves endothelium-dependent coronary dilation in hypertensive patients. J Am Coll Cardiol 2007;50(12):1144–9.

71. Prospective Studies Collaboration, Whitlock G, Lewington S, Sherliker P, et al. Body-mass index and cause-specific mortality in 900 000 adults: collaborative analyses of 57 prospective studies. Lancet 2009;373(9669):1083–96.

72. Quercioli A, Pataky Z, Montecucco F, et al. Coronary vasomotor control in obesity and morbid obesity: contrasting flow responses with endocannabinoids, leptin, and inflammation. JACC Cardiovasc Imaging 2012;5(8):805–15.

73. Valenta I, Dilsizian V, Quercioli A, et al. Impact of obesity and bariatric surgery on metabolism and coronary circulatory function. Curr Cardiol Rep 2014;16(1):433.

74. Campisi R, Camilletti J, Mele A, et al. Tibolone improves myocardial perfusion in postmenopausal women with ischemic heart disease: an open-label exploratory pilot study. J Am Coll Cardiol 2006;47(3):559–64.

75. Hunt SA, Abraham WT, Chin MH, et al. Focused update incorporated into the ACC/AHA 2005 Guidelines for the Diagnosis and Management of Heart Failure in Adults a report of the American College of Cardiology Foundation/American Heart Association Task Force on Practice Guidelines developed in collaboration with the International Society for Heart and Lung Transplantation. J Am Coll Cardiol 2009;53(15):e1–90.

76. Marshall RC, Tillisch JH, Phelps ME, et al. Identification and differentiation of resting myocardial ischemia and infarction in man with positron computed tomography, 18F-labeled fluorodeoxyglucose and N-13 ammonia. Circulation 1983;67(4):766–78.

77. Tillisch J, Brunken R, Marshall R, et al. Reversibility of cardiac wall-motion abnormalities predicted by positron tomography. N Engl J Med 1986;314(14):884–8.

78. Ghosh N, Rimoldi OE, Beanlands RS, et al. Assessment of myocardial ischaemia and viability: role of positron emission tomography. Eur Heart J 2010;31(24):2984–95.

79. Bax JJ, Schinkel AF, Boersma E, et al. Early versus delayed revascularization in patients with ischemic cardiomyopathy and substantial viability: impact on outcome. Circulation 2003;108(Suppl 1):II39–42.

80. Allman KC, Shaw LJ, Hachamovitch R, et al. Myocardial viability testing and impact of revascularization on prognosis in patients with coronary artery disease and left ventricular dysfunction: a meta-analysis. J Am Coll Cardiol 2002;39(7):1151–8.

81. Rahimtoola SH. Hibernating myocardium has reduced blood flow at rest that increases with low-dose dobutamine. Circulation 1996;94(12):3055–61.

82. Rahimtoola SH. Clinical aspects of hibernating myocardium. J Mol Cell Cardiol 1996;28(12):2397–401.

83. Schinkel AF, Bax JJ, Poldermans D, et al. Hibernating myocardium: diagnosis and patient outcomes. Curr Probl Cardiol 2007;32(7):375–410.

84. Partington SL, Kwong RY, Dorbala S. Multimodality imaging in the assessment of myocardial viability. Heart Fail Rev 2011;16(4):381–95.

85. Di Carli MF, Asgarzadie F, Schelbert HR, et al. Quantitative relation between myocardial viability and improvement in heart failure symptoms after revascularization in patients with ischemic cardiomyopathy. Circulation 1995;92(12):3436–44.

86. Carrel T, Jenni R, Haubold-Reuter S, et al. Improvement of severely reduced left ventricular function after surgical revascularization in patients with preoperative myocardial infarction. Eur J Cardiothorac Surg 1992;6(9):479–84.

87. Di Carli MF, Davidson M, Little R, et al. Value of metabolic imaging with positron emission tomography for evaluating prognosis in patients with coronary artery disease and left ventricular dysfunction. Am J Cardiol 1994;73(8):527–33.

88. Auerbach MA, Schoder H, Hoh C, et al. Prevalence of myocardial viability as detected by positron emission tomography in patients with ischemic cardiomyopathy. Circulation 1999;99(22):2921–6.

89. D'Egidio G, Nichol G, Williams KA, et al. Increasing benefit from revascularization is associated with increasing amounts of myocardial hibernation: a substudy of the PARR-2 trial. JACC Cardiovasc Imaging 2009;2(9):1060–8.

90. Elsasser A, Muller KD, Skwara W, et al. Severe energy deprivation of human hibernating myocardium as possible common pathomechanism of contractile dysfunction, structural degeneration and cell death. J Am Coll Cardiol 2002;39(7): 1189–98.

91. Bonow RO, Maurer G, Lee KL, et al. Myocardial viability and survival in ischemic left ventricular dysfunction. N Engl J Med 2011;364(17): 1617–25.

92. Elsasser A, Vogt AM, Nef H, et al. Human hibernating myocardium is jeopardized by apoptotic and autophagic cell death. J Am Coll Cardiol 2004; 43(12):2191–9.

93. Bax JJ, Schinkel AF, Boersma E, et al. Extensive left ventricular remodeling does not allow viable myocardium to improve in left ventricular ejection fraction after revascularization and is associated with worse long-term prognosis. Circulation 2004; 110(11 Suppl 1):II18–22.

94. Schwarz ER, Schoendube FA, Kostin S, et al. Prolonged myocardial hibernation exacerbates cardiomyocyte degeneration and impairs recovery of function after revascularization. J Am Coll Cardiol 1998;31(5):1018–26.

95. Iannuzzi MC, Fontana JR. Sarcoidosis: clinical presentation, immunopathogenesis, and therapeutics. JAMA 2011;305(4):391–9.

96. Sekhri V, Sanal S, Delorenzo LJ, et al. Cardiac sarcoidosis: a comprehensive review. Arch Med Sci 2011;7(4):546–54.

97. Silverman KJ, Hutchins GM, Bulkley BH. Cardiac sarcoid: a clinicopathologic study of 84 unselected patients with systemic sarcoidosis. Circulation 1978;58(6):1204–11.

98. Mc Ardle BA, Leung E, Ohira H, et al. The role of F(18)-fluorodeoxyglucose positron emission tomography in guiding diagnosis and management in patients with known or suspected cardiac sarcoidosis. J Nucl Cardiol 2013;20(2):297–306.

99. Blankstein R, Osborne M, Naya M, et al. Cardiac positron emission tomography enhances prognostic assessments of patients with suspected cardiac sarcoidosis. J Am Coll Cardiol 2014;63(4):329–36.

100. Osborne MT, Hulten EA, Singh A, et al. Reduction in 18F-fluorodeoxyglucose uptake on serial cardiac positron emission tomography is associated with improved left ventricular ejection fraction in patients with cardiac sarcoidosis. J Nucl Cardiol 2014;21(1):166–74.

101. Youssef G, Leung E, Mylonas I, et al. The use of 18F-FDG PET in the diagnosis of cardiac sarcoidosis: a systematic review and metaanalysis including the Ontario experience. J Nucl Med 2012;53(2):241–8.

Moving?

Make sure your subscription moves with you!

To notify us of your new address, find your **Clinics Account Number** (located on your mailing label above your name), and contact customer service at:

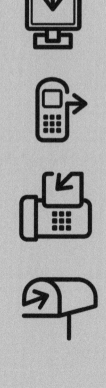

Email: journalscustomerservice-usa@elsevier.com

800-654-2452 (subscribers in the U.S. & Canada)
314-447-8871 (subscribers outside of the U.S. & Canada)

Fax number: 314-447-8029

Elsevier Health Sciences Division
Subscription Customer Service
3251 Riverport Lane
Maryland Heights, MO 63043

ELSEVIER

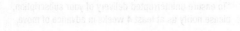

Printed and bound by CPI Group (UK) Ltd, Croydon, CR0 4YY

03/10/2024

01040376-0018